Eat to Thrive

or

Life Force Energy
The Hippocrates Approach to Optimum Health

by
Betsy Bragg, M.Ed., M.A.

Acknowledgements

This manual has grown out from my passion with Life Force and the Tao that flows through me. My desire is to have this universal energy flow freely through everyone until the whole world is in harmony and everyone fully participates in compassion, love and joy.

I've been inspired by Hippocrates, who in 400 BC is quoted to have said:

- Let food be thy medicine and medicine be thy food.

- Natural forces within us are the true healers of disease.

- As to diseases, make a habit of two things—to help, or at least to do no harm.

Those who have contributed to my life and this manual will find their afterglow in these pages and realize how many they are helping. My unending thanks go to the following people:

- Brian Clement, who is the essence and spirit of the Hippocrates Health Institute. We are honored to have him as a board member of Optimum Health Solution. Brian and Hippocrates Health Institute transformed my life, as I describe in my testimonial elsewhere in Chapter 10. He mentored the development of the "Life Force Energy: The Hippocrates Approach to Optimum Health"course, which I wrote while taking the HHI Health Educator Program and for which I was awarded the Derrick Brockie Memorial Scholarship. The 10-week course is based on the HHI DVD series, which is the core of the OHS DVD library, funded by this scholarship.

- Tom Lindsley, my son, for his life-long deep interest in health since his college days (especially spiritual), inspiration, continuous teachings and encouragement, culminating in paying and sending me for the Life Changing three-week program at the Hippocrates Health Institute in West Palm Beach, Florida, in 2006, and for inviting me to be the Director of pHat Free Nation, a non-profit, which he helped me rename Optimum Health Solution. He has been the guest speaker on Cleansing since the inception of the 10-week Health Educator course, "Live Force Energy – The Hippocrates Approach to Optimum Health" and has been my guiding light.

- Carla Finn, who spent hour upon hour taking pages from a three-ring binder and creating the first edition. Without her, this manual would not exist. She wrote Chapter 7 "Enzymes, vitamins and Minerals" and has been a guest speaker on this topic.

- Jeff Plotkin and Richard Weisbach, my dedicated volunteer Brandeis interns in the summer of 2010 and 2011, who wrote to all the contributors for permission to reprint their works and helped to write and revise the manual.

- Peggy Dougherty, who compiled all the information about the kitchen and food into Chapter 2 and made the charts.

- Miryam Wiley, who has edited many articles for the manual and photographed the children during activities, also made the collages and wrote the program descriptions for www.realkidsrealfood.org.

- Dr. Lorraine Hurley, for her incredible knowledge and inspirational manner of conveying her expertise on internal awareness, body ecology, the gastrointestinal system, and mind/

body issues in Chapters 4 and 8. Lorraine is a scientifically oriented MD with substantial self-directed continuing education and experience in the field of holistic, functional, environmental, nutritional and energetic medicine. She is a certified quantum biofeedback specialist and functional physician. As a visionary, she holds the belief that the medicine of the future will be based on the science of progressive physics and what it is teaching us about human abilities and potential. She is an avid researcher and student of the "quantum age" with a distinct ability to synthesize complex information and translate it into practical communication and application. She particularly enjoys working with groups and is an advocate of empowering others toward greater personal responsibility in the care of their health as a means of living a more satisfying, harmonious and creative life.

- Barry Harris, for his tireless editing of this manuscript that needed his constant attention. He has also ghost-written many of the articles. As past editor for Ann Wigmore and Viktoras Kulvinskas, co-founders of Hippocrates Institute, his skills, knowledge and understanding have been invaluable and greatly appreciated.

Foreword
by Dr. Brian Clement, Ph.D. N.M.D., L.N.

LIFE FORCE ENERGY – The Hippocrates Approach to Optimum Health.is a work from the heart that will transfer knowledge, health, and strength to those who read it. As Betsy's words permeate your awareness, make sure that you apply their meaning in your everyday life. Ms. Bragg's history is one that bounced from lows to highs. Her nemesis for a good part of her life was self-doubt, which perpetuated physical disorder. When she first arrived at Hippocrates Health Institute, we discovered a broken woman who sorely needed change. Not only did she pull herself up by her bootstraps, but she also went further by attending and being certified as a Health Educator. Her contributions as a student earned her an award as the most promising teacher.

Little did we know that she possessed a powerhouse of energy, passion and heartfelt sincerity. Putting together this manual for well-being is one of her many accomplishments, which is touching as well as helping to save the lives of many. Betsy's unwavering commitment and integrity makes her a force of nature to be reckoned with. We are proud of her work with underprivileged children and her courses that lay out a roadmap for success.

Life Force Energy brings you the concepts and tools that have helped hundreds of thousands to slow the premature aging process, prevent disease and even help to reverse disorders. Betsy's clear and concise way of expressing her thoughts affords the reader an opportunity to gain innate wisdom in the simple steps required to build health. There is no doubt that her book is one of the most important ever penned on lifestyle change and healing.

Chapter 1

Life Force Overview

Chapter 2

The Living Food Kitchen

Chapter 3

Indoor Sprouting

Chapter 4

Internal Awareness - Fasting

Chapter 5

Cleansing

Chapter 6

Mind Body Connection

Chapter 7

Enzymes andVitamins

Chapter 8

Holistic Medicine

Chapter 9

Master Your Destiny

Chapter 10

Testimonials

Chapter 11

Recipes

Chapter 12

Resources

Appendix

DVD Questions and Answers

Chapter 1
Life Force Overview

Overview

The underlying spirit of this book is directly reflected in the title, *"Life Force Energy – The Hippocrates Approach to Optimum Health."* The goal of The Hippocrates Approach to Optimum Health is to raise your level of Life Force Energy. This includes your mind-body connection, cleansing and nourishing the body through proper eating, juicing, limiting exposure to toxins, exercising, meditating and journaling, opening your heart, deep breathing and giving to others. Most important, however, is the empowerment that results from taking the responsibility for your beliefs. In other words, the mind, or soul, is the primary source of your optimal health. Remove any blockages preventing your ability to tap into your true self and you will unlock your innate potential to achieve optimum health.

Therefore, the first place where health starts is in your head. Our beliefs and thoughts, which result in our habits, rule our current state of health. Mark Twain said, "It's not what we don't know that hurts us, it is what we know for sure that just ain't so." For example, TV commercials tell us milk "does the body good." Science shows us this "just ain't so."

Congratulate yourself on doing research to change your thoughts and beliefs.

What is "Life Force Energy?"[1]

When you think about yourself, life in general, or your health, have you ever thought, "there's more to all this than meets the eye"? You're right. Humans—indeed, all living things—are more than mere collections of systems and cells. In addition to our physical selves, each of us also has a "Life Force."

Descriptions vary, but this Life Force is recognized in every religion and belief system throughout human history. Richard Anderson describes the Life Force as "… the potency of innate intelligence that gives life to everything that lives. It is the only healing force there is or ever will be, and is the most powerful and effective contributor towards your health."[1]

This Life Force resides in the atoms of every cell in our bodies. Each atom includes energy in the form of electrons (negatively charged) and protons (positively charged): The greater the "charge" of each cell, the more power it can generate to be healthy, according to Anderson. Cells that are highly charged with this life force energy can become radiant light, and it is this light that repels disease, he adds.

When the Life Force of highly charged cells flows unimpeded through our bodies' physical and emotional channels, "happiness and joy surface more readily," and "we ward off disease, handle stress effectively, stay healthy longer, and our aging is slowed," he states.

How Do We Begin This Journey?

We must naturally start with understanding ourselves. Ann Wigmore, who in 1968 founded the

---

[1] Anderson, R. (2002). *Cleanse and Purify Thyself (Book Two)*. Mt. Shasta, CA: Christobe Publishing (pg. 272).

Hippocrates Institute at 25 Exeter Street in Boston, wrote the following in her Health Digest publication No 152,*Spiritual Diet:*[2]

"Look into the human aspect of the self. Learn to know our inner self the mature way. Seek to understand what we really are and what our relationship to others is. Learning to understand why we are here on this planet and what our <u>mission </u>is. All of this is part of what it means to be working towards self-realization.

The first thing we must do is to analyze our actions, to really observe what our failures are and resolve to do something about them. Purification is also vital. The mind and the body must be purified from the stagnation of pollutants. The body must be cleaned of the accumulation of toxins caused by eating unnatural, cooked food containing synthetic chemical additives. These foods are completely lacking in the natural elements needed to keep the cells functioning vigorously in their work of renewing and repairing the body and cleansing it of waste. The mind also must be purified –from the inner stagnation of fears, doubts and confusion. We must overcome these blockages that prevent us from getting in touch with the universal law of harmony and feeling the unity of all of life.

*The most valuable realization we can come to is the awareness of our oneness with all life. We and everything else in the universe are expressions of the one divine Mind of God. (*You can substitute words for "God," such as Life Force Energy, Higher Power, the universal laws of nature, chi, prana/breath – whatever you believe is greater than yourself.)

When we can view all of life as one great family belonging to our Creator – with everything no matter how big or small being important and great because it is a manifestation of the divine Mind –then we are on the road to self-realization. God's spirit is in all things. Great teachers such as Moses, Buddha, Jesus and many others had this understanding. The invisible world of splendor was always present with them, and they left us so many wonderful gifts of truth to help free us from fear and doubt that only result from the ignorance of the value of our true self.

With inward self-realization one has the capacity to respond to the outward chord of beauty – the plants, flowers, mountains, rivers, seas, the animals, birds, sound in the form of music – are all striving to manifest themselves in different forms in the great Creation of the one Spirit. There is <u>no </u>separation of the One. All are beautiful revelations of the attributes of the one Great Spirit called God or the Creator

As we become increasingly aware of our true nature, our problems will be solved through the guidance of the spiritual self and through working together as one human family, with each individual placing on the altar the gift of his sincere effort. As we become aware of our physical and spiritual strength and the vast possibilities of our minds, nothing will be impossible. This awareness diminishes the gap between all peoples and nations. Self-realization develops with the understanding of one's true self and one's connection to the whole.

When we cleanse our bodies, our minds become clearer and we become open to receive more and more knowledge that will help us progress along the path of self-realization. The body needs

---

[2]Wigmore, A. Spiritual Diet.*Health Digest, No.*

to be purified and well-nourished in order to become a more fitting instrument for the higher Self. We need to remember that desire, will, universal love, wisdom and understanding come from the training and control of the mind. This can only come about when the mind is healthy, and a healthy mind can only come from a healthy and clean body.

So, how do we purify and strengthen our bodies according to the Hippocrates Approach? It starts with beliefs.

Mahatma Gandhi said,

Your beliefs become your thoughts.

Your thoughts become your words.

Your words become your actions.

Your actions become your habits.

Your habits become your values.

Your values become your destiny.

I want to congratulate you for taking this journey, not only for your body, but for your emotions and your spirit as well. You may find as you face and overcome health obstacles that certain emotional challenges also come up, and that by shedding new light on these emotional challenges, it allows us the strength to develop a better lifestyle of affirming habits, thoughts, and beliefs.

To make a shift from being sick (or having illness-producing thoughts) to becoming healthy requires adopting positive beliefs. Healing requires mental toughness and an outright refusal to remain trapped in negative thought patterns that undermine us. **Our thoughts do indeed create our reality, or our experience of reality.** From many years of working with people who are right on the edge of giving up, we have concluded that the primary element of healing is **self-responsibility.** When we proceed with positive intention, we reconstitute our resources from within, tapping that deep well of healing wisdom to forge a brighter future.

To bring about any change, in both your life and the world, you need to be aligned with your true self, and then be able to help others also find their true selves. This is essential to healing yourself and healing the planet. The steps toward self-actualization are:

I.   1. Faith – a set of beliefs with which the impossible becomes possible

2. Commitment – vow to take action

3. Practice – follow-through

4. Accomplishments – steps toward your final goal

My personal mission is to heal myself and heal the planet. The belief system underlying this mission is based on decades of trial and error experimentation in the field of nutrition.

Preface: These beliefs are based on my personal experiences, acquired throughout my life and reaffirmed at the Hippocrates Health Institute, in an effort to achieve optimal health.

Belief 1: Return to your Sincere Heart, your True Self. This means surrender your ego to something greater than yourself: Life Force Energy, God, chi, Love, Jesus Christ, Buddha, or other enlightened beings – all synonyms for the un-nameable, or the breath of life.

Belief 2: In order to return to our original state, our true selves, we need to abide by natural laws, adhering to an organic, plant-based diet.

Belief 3: To function optimally, we need to balance sleep, exercise, work and relationships.

Belief 4: We thrive when we embrace cleansing practices, removing the blockages in our bodies, and therefore in our lives.

Belief 5: A positive mindset is essential to health, because our mind and body are interconnected. As psycho-immunology shows us, our bodies reflect our minds. Gratitude contributes greatly to a healthy, balanced body.

Belief 6: Embrace acceptance, rather than resistance. "When you can't fight, and can't flee, flow." Whatever you resist will continue to recur until it has been resolved and accepted. Avoid expectations: They prevent acceptance and lead only to disappointment. Forgive yourself and others.

Belief 7: Self-reflection leads to self-actualization. We need to continually stop and reflect on whether we are on the right track, and adjust our path accordingly. Discern what is divine and what is ego. See the world for what it really is, reflect on it, understand it more deeply and truthfully, and be transformed.

Belief 8: A consistent, daily routine creates habit. Habit creates destiny. It takes twenty-one days to break or make a habit. Consistency, not perfection, will get you where you need to go. The answer to consistency rather than perfection lies in humility. If you have a bad day, let it go and get back on track the next day. Do this however long it takes to develop consistency. Grace, i.e. Life Force Energy, the Tao or whatever it is from your tradition, will allow us to do this.

Belief 9: We strengthen life force through doing what we are called to do. The true nature of reality is that we are indeed One. When we are involved in giving to others we are in actuality giving to ourselves; it is a fundamental spiritual law that in giving we receive.

Belief 10: Empowerment is a path, not a destination. If you are passionate about your commitment, you will be empowered to take moment-to-moment responsibility for your life choices. This includes an assessment of your current health and an assessment after completing the course. Celebrate your transformation, but realize it is just a beginning. You are now prepared to embrace the challenge of living a full, learning, joyous, and predictable life.

Transition from a Western Diet to a Living Food Diet[3]
by Brian R. Clement, PhD

It's about commitment; people have to make a decision based upon their own desire to want the best. If you come about this change through fear, it will never seat itself well in your heart and soul. So come to this because of interest and complete commitment.

If a person is facing an imminent problem, a disease of magnitude, he or she must rapidly and readily embrace the living food program. It will boost the immune system and give him or her back the army that has been weakened, so he or she can fight that disorder and disease.

If you are on the most horrific diet in the world, the type I used to be on, where I ate nothing with any health value or nutritional value, all you would have to do is reduce 8 percent of that dangerous diet each month and add 8 percent of the Hippocrates living food program. I don't think anyone would have a difficult time doing that.

At the end of the year, you will be eating a 100percent living food diet. Remember what we have learned from all the work we did many years ago in research: When a person is in a conquest of disease, she or he must be on 100percent living food, excluding fruits and including large amounts of high-density foods such as sprouts, sea vegetables, and freshwater algae.

A person who has conquered a disease and placed it in remission, or who has come to this place without being sick, could literally eat up to 15, 20,or even 25percent organic cooked vegan food. This makes it far more realistic for most people. Remember, this is not a religion.

We did work and looked at the immune system and discovered that a healthy individual with all functional differentials of immunity can literally eat up to that much cooked food, organic and vegan. Not polluted foods, but foods like steamed vegetables, alkaline grains, squash, etc., and not have any impact on the immune system.

Once we go beyond that, from 25 percent to 30 percent, we now lose 17 percent of our immune function. If we go up to 35 percent, we literally lose 48.6 percent, or approximately one half of our immune function. The immune system is now attacking the cooked food.

---

[3]Clement, B. Transition from a Western Diet to a Living Food Diet.*Hippocrates News.*

How to Get a Good Night's Sleep[4]

If you want to have a good night's sleep, I recommend reading *Sleep Disorders: Clinically Proven Alternative Therapies To Help You Get a Good Night's Rest* by Herbert Ross, D.C., Keri Brenner, L.Ac.,and Burton Goldberg. (Tiburon, CA: AlternativeMedicine.com Books, 2000). Before you can again enjoy the kind of sleep that children are blessed with, you need to know where your problems lie. It is helpful to examine your sleep habits, including such areas as your sleep history, your sleep environment, how many hours of sleep you get per night, difficulties getting to sleep, fatigue during the day, snoring or sleepwalking, dozing off while driving, exercise patterns, nutrition patterns, smoking and drinking habits, and history of sleep medications. An unbalanced diet, as reflected in ailments such as insulin problems, food addictions and hypoglycemia, often plays a role in sleep disorders.

So what can you do?

- Use detox diets and purifying colonics to cleanse the organs. Bacterial overgrowth in conditions like candidiasis, and certain internal parasites can interfere with the intestine's ability to rid itself of toxins, which can disrupt sleep.
- Have a set bedtime and waking up time each day- even on weekends
- Eat at least 3 hours before bedtime
- Avoid TV, computers and phones etc. an hour before bedtime
- Insure your room is less than 70 degrees and open your window
- Avoid liquid a couple of hours before bedtime so you don't have to get up at night
- Exercise during the day; morning is best
- If you have things on your mind, write them down before bedtime
- Sleep in total darkness
- Avoid caffeine and alcohol (caffeine can make it difficult to fall or stay asleep; alcohol will wake you early in the morning and keep you from the deep stages of sleep)
- Move electromagnetic objects (TVs, electric clocks, computers, portable and cell phones)at least 3 feet away from your bed. Check electromagnetic fields with a Gauss meter.

---

[4] Recommended Reading:

Ross, H., Brenner, K. & Goldberg, B. (2000).*Sleep Disorders – Clinically Proven Alternative Therapies to Help You Get a Good Night's Rest*. Tiburon, CA: AlternativeMedicine.com Books.

Ortner, A. (February 15, 2012). How Your Sleeping Habits Are Affecting Your Health. *Raw for Thirty*. Retrieved from http://www.rawfor30days.com/blog/?p=2006on February 16, 2012.

Dr. Mercola, (August 23, 2011). Avoid This Before Bed if You Want a Good Night's Sleep. http://articles.mercola.com/sites/articles/archive/2011/08/23/is-this-one-of-natures-simple-answer-to-sleepless-nights.aspx Accessed August 28, 2012.

Oil Pulling:
A gentle way to cleanse your teeth with added benefits[5]
by Miryam Wiley

If you haven't heard of oil pulling – the art of swishing oil in your mouth to get rid of harmful bacteria – you are certainly not alone. I, for one, just heard of it recently. But it is indeed an old practice which has its roots in Ayurvedic medicine, and it has been part of a daily regimen for a lot of people all over the world.

One is best advised to create a practice of oil pulling first thing in the morning, using a tablespoon or two of sesame or coconut oil and swishing it around the mouth for several minutes. At the end, it's best to spit the oil into the trash, as the repeated routine may pose a risk to the plumbing system if the oil becomes saturated at room temperature, as is the case with coconut oil.

Traditionally, sesame oil has been the first choice, but coconut oil is also used with success. Benefits include the cleansing of teeth and gums in ways that can capture whatever bacteria are not caught by daily brushing. It is also supposed to strengthen gums, teeth and jaws.

One full-length research paper printed in the *African Journal of Microbiology* in March 2008 states that "there was a remarkable reduction in the total count of bacteria" in an experiment to check the effect of oil-pulling. "The in-vitro antibacterial activity of sesame oil against dental caries* causing bacteria was determined. Streptococcus mutans and lactobacillus acidophilus were found to be moderately sensitive to sesame oil."

There are reports of many more benefits that come from this simple habit, thanks, some say, to the large vein under the tongue, which is a connection to help pull toxins from the body.

The website healingcancernaturally.com reports on a survey conducted among 1,041 readers of an Indian newspaper (*Andhra Jyoti*) on the effects of oil pulling on various diseases: 927 people (89 percent) reported healing effects curing one or more diseases, while 114, or 11 percent, did not report disappearance of symptoms or illnesses. Cases of cures included polio, polycystic kidneys, neural fibroma, diabetes, arthritis, skin problems and allergies.

The same site mentions a physician from India who reported three cancer cases healed within two months of oil pulling, with an added quote that "confidence/faith contributes to cure more than medicine."

*"caries" are also known as cavities or tooth decay.

Tongue Scraping

---

[5] Recommended Reading:

http://www.oilpulling.com/ayurveda.htm accessed January 20, 2012.

http://www.healingcancernaturally.com/detoxification-oil-pulling.html accessed January 20, 2012.

http://www.healingteethnaturally.com/oil-pulling-dental-healer.html#scientific-research-studies-oil-pulling-dental-health-benefits accessed January 20, 2012.

Asokan S. Oil pulling therapy. Indian J Dent Res 2008;19:169. Retrieved from http://www.ijdr.in/article.asp?issn=0970-9290;year=2008;volume=19;issue=2;spage=169;epage=169;aulast=Asokan on July 5, 2008.

Tongue scraping, an ancient Ayurvedic technique, is one of the best ways to aid in your oral hygiene. Bacteria and fungi tend to collect on your tongue and cause a large number of issues ranging from halitosis (chronic bad breath) to an increased risk of tooth decay or gum disease. Moreover, recent studies have shown that oral bacteria have a link to several systemic diseases such as an increased risk of diabetes or pneumonia due to inhaling bacteria in the mouth. Simply by using a tongue scraper (don't use a toothbrush since those are made for brushing your teeth, not for scraping your tongue) every morning before you brush your teeth, you can limit all of these issues and greatly aid your oral health.

In addition to helping optimize oral health, tongue scraping is also an important aspect of detoxing. Your tongue is one of the escape routes for toxins in the body. Bad breath can often be a detox side effect. As the body cleanses itself, mucus and bacteria accumulate at the back of the tongue and create a white film. Within this film are millions of sulfur-producing bacteria that lead to foul-smelling breath. It can also, over time, compromise oral hygiene and the functioning of your taste buds. Your body does most of its detoxification work during the night as you sleep. Some of the toxins removed during this process end up coating the tongue, which is why you may sometimes have a thicker coating on your tongue or a strange taste in your mouth when you first awake. If you gently scrape this coating off in the morning, you prevent your system from reabsorbing the toxins and also improve the smell of your breath.

Tongue scrapers start at around $4, and you can purchase them online at www.amazon.com. There is an abundance of videos on www.youtube.com demonstrating how to use them.

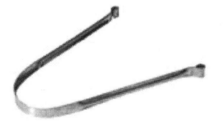

Components of a Sound Exercise Program
by Betsy Bragg

Adopt a regular exercise routine; proper exercise increases energy reserves and assists the body in eliminating waste and toxins.

When developing a routine, emphasize overall body conditioning and the development of all major muscle groups.

Three Types of Essential Exercice:

1. **Stretching** (Yoga, Tai Chi, Qigong, etc.) Enables your joints and muscles to become more limber and flexible.

2. **Aerobic** (walking, swimming, cycling, rebounding, jogging, etc.) Increases oxygen levels in every cell of the body and facilitates greater utilization of available nutrients, neutralizes toxins throughout the body and improves elimination.

3. **Resistance** (lifting, pulling, weight training, etc.) Free weights and machines are most common. Few repetitions using heavy weights increase muscle mass. More repetitions with lighter weights tone rather than build muscle mass.

Frequency:

- **Warming Up**: 3-5 minutes of brisk walking, jumping rope, stationary cycling and/or mild calisthenics, all of which increase respiration, elevate body temperature and stretch ligaments and connective tissue.

- **Stretch:** Every day; try to do this once in the morning and once in the evening for 10-15 minutes.

- **Aerobic** exercise 5 - 6 times per week for at least 35 minutes (walking, swimming, rebounding, and/or jogging). Finish with a short stretching routine.

- **Resistance** exercise 3 times per week every other day for at least 45 minutes. Open and close each session with appropriate stretching. Use only safe equipment.

Rebounding[6]
by Richard Weisbach

Rebounding (jumping on a mini trampoline for about 15 to 30 minutes daily) may be the healthiest, and most fun way to lose weight. Not only does rebounding facilitate weight loss by increasing the pull of gravity on the body – which conditions, tones, and strengthens each body cell – but it also has some phenomenal health benefits. The large amount of motion that comes with Rebounding facilitates the lymphatic system, allowing it to bathe every cell in lymph, which helps to remove toxins from the cells.

Unlike our blood, most cells in our immune system do not have the ability to move on their own. Lymph cells need lots of motion from the body in order to move. ... The increasing forces affecting the body as a result of continual jumping only exacerbates this phenomenon allowing for greater benefits.

In fact, daily rebounding can do the following:

- Increase the capacity for breathing
- Circulate more oxygen to the tissues
- Help combat depression
- Help normalize your blood pressure
- Help prevent cardiovascular disease
- Increase the activity of the red bone marrow in the production of red blood cells
- Aid lymphatic circulation, as well as blood flow in the veins of the circulatory system
- Lower elevated cholesterol and triglyceride levels
- Stimulate the metabolism, thereby reducing the likelihood of obesity
- Tone up the glandular system, especially the thyroid to increase its output
- Improve coordination throughout the body
- Promote increased muscle fiber tone
- Relief from neck and back pains, headaches, and other pain caused by lack of exercise
- Enhance digestion and elimination processes
- Allow for easier relaxation and sleep
- Result in a better mental performance, with sharper learning processes
- Relieve fatigue and menstrual discomfort for women
- Minimize the number of colds, allergies, digestive disturbances, and abdominal problems
- Possibly slow the aging process

---

[6]http://www.healingdaily.com/exercise/rebounding-for-detoxification-and-health.htm accessed August 15, 2010.

Skin Brushing[7]

One of the best detoxifying therapies is dry skin brushing. Your skin is your largest elimination organ and eliminates a quarter of the toxins in your body. Skin brushing allows for the blood and the lymph to carry away toxins from the skin. By putting these toxins into the bloodstream, one allows them to go to the colon for elimination. Blemishes on your skin (dead skin cells, dirt, etc.) make it so your skin cannot effectively release toxins and can result in acne, rashes, or even psoriasis.

How to skin brush:

1. Brush your dry body before you shower or bathe, preferably in the morning.

2. Start at your feet and always brush toward your heart. Use brisk circular motions or long, even strokes.

3. Brush all the way up your legs, then over your abdomen, buttocks, and back. If you have cellulite on your hips and thighs, concentrate there a little longer. To completely dissolve cellulite, brush for 10 minutes daily for several months.

4. Brush lightly on sensitive areas like breasts and more firmly on areas like soles of the feet.

5. When you reach your arms, begin at your fingers and brush up your arms, toward your heart. Brush your shoulders and chest down, always toward your heart.

6. Avoid brushing anywhere the skin is broken or where you have a rash, infection, or wound.

7. Finish by taking a shower and if you choose, use cold/hot therapy to further stimulate the lymphatic system and improve circulation.

8. Dry off vigorously and massage pure plant oils into your skin such as almond, sesame, avocado, coconut, olive or cacao butter.

Skin brushing provides tons of benefits, from removing irritants from the skin to actually strengthening the immune system through increasing blood flow and to the skin and helping our lymphatic system work. Skin brushing can also decrease cellulite buildup over time and tone muscles along with the other external benefits that come from exfoliating – such as having softer, more beautiful skin.

---

[7] Recommended Reading:

http://www.whole-body-detox-diet.com/dry-skin-brushing.html accessed July 26, 2011.

Go to www.youtube.com/watch?v=AZfMhXsjXeQ&feature=youtube_gdata_player to see a video with directions for skin brushing. Accessed August 24, 2012. .

Life Force Energy Class
Health and Wellness Practices Record

Record For (name): _____

Time Period (dates): _____

Daily	Sunday	Monday	Tuesday	Wednesday	Thursday	Friday	Saturday
Oil Swish							
Skin Brush							
Water/Supplements							
Stretching							
Meditation							
Wheatgrass							
Juicing							
Leafy Greens							
Exercising							
Journaling							
Sleep							

Your Physical Health[8]

Your immune system's healthy function is intertwined with your psychological well-being. It's no coincidence that many people encounter health issues—adverse immunological changes—when they undergo stressful situations such as college exams, divorce, job loss, or the death of a loved one. However, there are things you can do to help safeguard your psychological health and maintain your physical health in the process.

Boost Your Immune System

… by *writing*? Yes! Keeping an online diary or personal journal regularly can have a very positive impact on the immune system. Simply writing about important experiences for as little as 15 minutes per day can not only reduce stress and anxiety, it also can decrease visits to the physician. Writing regularly in a journal can also increase antibody response, lower heart rate and electrodermal activity, and lower pain and medication use. This is especially the case if you write in your diary about traumatic life experiences and feelings. In fact, by writing about emotional thoughts that are actively hidden from others, you can achieve significant health improvement.

Lose Weight

Keeping a daily food diary can double a person's weight-loss, according to a 2008 study conducted by Kaiser Permanente's Center for Health Research. "Those who kept daily food records lost twice as much weight as those who kept no records," stated author Jack Hollis Ph.D. "It seems that the simple act of writing down what you eat encourages people to consume fewer calories."

Keeping a food journal, combined with healthy eating and moderate exercise, enabled more than 1,700 patients in the study to lose an average of 13 pounds, according to the study, which was published in the August 2008 issue of the *American Journal of Preventive Medicine*.

Apparently, the pen is mightier than the sword ... *and* our eating habits. Even in today's information-overloaded world, written words carry real weight. If losing as little as five pounds can reduce your risk of developing high blood pressure by 20 percent, why not start a food diary?

---

[8]http://penzu.com/content/why/health#boost accessed August 24, 2012.

The Benefits of Keeping a Journal Are Endless
by Francis A. Goldstein

The health benefits of keeping a personal journal or diary are proven and highly recommended by therapists.

The pioneer of journal therapy, Dr. James W. Pennebaker, has been researching the effects of expressive writing for decades. He, and other researchers and scientists around the world, have found that actively holding back feelings from others is extremely stressful. By simply expressing yourself through writing, you could potentially experience immediate life improvements. His research suggests that journal writing, especially expressive writing, over short periods of time (specifically, four days in a row for 15 minutes each day) will generate health improvements.

Suggestions for Journaling

If you are new to journaling or just looking for a fresh approach, start by answering these questions in your journal today.

Remember, anything goes! Some of you may answer one question at a time and others in one sitting, whichever resonates with you. What is important is that you download both the positive and negative chatter that's in your head.

HAPPY JOURNALING!

1. Who I am today:

2. What I did well (today, yesterday, this week etc.):

3. What I am grateful for:

4. Cravings I am having:

5. Favorite new recipe:

6. What I did (or commit to do) for exercise:

7. My meditation today:

8. My mantra for today:

9. If I need support I will reach out to:

10. Today's intention:

You can begin with any question – you can w*rite as much or as little as* you are comfortable writing. If you have questions, feel free to reach out! Let it flow, no judgment, have fun with this!

PS: One of my favorite mantras from Deepak Chopra is "**I am no better than anyone else. I am no worse than anyone else.**"

Francis A. Goldstein is President and CEO of Gold Staff Consultants (Empowering Personal Performance) and a Life Force graduate / Health Educator. See her website: www.goldstaff.com. Contact number: 781-956-8810.

Promote Healthy Change with a Health Assessment

"Motivating and sustaining health behavior change is the key to improving population health and productivity and controlling health care costs. A health risk appraisal can lead to health risk reduction. Health behavior research has shown that helping people identify threats to their health facilitates the process of healthy change." –*MayoClinicHealthSolutions.com website*

Who is responsible for our health and well-being? Our doctor? Our insurance company? Ourselves? Your health – in fact, your life – depends on the knowledge you accumulate, the choices you make and the habits you develop. Assess your health so you are knowledgeable about the health of your body. Then learn and practice what you can do to optimize your health. Check your health before you start the 10-week program and again, three months later, after you have been practicing the Hippocrates Approach to Optimum Health. See and feel the difference!

When you attend the Hippocrates Health Institute, you not only have a live blood analysis, but the following Chemical 24 Blood Test. For the rest of one's life, graduates of the Hippocrates program can send their semi-annual or annual Chemical 24 Blood Test and have it assessed.

Many may benefit from a food allergy panel in addition to the preceding lab work. The Spectrum Food Allergy Assay is highly recommended. A wide array of practitioners can make this test available for you.

Besides having objective laboratory testing, it is just as important to take subjective tests. Go to www.metagenics.com to take their health assessment questionnaires.

Health Assessment

Have your blood tested before and after the course filling in the following chart. Please give Optimum Health Solution a copy of both pre and post blood tests. This will be kept absolutely confidential. Only your statistics will be used for research purposes. Most people's medical insurance will cover this. This will be helpful for you to see your progress and helpful for Optimum Health Solution's research.

Your Health Scores

Risk factors	Your results	Desirable	Borderline Risk	Elevated Risk
Systolic Blood pressure		119 or below	120-140	Greater than 140
Diastolic Blood pressure		79 or below	80-90	Greater than 90
Total Cholesterol		Less than 200	200-240	Greater than 240
HDL Cholesterol		40 or higher (Most sources say 60)	Less than 40	
LDL Cholesterol		70-129	130-159	Greater than 159
Total/HDL Cholesterol Ratio		Less than 4.0	4.0 or higher	
Non-fasting glucose level		Less than 150	150-200	Greater than 200
Fasting glucose level		Less than 100	100-126	Greater than 126
HgA1C (A1C)		Less than 6.1	6.1-6.5	Greater than 6.5
Body Mass Index (BMI)		Less than 25	25-30	Greater than 30
Ht: _____ Wt:		Less than 35		
Waist circumference		Less than 40		
Ratio				

Blood Pressure Screening Results

Your heart is a muscle. When it beats (sends out blood) – this is your systolic reading. When your heart relaxes or fills back up with blood – this is your diastolic reading. Blood pressure is the force of your blood pushing against the walls of your arteries. When your blood pressure is high, your arteries become weak and you are at great risk for heart attack and stroke. One elevated measurement does not diagnose hypertension.

Hypertension is diagnosed when the average of multiple measurements on more than one occasion is consist-ently greater than 120/80. Blood pressure is affected by many factors such as over the counter medications (i.e., sinus or cold/flu medicines) weight, salt intake, caffeine diet, smoking, exercise, stress, and family history. High blood pressure may be controlled by some combination of diet, exercise, smoking cessation and medication.

Many may benefit from a food allergy panel in addition to the preceding lab work. The Spectrum Food Allergy Assay is highly recommended. A wide array of practitioners can make this test available for you.

Besides having objective laboratory testing, it is just as important to take subjective tests. Go to www.metagenics.com to take their health assessment questionnaires.

If you have health concerns and want a super diagnosis, request a consultation at Hippocrates with Dr. Brian Clement by calling 561-471-8876. You will be required to send a health history and a list of your questions along with the following blood test.

Hippocrates Institute offers free lifetime health diagnoses based on your blood test, twice a year or whenever you are ill.

Chemical 24 Blood Test at Hippocrates

1- LDH
2- Phosphorus
3- Sodium
4- Potassium
5- Chloride
6- Carbon dioxide
7- Glucose
8- BUN
9- Creatinine, serum
10- BUNcreatinine ratio
11- Uric acid
12- Calcium
13- Bilirubin total
14- Total protein
15- Albumin
16- Globulin
17- A/G ratio
18- Cholesterol
19- Triglycerides
20- HDL
21- VLDL (calculated)
22- CHOL/HDL
23- LDL (calculated)
24- AST

Why is Alkalinity Important?
by Barry Harris

- Why is osteoporosis promoted by eating acidic foods?

- Why is acidity harmful in your body?

- Which foods are the most acidic versus most alkaline?

- Why does consuming large amount of dairy do nothing to prevent osteoporosis?

- What is the real cause of osteoporosis and how do you reverse the condition through dietary change?

- How do we accurately test our pH levels?

- How does our overconsumption of meat and grains result in an overly acidic body?

Michael Adams, the Health Ranger, in his *Natural News*, says: "Back in high school chemistry, we learned about pH: Acids had low numbers, alkalines had high numbers, and a pH of 7.0 was neutral. And it all meant absolutely nothing in terms of day-to-day life.

"It now turns out that we have a better shot at long-term health if our body's pH is neutral or slightly alkaline. When we tilt toward greater acidity, which can be measured easily, we have a greater risk of developing osteoporosis, weak muscles, heart disease, diabetes, kidney disease, and a host of other health problems.

"The solution, according to scientists who have researched 'chronic, low-grade metabolic acidosis,' is eating a diet that yields more alkaline and less acid. Just what kind of diet is that? One that's high in fruits and vegetables."

"After digestion, all foods report to the kidneys as either acidic or alkaline. The kidneys are responsible for fluid balance and maintaining a relatively neutral pH in the body..." states Loren Cordain, Ph.D., professor and researcher in the Department of Health and Exercise Science at Colorado State University.

Long-term, excess acidity leads to thinner bones and lower muscle mass, points out Anthony Sebastian, M.D., of the University of California, San Francisco. These problems are compounded by normal aging, which increases acidosis, bone loss, and muscle wasting. Along the way, calcium and magnesium losses can equate to deficiencies, with many ramifications. Both minerals play essential roles in bone formation and normal heart rhythm. Low magnesium levels can cause muscle cramps, arrhythmias, and anxiety."[9]

We cannot fully understand our body's functioning, or be motivated to the practices that will result in super-health, until we understand the importance of alkalinity in the cells of our body and, therefore, in our bloodstream. Unfortunately, this basic building block for optimal health has been almost entirely neglected by Western allopathic medicine.

We can begin to appreciate the crucial importance of alkalinity in the cells of the body, once we recognize that each cell operates very similar to the battery in your car. Your car's battery stops

---

[9]http://www.naturalnews.com/report_acid_alkaline_pH_1.html Accessed April 26, 2012.

working when there is no longer an opposite polarity created with one side producing positive charge, and one side producing negative charge. If that clear distinction is lost, the spark that operates your battery can't jump from one side to the other, and the battery dies. Likewise, the cells of your body collect toxins, and become unhealthy when the opposite polarity is lost. A bloodstream with the optimal acid/alkaline balance feeds cells ensuring their optimal acid/alkaline balance, and this results in cells with a potential for maximum energy flow and minimal toxicity. On the other hand, if the bloodstream doesn't have the proper acid/alkaline balance, toxins collect in the cells, energy flow within the cell is blocked and weakened, and sick cells create a weakened, sick body.

Responsibility for a natural diet and lifestyle is the key for achieving optimal acid/alkaline balance, and, thus, for maximizing cellular energy, and minimizing acid-waste products. When the charge between the nucleus and cytoplasm decreases, cellular energy is diminished, and additional metabolic acids, other than those just created by a poor diet, result in a cellular environment even more conducive to degeneration and disease. Once begun, only a radical new lifestyle can reverse the trend.

Testing pH To Determine Acid/Alkaline Balance:

PH paper is often used to diagnose the acid/alkaline balance of the body. The pH of the urine and saliva should be tested, over a period of time, for the most accurate results. A pH reading of 6.5, -7.5 or thereabouts, is considered normal, and a sign of good cellular alkalinity. To achieve this optimal pH, a diet of 80 percent of foods from alkaline sources, and 20 percent of foods from acidic sources is highly recommended.

What to Eat:

Dr. Young's excellent book, "The pH Miracle," clarifies for us the acidic or alkaline effect on the body produced by a large variety of foods. Most vegetables and low-sugar fruits have an alkaline effect on the body. These include: Peas, asparagus, artichokes, comfrey, green cabbage, lettuce, onion, cauliflower, white radish, rutabaga, white cabbage, savoy cabbage, kohlrabi, zucchini, red cabbage, rhubarb, horseradish, leeks, watercress, spinach, turnip, lime, chives, carrots, lemon, French cut beans, red beets, sorel, garlic, celery, tomato, endive, avocado, red radish, cayenne pepper, dandelion, kamut grass, barley grass, soy sprouts, chia seeds, alfalfa, wheatgrass.

Several kinds of nuts and seeds are alkaline. These include: almonds, soy nuts, sesame seeds, etc. Among alkaline producing fats are olive oil, flax seed oil, and coconut. Most grains and legumes (i.e. beans) are slightly acidic, which means they should be eaten in moderation, but are still part of a healthy diet. These include: brown rice, wheat, buckwheat groats, millet, lentils, tofu, lima beans, white beans, etc.

Almost all meat products, poultry, fish that isn't freshwater fish, white breads, peanuts, cashews, pistachios, all cheeses, and milk products, all forms of sugar, all condiments such as vinegar, soy sauce, mustard, mayonnaise, and ketchup, as well as most beverages, such as beer, coffee, wine, or fruit juice, are so high in acidity that they can't be balanced, and should, as a rule, be avoided if one is facing health challenges.

In addition to diet, the quality and quantity of the water we drink is a major component in creating the optimal acid/alkaline balance, since our bodies are almost 70 percent water, and our brains are 90 percent. There is now a new technology, as described in Chapter 2, which ensures that our water has the highest alkalinity.

Of course, the foods we eat are only part of the story. The idea that our emotional state, or our choice of activities, could affect one's pH, making it more or less acidic, was considered quite a controversial theory. This is no longer the case. There is now overwhelming scientific evidence that achieving a state of consciousness commonly associated with a spiritual outlook on life is very beneficial to one's health. Alkaline forming activities include: moderate sunshine, rest/sleep, deep breathing, fasting and under-eating, relaxation, soothing music, laughter, emotional release processes, self-esteem. Not surprisingly, acidic forming activities include: lack of rest, overeating, stress, noise, anger, denial, confusion and fear.

Unfortunately, taking the responsibility to rebalance one's acid/alkalinity ratio, and, thus, restoring one's body to the optimal balance that promotes optimal health, will often result in withdrawal symptoms similar to those experienced by an alcoholic or drug addict. As long as one knows what to expect, this shouldn't cause undo alarm nor be a major handicap to the process of detoxification.

After a period of time, one's body will regenerate to a state of health, and thus level of happiness and joy, never before experienced. Doesn't this make one's struggles for self-discipline all worthwhile?[10]

Do You Have an Addiction?

By Barry Harris

"Food is the earliest addiction, the basic prejudice, starting with the newborn's first mouthful. Food is more controversial than sex, politics, religion, or drugs. Many people feel that their lifestyle is questioned and discredited if you refuse, on philosophical grounds, to eat certain foods at their home.

"People generally have no instinctual or rational basis for their diet; as a result, they can become very emotional about it. The average person has no idea what natural food is, or how to maintain good health. Doctors know a great deal about disease, but very little about health-promoting nutrition."

The above quote claims that we can become very emotional about our food choices. Perhaps the major reason is that we expect food to compensate for the emptiness we feel inside because of our separation from spirit. We try to distract ourselves from the pain resulting from this separation, which is actually a separation from the experience of love. The pattern is set in infancy, when we are taught that candy, cookies, and ice cream mean love. Our craving for love is soon replaced by these symbolic stand-ins.

---

[10] Recommended Reading:

Kulvinskas, V. *Survival Into the 21st Century.* pg. 21.

Baroody, T. *Alkalize or Die.*

Worter, M.T. *Your Health, Your Choice.*

The addiction stemming originally from a psychological and spiritual need now becomes reinforced by disturbed blood chemistry and inadequate nutrition, as an actual physiological need. Once we have an imbalanced blood chemistry and a body that is not getting enough nutrition, we can no longer trust the feedback of our natural instincts.

As an example, we can trace the addictive process that so innocently began with the morning cup of coffee, to see how this works. At first, coffee gives us energy, and this is mistakenly interpreted as having a positive effect on our health, whereas stopping our addiction to coffee temporarily depletes our energy, and we interpret this occurrence as proof that withdrawal from caffeine has a negative effect. We don't realize that the misperception of energy only came from a weakened body marshaling all its forces to respond to a crisis created by the introduction of a powerful toxin. The crash after the morning coffee would make this evident, if it were not prevented by drinking an afternoon cup of coffee.

As long as we keep our bodies acidic and addicted, we will experience the negative effects of a toxic body as the norm, and the drug companies selling us their antacids and poisonous chemicals will be happy, but the important question is, "Will you be happy?"

In summary, many addicted individuals don't realize that human beings only experience addictions when the body is acidic, and there is a chemical imbalance present. The Hippocrates Institute has seen the demonstration of this truth time and time again. Its program, when followed faithfully, results in alkalizing the body, and restoring its chemical balance, and it has been observed as a side benefit, that it frees one from the slavery to cravings and addictions.

However, one must be patient, and allow the alkalinizing process enough time to achieve its optimal results. Not being informed about what to expect during this process often interferes with this patience, for the withdrawal symptoms that arise can lead to discouragement. All of the symptoms of detoxification may arise, and the most distressing symptom is craving for the very substance to which one has been addicted. As a result, there is motivation to rationalize, again, choosing the addictive behavior, and this only compounds the discouragement.

If we are prepared for the emotional and mental changes, which accompany alkalizing the body, then we can "weather the storm." Keep your eyes on the prize, and a new "you" will emerge, free not only from addictive behaviors, but, most importantly, free from addictive emotions and addictive mind patterns. Then you will know true power, true self-esteem, and true happiness. For a personal experience of this, see Betsy Bragg's "The Turning Point to Vitality, Inner Peace & Mindfulness – Arthritis, Substance Cravings, ADHD" in Chapter 10.

The legendary Jack LaLanne once said, "People don't die of old age, they die of neglect." Go to http://articles.mercola.com/sites/articles/archive/2009/08/11/Do-You-Want-to-Look-Like-This--Great-Reasons-to-Exercise-and-Eat-Right.aspx accessed February 22, 2012.

DVD: Principles of Health

Hippocrates DVD Health Series: Lecture 1

www.hippocratesinst.org

12-part series DVDs ($299) or CDs ($149)

A brief history of how Hippocrates came into being. A comprehensive explanation of the food groups in the living foods diet. Check your answers in the DVD Questions and Answers Appendix.

Questions:

1. Who was the Hippocrates Institute named after and why (what were his primary beliefs)? (Feel free   to use outside sources to further your research)

2. Who was the founder?

    a. What was her country of origin?

    b. How was she healed and from what?

    c. When and where did she found Hippocrates?

    d. What great book inspired her?

3. Who were the key people who helped the founder make the Hippocrates Institute what it is today and   what were their roles?

4. What are the three major food groups of the Living Foods Diet?

5. Why are wheatgrass and sunflower greens the No. 1 food group at Hippocrates?

6. How much wheatgrass is the recommended amount to have per serving per day?

7. How many pounds of vegetables is 2 oz. of wheatgrass said to be equivalent to?

8. Name the five of the second group of healing sprouts with half the amount of chlorophyll?

9. What is in the Hippocrates Green drink?

10. What is the third group of living food?

11. What is the process of sprouting grain?

12. How is the pulp from juicing wheatgrass used and why?

13. .What are the 5 most highly recommended grains?

14. How should beans be eaten and why?

15. .What are the two types of beans not to be eaten?

16. What are two unique beans from Asia? What are their benefits?

17. What sprout makes your body odor disappear?

18. Should sprouting be taken place inside or outside?

19. Which sprouts create more alkalinity in the body?

DVD: Eating
by Michael Anderson

1 hour 50 min.

"Eating" frames a low-fat vegan diet as a cure-all for just about every physical malady.Check your answers in the DVD Questions and Answers Appendix.

Introduction

1. Health conditions caused by eating kill 2 out of 3 Americans each year. True or False?

2. What condition was not even included in medical textbooks in the 1800s?

3. Name 3 foods that were a major part of the diet of the people in the 1800s.

4. What foods were uncommon on the plates of the working class in the 1800s?

    a. Why were they uncommon?

5. What was the biggest dietary change in human history? Why?

Heart Disease

6. What became our #1 killer?

7. An animal based diet causes arteries to open/close while a vegetable based diet caused arteries to open/close.

8. What percentage of the population will get some form of cancer?

9. The one thing an animal based diet does best is _____.

10. What happens when you deprive the heart of oxygen?

11. What happens when you deprive the brain of oxygen?

12. What happens when you deprive your tissues and cells of oxygen?

13. The vast majority of diseases today are caused by _____.

14. More people die of _____ than from all other causes of death combined.

15. The primary cause of clogged blood vessels is _____.

16. What is the only dietary source of cholesterol?

17. What is estimated to be more deadly than all the wars of the 20th century, all natural disasters and all automobile accidents combined?

18. How many varieties of fruits and vegetables did ancient humans eat?

19. What has been called "animals revenge"?

20. How much cholesterol is required in our diets?

21. The Atkins diet causes a _____ reaction.

22. What is the only thing that can reverse heart disease?

23. According to US Health Standards, a cholesterol level under 200 is safe. What is the only safe level?

24. It is not the type of fat (good or bad) but the _____ in your body.

Cancer

25. What are two hallmark diseases of an animal-based diet?

26. What strengthens our immune system?

27. An animal-based diet has caused abnormal _____ levels in men and increased risks for _____.

Food Myths

28. Is protein deficiency a problem in the United States?

29. True or False: Fruits and vegetables have protein.

30. Is calcium deficiency of dietary origin?

31. What is the primary cause of osteoporosis?

32. How do you make your bones stronger?

33. Three glasses of milk have the same amount of cholesterol as ___ pieces of bacon.

Food Politics

34. In United States, what percent of raw materials and fuels are used to raise animals _____.

35. What would be the cost of beef, per pound, without subsidies?

36. What percent of food subsidies are given for fruits and vegetables_____.

37. Who said "Let food be your medicine and medicine be your food"?

38. What does the acronym R.A.V.E. stand for?

39. Name 3 of the long-term changes caused by a plant food diet?

40. Is a plant-based diet old or new?

41. What is the leading cause of kidney failure in the United States?

42. How many wild animals are slaughtered each year to protect cattle in United States?

43. What is Mad Cow Disease often misdiagnosed as?

44. What is the cause of 75 percent of all new infectious diseases?

Summary Questions

1. What are the nine basic Hippocrates beliefs?

2. Name at least 5 alkaline and acid forming activities.

3. Why is it important to be consistent with following the Hippocrates approach to Optimum Health?

Chapter 2
The Living Food Kitchen

Overview

Our bodies need live food to fuel energy and to fight off infections and disease. Transitioning can be overwhelming at first, so plan to transition slowly to a living food (raw, vegan), plant-based diet. Consider consuming 50 percent living foods and slowly increasing to 80 percent living foods. This slow transition allows your body and your mind to adjust to the changes. Eating a living food diet is one of the necessary steps to achieving optimum health for the long term. You can optimize health by lowering cholesterol levels, blood pressure, blood sugar levels, and reducing the overall degree of disease in your body. The goals of optimum health include a mental, physical and spiritual approach along with a living food lifestyle.

What you will find in this week's lesson is how to set up your living food kitchen. You will have a guide on how to select fruits, vegetables, grains, seeds and nuts.

You will learn:

- What living food is.
- To set up a living food kitchen.
- How to combine your food when planning your menu.
- How to create a weekly menu and shopping list.
- How to select living food equipment.
- To differentiate organic, conventional and genetically modified foods.

What is plant-based living food?

Live food adherents consider food to be raw/living if it has not been heated beyond 118 degrees. Pasteurized products, canned foods, and frozen vegetables have been heated beyond this point, but most frozen fruit have not. The living food diet also emphasizes live sprouts, and unpasteurized probiotic foods such as miso and pickled vegetables.

Extras: Foods that are common to the raw food diet, but might be unfamiliar to you, include chia seeds, goji berries, medjool dates, hemp seeds and coconut butter.

Shopping the Life Force Way

Shopping with "Life Force" in mind, will lead you straight to the fresh vegetable section of health food stores and supermarkets. But, this is just the beginning of the considerations that should guide you in your food shopping choices.

It should be obvious that, whenever possible, you should choose organic. If the higher cost takes away your motivation for choosing organic, remembering the cost of your future medical bills should bring it back. And, of course, if one is serious about restoring or retaining one's health, as soon as one knows that produce has been irradiated or genetically modified, one will just pass it by.

There are other criteria determining the contents of your shopping cart, which might not be so obvious. Is the produce still fresh? Are you healthy enough that metabolizing sugar is not a problem? If the answer is "no," even organic fruit cannot be tolerated. If the answer is "yes," and you don't suffer from candida, then 15 percent of your daily dietary intake can be fruit.

You also may not know about the superiority of locally grown produce. Shopping at farmers markets ensures that you are purchasing locally grown produce still retaining its nutrition, because locally grown produce is picked at its peak and is usually sold within 24 hours of harvesting.

As final considerations, make sure that your produce purchases cover all the colors of the rainbow, and that you never forget to purchase the highest-quality sea vegetables, thus guaranteeing you will get all the minerals your body needs.

Once you have collected the healthiest ingredients for your daily food intake, what kind of preparation will optimally retain all their health giving goodness? Some of the options include: (1) salads, (2) green vegetable drinks, (3) occasional blended soups and sauces, (4) dehydrated snacks and (5) vegetable dips and loaves.

Shopping List (organic, whenever possible):

Vegetables		Leafy Greens
Asparagus	Green Beans	Arugula
Avocado	Jerusalem Artichoke	Bok Choy
Beets	Jicama	Chicory
Broccoli	Mushrooms	Collard Greens
Burdock Root	Parsnip	Dandelion Greens
Cabbage	Radishes	Kale
Carrots	Rutabaga	All Lettuces
Cauliflower	Snow Peas	Mustard Greens
Celery	Sweet Potato	Spinach
Celery Root	Squash - all varieties	Swiss Chard
Corn	Tomatoes/Sun dried	Watercress
Cucumber	Turnip	
Garlic	Zucchini	
Ginger		

There are numerous reasons to eat vegetables and since their nutritional value varies, it is important for us to eat a variety of them. Following is a short list of some of the known specific reasons to consume certain vegetables. See chapter 7 for the Hippocrates charts with more detailed health benefits.

Asparagus is very good for kidney and bladder conditions.

Bell Peppers are a good source of vitamin C. Use red, orange or yellow; these are mature, ripe peppers. (Green bell peppers are unripe. That is why they are less expensive.)

Broccoli and cauliflower are cruciferous vegetables that contain a phytonutrient that inhibits the development of cancer. Sprouted broccoli seeds are several dozen times more effective in combating cancer than other vegetables in this family. They have only been in existence for about 100 years; they have been hybridized into existence.

Cabbage, both green and purple, helps to heal the digestive tract, ulcers, cancer, osteoporosis and osteoarthritis. It's also effective to heal sore throats. Purple has a bit more minerals because of its darker color. (See John Duffy's testimonial in chapter 10 to read how he recovered from ulcers with cabbage juice. Also read Judith Hiatt's book, *Cabbage, Cures to Cuisine.*)

Carrots and beets are higher in sugar than the other veggies. If you are eliminating sugar in your diet, you don't have to stay away from them completely but be mindful that they do have more sugar. It's not a good idea to juice a lot of carrots or beets, because that would be too much sugar.

Frozen Veggies – Cascadian Farms has only organic vegetables. If you can't find something that is fresh and organic, it might be worthwhile getting some frozen vegetables now and again. The company flash freezes them and this helps to protect some of the nutrients.

If you grow vegetables yourself and you put them in the freezer for storage and use them within three months, then you do not have to blanche them. Blanching is quickly putting the vegetables in boiling water. The reason you do that is to kill the enzymes because that quick dunk in the boiling water stops the enzymatic process and preserves the food for a longer period of time. However, you have lost the benefit of having the enzymes alive. If you are going to use fresh vegetables within three months, you do not have to blanch them before freezing. If you want to preserve them for a longer time, you'll have to blanch the vegetables. Otherwise, the enzymes, even in the freezer, will start to break down the vegetables and they will not last as long.

Greens offer a large range of phytonutrients, which are chemical substances that help you fight and heal disease. Select a wide variety of vegetables because every vegetable has a different nutritional gift.

All dark leafy greens are excellent for health. (See Dr. Joel Fuhrman's ANDI list – Aggregate Nutrient Density Index at http://www.eatrightamerica.com/andi-superfoods)

The Hippocrates Health Institute green drink consists of 50 percent cucumber and celery and 50 percent sunflower and pea sprouts. When you are making your own juice, you can use other greens such as kale, chard, lettuce, carrot and beet tops.

Radishes are high in anti-cancer phytonutrients and very low in sugar.

White potatoes are low in nutritional value. You are better off choosing something with more color, which means a higher mineral content. In general, the darker the vegetable is, the more minerals and nutrition it possesses. White potatoes have been shown to help arthritis. If you're dealing with arthritis, juice white potatoes and let the starch settle to the bottom of the cup, then drink the clear liquid.

If you are on the HHI maintenance diet, which is 80 percent raw and 20 percent cooked, then good cooked choices are baked squash, yams and steamed veggies. Yams and sweet potatoes can also be used raw shredded in salads or used in dressings and sauces.

<u>Zucchini and yellow squash</u> are good for blending into your salad dressing to give it hearty substance.

Sprouts		Alkaline Grains
Adzuki Beans	Lentils	Amaranth
Alfalfa	Mung Beans	Buckwheat Groats
Broccoli	Onion	Millet
Buckwheat greens	Pea Greens	Quinoa
Cabbage	Radish	Teff
Chickpeas	Sunflower Greens	
Clover	Wheatgrass	
Fenugreek		

Nuts & Seeds	Sea Vegetables	Salt Substitutes
Almonds	Alaria	Braggs Liquid Aminos
Brazil Nuts	Arame	Dehydrated celery powder Miso
Chia Seeds	Bladderwrack	Nama Shoyu
Flax Seeds	Digitata	Olive water/Brine
Hemp Seeds	Dulse	Tamara
Macadamia Nuts	Hijiki/Hiziki	Seaweeds: kelp, dulse
Pecans	Kelp/Kelp Noodles	**Sugar Substitutes:**
Pine Nuts	Laver	Coconut Water
Pistachios	Nori	Dates
Pumpkin Seeds	Sea Lettuce	Figs
Sesame Seeds	Sea Palms	Lucuma
Sunflower Seeds	Wakame	Stevia
Walnuts		Yacon

Raw seeds, nuts, grains and legumes must be kept in freezer or they go rancid.

Please note that the cashews we consume are never truly raw, even if labeled as such. Cashews are actually a seed, not a nut, and are surrounded by a double shell. This outer shell contains a resin called urushiol, which can cause skin rashes and allergic reactions, especially in those who are allergic to poison ivy and therefore have an increased sensitivity. Because of this potential toxin, "raw" cashews are still steamed to release the urushiol and make them safe to eat.[11]

Grains, nuts, seeds and beans. Buckwheat groats are served as a raw cereal in the morning. These have been soaked, sprouted for a couple of days and then dehydrated. There are five varieties of oats: whole oat groats, steel cut oats, oat bran, quick oats, and rolled oats.

The only oat type that that has a life force and will sprout is the groat, so that would be your best choice. The more the oats are processed, the more nutrition is lost along the way. By the time you come down to instant oatmeal, you just have some fiber. You can make nice grain milk by sprouting the grain and putting it in the blender with some water and then straining it. You can add some stevia, cinnamon and vanilla to make sweet tasting milk. Then you can put it over a grain cereal.

[11]http://www.wisegeek.com/are-raw-cashews-really-poisonous.htm accessed on August 29, 2012.

Grains like kamut, spelt, oats, wheat berries, quinoa, and millet can be sprouted and eaten raw. What we serve cooked cereal at HHI, we soak quinoa or millet overnight, pour off the soaked water, add water that is about twice the amount of the grain, bring it to a boil, shut it off and let it absorb all water in about a half an hour. Then it is ready.

Vegetables		Leafy Greens
Asparagus	Green Beans	Arugula
Avocado	Jerusalem Artichoke	Bok Choy
Beets	Jicama	Chicory
Broccoli	Mushrooms	Collard Greens
Burdock Root	Parsnip	Dandelion Greens
Cabbage	Radishes	Kale
Carrots	Rutabaga	All Lettuces
Cauliflower	Snow Peas	Mustard Greens
Celery	Sweet Potato	Spinach
Celery Root	Squash - all varieties	Swiss Chard
Corn	Tomatoes/Sun dried	Watercress
Cucumber	Turnip	
Garlic	Zucchini	
Ginger		

Quinoa and millet are whole grains. They are alkaline. Couscous looks similar to millet, but is NOT a whole grain: It is actually tiny pasta, so we do not recommend couscous.

Organic popcorn is one of your better choices when you want a crunchy, munchie kind of snack. Use an air popper to avoid popping the corn in oil. You can make a topping from sesame oil with seasonings like garlic powder and Bragg's. FYI, corn is one of the most genetically modified crops in this country so Hippocrates does not recommend consuming corn at all. This is a transitional food, not found at Hippocrates.

Two beans HHI does not advise using are soybeans and black beans, unless you grew up eating black beans. The density of the protein in these beans is hard to break down and digest well. All other beans are fine. Remember to soak them before you use them.

Flax seeds are very nutritious. Mix 1/5 of flax seed to 4/5 water and let the mixture stand until it gains a mucilage consistency. It is good for helping you to eliminate.

Hemp seeds are an excellent source of protein. You can sprinkle them on your salad or take a handful when you want a little snack.

Grain-Seed-Nut Rotation Chart created by Sally Lukez

This is transitional because HHI does not recommend combining carbohydrates and protein. They require different enzymes and take different times to digest, which causes indigestion.

Day of the Week	Grain	Seed/Nut
Sunday	Quinoa	Macadamia
Monday	Rice	Almond/Sunflower/Pumpkin
Tuesday	Buckwheat	Pecan
Wednesday	Millet	Walnut
Thursday	Flax	Hemp
Friday	Oat	Almond/Sunflower/Pumpkin
Saturday	Millet	Chia
Herbs, Spices & Flavorings		
Allspice	Cloves	Marjoram
Basil	Coconuts	Mesquite
Bay leaves	Coconut Flakes	Mustard – dried
Caraway Seeds	Coriander	Peppermint Extract
Cardamom	Cumin	Poppy Seed
Carob	Curry	Rosemary
Celery Seed	Dill	Sage
Cayenne Pepper	Garam Masala	Saffron
Chervil	Garlic Powder	Salt - Celtic & Himalayan
Chile Powder	Ginger	Slippery Elm
Chipotle (2)	Italian Seasoning	Tarragon
Chives	Juniper Berry	Thyme
Cinnamon Sticks	Lecithin Granules	Turmeric
Cinnamon Powder	Maca	Vanilla Extract

Extracts such as vanilla extract and maple extract can be used to add flavor, but HHI chefs emphasize vanilla and other "flavors" rather than the extracts, to avoid the alcohol. Frontier is a good brand, especially for organic spices and extracts.

Herbs such as parsley, cilantro and basil have a strong taste that repels insects. Therefore, farmers do not have to use a lot of pesticides on them. They might be organic even if they are not labeled organic. These are one of your better choices if you are traveling and are unable to find organic greens.

Seasonings should be organic and fresh. Be aware of their limited shelf life, which is generally one year.

Where To Buy:

(1) South River Miso:www.southrivermiso.com

(2) Mountain Rose Herbs:www.mountainroseherbs.com

Oils	Butters	Dried Fruits
Extra Virgin Olive Oil	Almond Butter	Apricots
Flax Seed Oil	Sesame Tahini	Coconut Flakes
Hemp Oil	Sunflower Seed Butter	Currants
Virgin Coconut Oil	Pumpkin Seed Butter	Dates-Medjool
Sesame Oil		Figs
Pumpkin Seed Oil		Goji Berries
		Prunes
		Raisins

Nut butter, such as almond butter or tahini, is recommended over peanut butter.

- Tahini is made from sesame seeds. Look for raw organic tahini.

- Hazelnut butter and macadamia butter are quite rich. They are fine for minimal use.

- Cashews, which are the nuts found inside the seeds of the tropical cashew fruit, have a tight shell and in most cases, the shell must be heated to come off. So even though it is a raw cashew, it has been exposed to heat and no longer has enzymes. Also, cashew shells have a poison that is similar to what is found in poison ivy – therefore, cashews are not recommended in the HHI diet.[1]

- Peanuts may develop a mold known as aflatoxin that grows quite readily and is carcinogenic. Peanuts also cause allergies. They are not recommended at HHI.

Oils should limited in your diet as these are the most carcinogenic items in the super-market. They turn rancid quickly with exposure to heat and light. Olive oil is best if it is extra virgin, and should be cold-pressed or expeller-pressed, where neither heat nor a chemical process is used. You do not need a lot of additional oils in your diet if you are eating nuts and/or avocados a few times a week. Use oils that come directly from plants such as olive, avocado, walnut, pumpkin, sesame and flax seed oil. Udo's Oil is an excellent source of omega 3, 6, and 9 and is found in the supplement, refrigerated section of Whole Foods and should be kept in the refrigerator or freezer. Dr. Tel-Oren highly recommends coconut oil because, he says, it *functions as a cardio-protective, immune-protective and cellular defense antioxidant, preventing the formation of dangerous fatty acid free radicals in rancidity-prone seed oils ... Coconut oil is perfect for improved fat-burning metabolic activity, so it is an excellent addition to any weight-loss program (remember, good fat is necessary for general health!). It is great for skin care, since "you don't want to put anything on your skin that you won't put in your mouth..."*[12] One reason saturated fat (when not derived from animals) is actually very good is that it is very stable (and does not go rancid as easily in heat, oxygen, and light).

(Dr. Tel-Oren does not necessarily agree with some of the statements or concepts or principles included by the Hippocrates Health Institute. For more information, please contact office@ecopolitan.com as well as his bio.)

---

[12]http://www.ecopolitan.com/healtheducation/ask-dr-t/96-coconut-oil-saturated-fat-myth accessed May 5, 2012.

Fruit, initially thought to be "the perfect food for health," has been reassessed as a result of our research, because it has too much sugar due to hybridization. HHI has discovered that most people can tolerate a small portion of fruit in their diets but it is not recommended for those who are dealing with health challenges. It is very important that all fruit consumed be unsprayed and preferably organically grown, and that it is tree-ripened (rather than gas-ripened or countertop-ripened off the vine). Learn to choose fruits in the prime of their season. Some choices of fruit follow:

Best	**OK Occasionally**	**Best Not Eaten**
Apples	Avocado	Apricots (unripe)
Bananas	Berries	Brown coconut (old)
Cherries (deep red only)	Cantaloupe	Dates (too sweet)
Grapes (when stems are brown)	Grapefruit (no green skin)	Dried fruit (too sweet)
Kiwi	Honeydew melon	Mangoes (unripe)
Lemons (juice with water)	Persimmons (very soft)	Oranges (unripe)
Papaya (must have some yellow)	Pineapple (amber skin only)	Peaches (unripe)
Pears	Star fruit	Plums (unripe)
Watermelon (with rind)	Tangerine (no green, loose skin)	

Berries are one of the best fruit choices because they are less hybridized, have lots of antioxidants and lower sugar content than other fruits. We recommend that you are healthy for at least two years before introducing fruit back into your diet.

Coconuts are almost like a green drink and are an excellent source of nutrition! However, when imported from Thailand, they have been taken out of their large greenish shells and cut in a cone shape for easier shipping. To keep them from turning brown, they are dipped in a fungicide bath, a solution of sodium metabisulfite. So Thai coconuts are not recommended. We do recommend the organic coconuts or a local coconut when one is lucky enough to be in Florida or on a tropical vacation. Baby coconuts are wonderful: The meat is very soft and can be scooped out with a spoon, unlike mature coconuts, which are quite thick and do not have that much water in them. It is the water of the green coconut that is so good and healthy!

How can you tell when a fruit is ripe? Sometimes the stem will come off easily, as in the case of a peach, for instance. Avocados will give slightly to the touch, but we do not want to keep pressing it a lot because it will bruise the fruit. The perfect situation would be to wait until the fruit fell off the tree and eat it right away. For practical reasons, however, fruit is picked unripe then transported and stored before getting to the market. Many times you are buying things that are not ripe yet and you will have to wait until for them to ripen. That is crucial: When the fruit is ripe, it gives you nourishment. When it is not ripe, it steals nourishment from you to complete its ripening process. Make sure your fruits are ripe before you eat them.

Dried fruits such as dates and raisins contain super-concentrated sugar. It is best to rehydrate dried fruits before using them or at least make sure you are very well hydrated when you eat dehydrated food, because it will absorb moisture from you.

Melons must be eaten alone, or combined with other melons, because they digest faster than other fruits. Combining melon with anything will slow it down, causing it to ferment instead of digesting properly. To know if a melon is ripe, the trick is to smell where the stem would be. When it smells like a ripe melon, then it's ripe.

Pineapples are ripe when you can pull the top leaf out easily.

Miscellaneous Living Foods Items:

Apple cider vinegar and all vinegars are very acidic and therefore, not supported by HHI. While they interfere with digestion, they have good medicinal uses. If you feel you have a scratchy throat, you can take a tablespoon of apple cider vinegar in a glass of water on arising and at bed time. It can get rid of that scratchiness. (But remember you may also use lemon juice or cabbage juice, this one about 2 ounces with a little lemon.)

Miso is made of fermented chickpeas or barley. You may buy it locally from http://www.southrivermiso.com/

Organic Herbal Tea Yogi and Traditional Medicinals are good brands because they use mostly organic ingredients. Good teas often can have a medicinal quality. Herbal tea is said to help your sore throat or help you sleep, as is the case with chamomile. Some others offer stress relief or joint comfort.

Stevia is a sweet herb but it is the only sweet food that does not become sugar in the body. It comes in different forms: white powder, and dark and light liquids. You might try a few different brands and see which one has a taste you like. They now have stevia with different flavors as well. HHI uses Stevita (http://stevitastevia.com) because members say it has the least after-taste. Betsy Bragg likes SweetLeaf SteviaClear, found at Whole Foods. She also says: "or grow it in your garden!" She was once offered a delightful dessert by Sparkle Richardson: a slice of banana with a stevia leaf on top from his garden.

Miscellaneous Living Food Kitchen Items:

Cleaning Products make a big difference in a green and healthy lifestyle. Products that are healthy for the earth and for you are a much better choice than commercial products that poison you and the environment. You can learn to the make inexpensive green cleaning products of the Vida Verde Cooperative, which is part of the Brazilian Women's Group.The recipes are at www.optimumhealthsolution.org/article_vida_verde_ecoproducts.htm. A group of Brazilian house-cleaners developed these preparations after getting sick from commercial products. Their "green cleaners" have been approved by the University of Massachusetts/Lowell's Toxics Use Reduction Institute.

Green produce bags are useful for extending the life of your produce. If you happen to be in a position where you can shop every three days for fresh produce, they might not be necessary. But if you want to store produce for more than a week or 10 days, this can be helpful for extending the life of your produce without any chemicals. These bags are reusable. Just rinse them out and use them again. Whole Foods and Amazon sell the Debbie Meyer brand.

NOT in a Living Foods Kitchen

Bottled dressings often have vinegar in them. Vinegar interferes with digestion, so avoid it in dressings. Annie's makes a lemon and chive dressing that is vinegar free. They also make green garlic dressing without vinegar. What is best is to make your own dressing or to discover the wonders of having your salads with a few squirts of fresh lemon.

Bottled Juices are pasteurized. What is in those bottles that are ready for a long shelf life? You have sugar and probably a few minerals left. Essentially, you have lost the life force, the vitality and the electromagnetic field you would have if you actually juiced the fruit fresh. As it stands, it's dead; it has no more enzymes in it. When making a juice/seltzer drink for the kids, keep diluting it. Add things like fresh lemon juice and stevia.

Cheese may be on your list to have every once in a while. In order to avoid animal foods, you may think: "I won't have a dairy cheese, I'll have a vegetarian, non-dairy cheese." This is where it is important to always read the labels. Whether you pick up sliced or block cheese, it is important to read the label because most cheeses have casein, which is a milk protein. There are a lot of different words you need to be aware of – whey is from dairy, casein is from dairy, so you want to look for those words and know that it still has dairy it and avoid it. Look for the word VEGAN or dairy-free. These can be used once in a great while such as at a special party. It won't hurt you in small quantities.

Food Bars are usually bad food combinations. They usually combine dried fruits and nuts, but fruits and protein digest at different rates. Fruits usually take one hour and proteins take four hours. So a bar that contains almonds and dates has a poor food combination because those ingredients digest at different times. If you are going to have them, because they are easy to pick up for traveling, look for ones that don't mix fruits and nuts or that don't mix nuts and a starch, such as quinoa. If you are going to get a food bar, Go Raw is a better choice. Its banana bread flax bar is 100 percent organic, gluten-free, wheat-free and nut-free. (See section on Food Combining later in this chapter.)

Soy Products we do not use because soy has been hybridized over the years until the protein in it is extremely dense and difficult to break down. Undigested protein is one of the things that can cause problems. The one soy product used at HHI is tempeh, perhaps only once a month. Tempeh is inoculated with food-grade bacteria that work on it, that has predigested and broken down some of that dense protein for you. You can add onions and celery to it and use it to make a mock chicken salad.

Since HHI advocates a vegan diet, we are not going to talk about meat or dairy. We do not advise you to use any of these products at all. However, if a mother cannot breast feed her baby, then goat milk can be used. It is much closer to human milk than cow milk. Cow milk is meant to grow a calf to 700 pounds within a year. So the proportions of the proteins and fats are much higher than in human milk and our bodies cannot break that down easily. Avoid cow's milk.

Food Combining for Health and Longevity
by Dr. Wayne Pickering

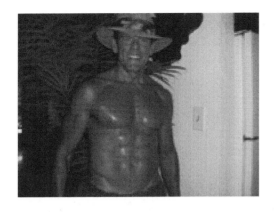

In my travels throughout 23 countries, and from my studies of people who have reached 90 years and upwards, as well as others acclaimed to be the healthiest individuals in the world, I have found seven common factors. All of these healthy people enjoyed plenty of fresh air, pure drinking water, ample sunshine, adequate rest, a fitness program for the body's cardiovascular and muscular systems which included some stretching, emotional stability, and diets of natural foods which were relatively free of toxic sprays.

The diets of these individuals varied. There were vegetarians, fruitarians, raw food eaters, fish eaters, and meat eaters. This puzzled me a great deal at first, and it was only after extensive research that I saw six common factors in the diets:

1. in all of them, foods were eaten in moderation;

2. the kinds of foods eaten were appropriate for the energy expended in the type of work the individual did;

3. the foods eaten were native to their environment;

4. they were foods to which the individuals were biologically adapted;

5. foods were eaten in season; and

6. foods were eaten in compatible combinations with the body's digestive chemistry, or other factors mitigated the effect of the breaches.

Most of the above needs little in the way of explanation. Food choices, especially American food choices, which are generally made (in a very competitive consumer's market) for taste, with a certain complacency of thought regarding nutritional value, do not encourage moderate eating.

Here is a phrase I wrote some time ago: "We must combine when we dine to get the correct effect!"

Another quote I coined some time ago: Most of us are serving food on the basis of taste and tradition and we do it in haste and forget nutrition!

Our food has been made to taste so unnaturally good, being visually (through various chemicals, including pesticides) and flavor enhanced and preserved with so many additives (many of which should never be placed in our bodies), that we heap more and more onto our plates, going far beyond the point of satiety.

It takes about 20 minutes for the signal from the stomach to reach the brain which lets us know that the stomach is full, hence the word "satisfaction," part of the meaning of the word "satiety." Studies have shown that undereating increases longevity, whereas overeating, which often leads to obesity, is certain to cause problems that will shorten life.

The formula for obesity is: O = U/8 orYOU OVERATE

A good rule of thumb is: Foods that are native to one's environment are those which should be eaten. This is because all foods are picked green for shipping purposes, and most will not ripen after they're picked, thus rendering no nutritional value. In the "Getting Started" booklet that accompanies our Perfect Diet MINI Program at the www.DefeatingBadEating.com website, there is a list of fruits that ripen at room temperature after picking!

A person who lives a sedentary life would surely not need to eat an abundance of heavy foods. It is generally accepted that a lighter diet might suffice for that individual, rather than one which might be chosen by a heavy laborer. This seems rational on the surface, unless the choice is emotional rather than necessary, especially when we consider that the strongest animals in the world — elephants, oxen, horses, mules, camels, and water buffalo —all eat leaves, grass, and fruit.

Each species of mammal (carnivore, herbivore, omnivore, graminivore, and frugivore) has a specific type of digestive system which biologically adapts to a particular type of food. According to Herbert M. Shelton in *The Science and Fine Art of Food and Nutrition*, every anatomical, physiological and embryological feature of man places him in the class of frugivore. This means, according to *Densmore's Medical Dictionary*, that he feeds on fruits, vegetables, nuts, seeds, and grains.

Although Shelton could cite no true frugivore, meaning mammals which subsist on fruits, seeds, and nuts alone, he was disparaging of the grains, and most nutritionists agree that grains can be troublesome. They are easily overeaten.

It is certainly indisputable that humans do not have all the different types of digestive systems. Yet, the folly of the human species, observe Harvey and Marilyn Diamond in their book, *Fit For Life,* is that we have attempted to eat the different diets of all the animals. Even worse, with no discrimination whatsoever, we eat it all in one meal. Our reason for eating so much food is that, ironically, we have become prisoners of our tiny taste buds.

I stated above that among the healthiest people I have ever met were some fish and meat eaters, and this had particularly puzzled me. I must qualify that the fish and meat consumption of these individuals was sensible, and that their diets consisted of plenty of those foods to which their bodies adapted.

Compatible Food Combining with respect to the body's digestive chemistry is a science that is becoming accepted. Its basic fundamentals were revealed from studies by Ivan Pavlov in his book, *The Work of the Digestive Glands*. Pavlov is perhaps better known for his experiments on conditional reflexes. Herbert Shelton's extensive research is notable among the many studies that have substantiated the validity of Proper Food Combining.

Compatible Combinations or Food Combining

Years of counseling the nutritional needs of thousands of people provided me with ample evidence that proper food combining is the sensible, logical way to eat for effective digestion.

The purpose of food combining is to uncomplicate the process of digestion, thereby eliminating digestive problems. No food value can be obtained from undigested foods.

Furthermore, when food doesn't digest, it rots in the intestines, resulting in the production of alcohols and poisons, thus creating a climate in the digestive tract that is conducive to illness. As long as we remain harmonious on the emotional level (strong negative emotions are physically debilitating), proper food combining will assure us of better digestion and, consequently, better nutrition.

Beyond that, precious energy will be freed up from dealing with a mess in our digestive tracts that can, instead, be utilized constructively for other activities. This can make a critical difference in our outlook and in all our endeavors.

Unquestionably, plenty of people have complacent attitudes about their "traditional" diets, and those individuals strenuously object to changing old eating habits, even when their bodies are screaming proof that they are out of kilter.

I would like to suggest that just because there are staples of a population, that doesn't necessarily give them any virtues.

It has been suggested that about two percent of all people think logically for themselves; eight percent think when they are in pain; and 90 percent would rather die than think. I am addressing those who think, with the hope that they will soon influence the rest who don't think.

A person will dedicate years of life to the training necessary to become an airplane pilot, electronics technician, architect, or some other professional; yet many, probably most, show little regard for the ONLY PERFECT MACHINE – THE HUMAN BODY. We may have considered that there may be laws and rules governing our universe and nature, but how many of us have reasoned that there might also be specific rules for the efficient operation of those perfect machines – our bodies?

Take the automobile, for example: It has an exhaust system, carburetor system, electrical system, cooling system, lubricating system, and a fuel system. All of these work together for smooth operation. We would never put oil in the radiator, gas in the battery, or water in the gas tank.

The human body has ten systems that work together harmoniously for normal function. These are the muscular, skeletal, nervous, lymphatic, excretory, respiratory, digestive, circulatory, glandular, and reproductive systems. Each is a separate entity, yet each is also dependent on each of the others. The system that we have the most control over is THE DIGESTIVE SYSTEM, through the way we feed ourselves; this, in turn, affects all the others.

The digestive system is the site of ongoing chemical activity, and different chemicals are needed for the digestion of the different types of food. For example, starch foods require an ALKALINE digestive medium which is supplied initially in the mouth by the digestive enzyme PYLATIN, and protein foods require an ACID medium for digestion – PEPSIN and HYDROCHLORIC ACID. Anyone with any knowledge of chemistry knows that acids and alkalines neutralize each other. Hence, when they are forced to go to work at the same time in the stomach, digestion is completely arrested.

Food will rot whenever it is allowed to remain for a prolonged period at a temperature of 85 degrees. Everyone has had occasion to see and smell food rotting. When it is improperly combined or overeaten, this rotting or fermentation is what happens to food that remains undigested in the stomach which has a temperature of 104 to 106 degrees during digestion. The body goes through a state of shock and tries to get rid of the unwanted matter by discharging more chemicals into the stomach. The symptoms which may occur are: gas, flatulence, heartburn, upset stomach, regurgitation, and diarrhea.

An antacid tablet can't get to the root of the problem of indigestion; it is not a remedy. The science of the body is the SCIENCE OF CAUSE AND EFFECT. We must deal with cause. Masking and pacifying symptoms with antacid tablets and other digestive aids really isn't rational treatment; it's downright irresponsible, in fact. Food rotting in the body can lead to a wide assortment of sickness and misery such as dysentery, headaches, colds, constipation, kidney and liver disorders, and huge medical expenses. This misery is not necessary.

Isn't it ironic that inhabitants of the best-fed nation in the world can have so much trouble digesting their food? The problem is compounded when we not only mix it all up improperly, but many of us eat with almost no discrimination. To be more blunt, we eat junk.

It boggles the mind in trying to fathom why intelligent human beings would attempt to subsist by eating JUNK, meaning all the processed, canned, and ultra-sweetened foods and drinks that are only available in our grocery stores because we buy them. We mix these in with everything else. There are consequences for eating junk foods; it affects behavior and thought processes, and we are the losers.

Here are the three categories of food to totally avoid from this point on in your life:

1) White Foods = "If it's White, it's not Right!"

2) FIZZY Drinks = "If it Fizzes, you'll Fizzle!"

3) Greasy Foods = If it Greasy, it's Sleazy!"

Somewhere I read, "The best way to lengthen your life is to avoid shortening it!" If you will refrain from overeating and combine your foods correctly as indicated below (an excerpt from *The Food Combining Guide,* at www.CombineWhenYouDine.com), YOU SHOULD NEVER AGAIN HAVE A PROBLEM WITH WEIGHT CONTROL OR EXPERIENCE THAT BLOATED FEELING.

Constipation will be eliminated, except for that which comes from eating too fast (not chewing food well enough), drinking with meals, or mismanaged stress (emotions), and the effects of the stress will be less with proper food combining. Your odds for avoiding illness will be greatly improved. Years will be added to your life, and, even more importantly, life will be added to your years.

Men don't die – they kill themselves. Similarly, age doesn't cause disease because if that notion were true then everyone who is old would be sick, and we know that is not the case. So I coined another phrase some time ago that I feel we need to remind ourselves of from time to time: "Age Is Not Our Cage!"

Remember, one of life's laws is replenishment. If we do not eat, we die. Just as surely, if we don't combine foods properly and eat the kinds of foods which will nourish our bodies, we will not only die prematurely, but we have to suffer along the way. So here are

Seven Proper Food Combining Rules

I. Proteins and Starches Should Not Be Eaten Together!

Mixing proteins and starches is one of the worst of the disease-producing habits. There is no way this combination will digest properly. You're thinking, "What about meat and potatoes, hamburgers, sub sandwiches, meat pizzas, macaroni and cheese, hot dogs, and all those other favorites?" Take, for example, the hamburger. The meat is a protein and the bread is a starch. It takes a series of acid digestive juices to digest the protein (pepsin, hydrochloric acid), and a series of alkaline digestive juices to digest the starch (ptyalin, maltase). When proteins and starches are combined, their digestive juices neutralize each other and digestion comes to a halt. Then, as we have learned, when food doesn't digest, it rots.

II. Fruits Should Not Be Eaten With Starches!

The digestion of fruits requires hardly any time at all in the mouth and stomach, while starches require most of their digestion in those areas. The fruit sugars are quickly absorbed into the intestines, while the starch requires chemical and mechanical digestion in the mouth and stomach. Incidentally, starch is the only food that begins to digest in the mouth with the enzyme ptyalin. When sugar, for which ptyalin is required, is combined with starch, the mouth fills with saliva and the signals get jumbled; impaired digestion is the result. If fruit sugars are held up in the stomach awaiting the digestion of starch, fermentation is inevitable.

The rule of thumb when eating fruit is to eat fruit as a fruit meal. This gives a new perspective to some old favorite combinations — the raisin bran products, fruit preserves on toast, bananas on cereal, carrot slaw with raisins. Oranges with rice is a bad combination that is easy to identify and doesn't even sound good.

III. Fruits Should Not Be Eaten with Proteins.

Here, too, the fruit sugars are absorbed directly into the intestines and the protein requires much time digesting in the stomach. If the sugars are held back in the stomach while the protein is digesting, fermentation will result. The only exception to this rule is the avocado, which combines well with acid and sub-acid fruits. Also, there is enough oil in seeds and nuts to prolong the protein digestive gastric juices in the stomach, while the fruit sugars of acid fruits are absorbed into the intestines.

IV. Fruits and Vegetables Should Not Be Eaten Together!

When these are combined, the digestion of the fruit is delayed and fermentation again occurs. Lettuce and celery are exceptions and may be combined with any fruit except melon. Tomatoes are a fruit and an exception to the rule, also. You can have tomatoes with the following vegetables – lettuce, celery, okra, cucumbers, eggplant, bell peppers, and summer squash.

V. Melons Should Be Eaten Alone or Left Alone!

Melons combine with NO OTHER FOOD. They are in their simplest form and require no digestion time at all in the stomach. If they are held back in the stomach while something else is being digested, again, fermentation will take place. Put a piece of melon outside in the sun at 80 to 90 degrees and see how quickly it decomposes. It's no wonder that so many people are bothered by melons. They eat them before, with, or directly after a meal. THERE IS NO EXCEPTION TO THIS RULE. Eat melons alone or leave them alone.

VI. Acid and Sweet Fruits Should Not Be Eaten Together!

These two food groups definitely should not be combined. Banana and grapefruit, oranges and raisins, tangerines and prunes don't even sound like good combinations, do they? NO EXCEPTION TO THIS RULE!

VII. Do NOT Mix More Than 4 to 6 Fruits or Vegetables at a Meal!

The simpler the meal, the better you feel.

***

Benjamin Franklin made the following observations regarding the eating habits of his time, showing that things haven't changed much:

- "I've seen few die of hunger, but 100,000 of overeating."
- "There's more that die from the platter than from the sword!"
-
- "When feasts are spread, the doctor rolls his pills, and in 50 dishes lie a hundred ills."
- "Think health. When you have it, you have everything. When you don't, nothing else matters."

Below is a favorite recipe excerpted from my recipe guide that you can see when you go to www.DefeatingBadEating.com. It's a great recipe to start the day or for a mid-morning snack instead of coffee.

Wayne's Banana-Dana

In 12 ounces of distilled water, soak 4 ounces of raisins and 4 ounces of dates for 24 hours. Then slice 6 bananas and pour the soaked raisins and dates, including the now very sweet liquid, over the top of the cut-up bananas and mix well. This is a fantastic treat and serves 2 people.

Wayne Pickering is an author, speaker, Nutritional Performance Coach, award-winning triathlete and double nominee for The Mr. Healthy American Fitness Leader Award. He can be reached at www.CombineWhenYouDine.com or 866-626-4662.

45

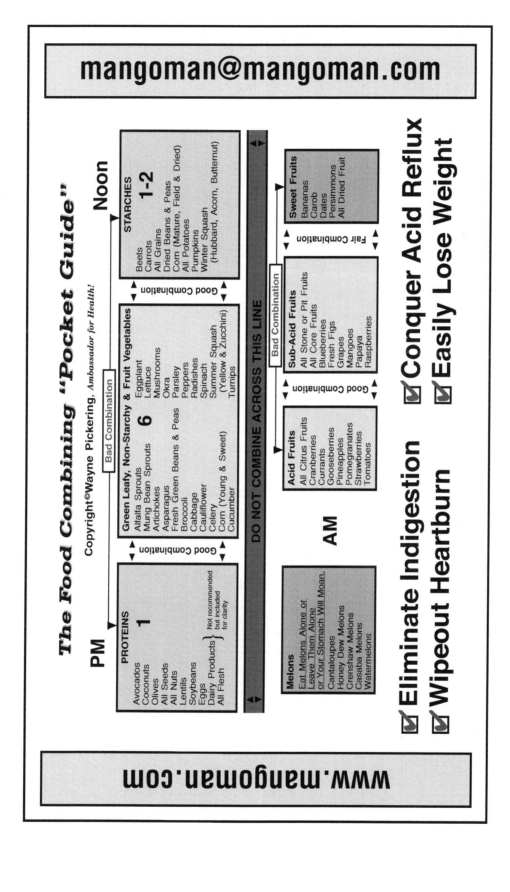

The Food Combining "Pocket Guide"

Copyright©Wayne Pickering, *Ambassador for Health!*

mangoman@mangoman.com

www.mangoman.com

PM — **Noon** — **AM**

PROTEINS 1
Avocados
Coconuts
Olives
All Seeds
All Nuts
Lentils
Soybeans
Eggs
Dairy Products } Not recommended but included for clarity
All Flesh

Green Leafy, Non-Starchy & Fruit Vegetables 6
Alfalfa Sprouts
Mung Bean Sprouts
Artichokes
Asparagus
Fresh Green Beans & Peas
Broccoli
Cabbage
Cauliflower
Celery
Corn (Young & Sweet)
Cucumber
Eggplant
Lettuce
Mushrooms
Okra
Parsley
Peppers
Radishes
Spinach
Summer Squash (Yellow & Zucchini)
Turnips

STARCHES 1-2
Beets
Carrots
All Grains
Dried Beans & Peas
Corn (Mature, Field & Dried)
All Potatoes
Pumpkins
Winter Squash (Hubbard, Acorn, Butternut)

Sweet Fruits
Bananas
Carob
Dates
Persimmons
All Dried Fruit

Sub-Acid Fruits
All Stone or Pit Fruits
All Core Fruits
Blueberries
Fresh Figs
Grapes
Mangoes
Papaya
Raspberries

Acid Fruits
All Citrus Fruits
Cranberries
Currants
Gooseberries
Pineapples
Pomegranates
Strawberries
Tomatoes

Melons
Eat Melons Alone or Leave Them Alone or Your Stomach Will Moan.
Cantaloupes
Honey Dew Melons
Crenshaw Melons
Casaba Melons
Watermelons

Good Combination
Bad Combination
Fair Combination

DO NOT COMBINE ACROSS THIS LINE

☑ **Eliminate Indigestion**   ☑ **Conquer Acid Reflux**
☑ **Wipeout Heartburn**   ☑ **Easily Lose Weight**

Menu Week One - RAW Menu

Breakfast	Lunches:
Green Juices (made from celery, sprouts, kale, cucumbers, etc.)	Salad and Sprouts
Dinner:	**Desserts:**
Mock Tuna (from Rawvolution)	Blueberry Pie (from 5 Alive)
Taco (from Rawvolution)	Chocolate Shake (from 5 Alive)
Cauliflower Couscous (from Rawvolution)	
Avocado Boats (from 5 Alive)	

Grocery List

Produce	Fruit	Seeds/Nuts/Bulk	Miscellaneous
Celery 3-4 stalks	Lemon juice 2 cups	Sunflower Seeds 3 cups	Dill – 1/4 cup
Scallions – 2	6 Avocado	Cashews 2 ½ cups	Thai coconut Water – 1 ½ cups
Garlic 10 cloves	4 Mangos	Walnuts 2 ½ cups	Stone-ground mustard – 1/2 cup
Collard Greens 3-4 leaves	2 Thai coconuts, meat and liquid	Dates, pitted ½ cup	Cumin
Romaine Lettuce 1 cup		Almonds 3 cups (milk)	Coriander
Cherry Tomatoes 2 cups			Nama Shoyu
Parsley 2 bunches	**Salad Stuff**		Olive oil
Cauliflower 2 heads	Spinach		Cayenne pepper
Mint	Cabbage	**Frozen:**	Pitted Greek olives, two 13-ounce jars
Tomatoes 2 cups	Tomatoes	Blueberries 4 cups (or fresh)	Mexican Seasoning
Onions	Jicama		Cinnamon
Jalapeno 1/2 cup	Beets		Vanilla
Celery for Juice	Carrots		stevia crystals or liquid
Cucumbers for Juice	Peppers		Coconut Oil
Kale for Juice			Cacao nibs 1 cup
			Carob Powder

Why Should You Care About Pesticides?[13]

The growing consensus among scientists is that small doses of pesticides and other chemicals can cause lasting damage to human health, especially during fetal development and early childhood. Scientists now know enough about the long-term consequences of ingesting these chemicals to advise that we minimize our consumption of pesticides.

Dirty Dozen Buy These Organic	Clean 15 Lowest in Pesticides
1. Apples	1. Onion
2. Celery	2. Sweet Corn
3. Strawberries	3. Pineapple
4. Peaches	4. Avocado
5. Spinach	5. Asparagus
6. Nectarines- imported	6. Sweet Peas
7. Grapes - imported	7. Mangoes
8. Sweet bell peppers	8. Eggplant
9. Potatoes	9. Cantaloupe - domestic
10. Blueberries - domestic	10. Kiwi
11. Lettuce	11. Cabbage
12. Kale/collard greens	12. Sweet potatoes
	13. Grapefruit
	14. Mushrooms
Environmental Working Group www.ewg.org 1436 U St. N.W., Suite 100 Washington, DC 20009	

---

[13]http://www.ewg.org/foodnews/ accessed February 15, 2012.

Pesticide Pestilence[14]
by Gabriel Cousens

Presently, more than 20 percent of the pesticides currently registered in the U.S. are linked to cancer, birth defects, developmental harm, and central nervous system damage.

Let us understand, pesticides are designed to kill living creatures, and human beings are living creatures. The organic movement is one of the most important things we have to begin to rectify the destruction of our soils, the very high rate of cancer in children and adults, and the literal poisoning of the planet. The only people who benefit from this pollution are the corporations that profit directly from the sale of chemicals and indirectly from the suffering of others.

Some research has shown that when children are put on an organic diet, there is a 50 percent cure rate of hyperactivity, without doing anything else. This is not surprising since most pesticides and herbicides are neurotoxins, and developing nervous systems are more vulnerable to these brain and nervous system poisons. More than 12,000 children in the U.S. are diagnosed with cancer every year. Cancer is now the second leading cause of death, after suicide, for children under age 15. These high cancer rates in children were unheard of before this era of pesticides, herbicides, and genetically engineered food.

One of the most significant effects of an organic vegan diet is the tremendous health benefit of stopping the chronic poisoning from pesticide intake. Unless one eats organic fruits and vegetables, one is continually exposed to pesticides. One of the most important pathological effects of these toxins, besides initiating cancer, is varying levels of neurotoxicity to the brain and the rest of the nervous system. These have more subtle symptoms such as reduced mental functioning, decreased mental clarity, poor concentration, and, the author believes, hyperactivity and Attention Deficit Disorder (ADD). Some recent re-search has linked a higher rate of Parkinson's disease, a brain disease, to those people who have a history of higher pesticide exposure. So we do have some very suggestive evidence that the use of pesticides and herbicides really affects our mental function and brain physiology, including increasing the incidence of Parkinson's. This is not exactly a surprise when you realize that pesticides are designed as neurotoxins. Does it surprise us to think that we are biologically similar to the pests that we are trying to eliminate? Our nervous systems are more sophisticated, and may take longer to poison, but it still happens.

Scientists can pretend to discern "safe" levels for an individual chemical, but in fact, there are no "safe" levels. Certain categories of dangerous chemicals, such as those that cause cancer and disrupt nervous system and hormone function, need to be immediately discontinued if we are to survive as a species.

The amazing observation is that pesticides do not even achieve their stated purpose, yet we still are willing to risk our lives to use them. Dr. David Pimentel of Cornell University, an entomologist and one of the world's leading agricultural experts, estimates that more than 500 species of insects are now resistant to pesticides. It is no accident that crops destroyed by insects have nearly doubled during the last forty years, in spite of an almost tenfold increase in the amount and toxicity of insecticides.

---

[14] Cousens, M.D., G. (1986). *Spiritual Nutrition.* Berkeley, CA: North Atlantic Books, pg. 501.

Even on a cost-benefit versus health approach, the use of pesticides comes out on the negative side of things. According to Dr. Pimentel, pesticides cost the nation $8 billion annually in public health expenditures, not to mention the unmeasured losses from groundwater contamination, fish kills, bird kills, and domestic animal deaths.

In summary, pesticides can affect every living organism: Humans are no exception. The more detrimental effects of pesticides, herbicides, and fungicides include: cancer, nervous system disorders, birth defects, alterations of DNA; liver, kidney, lung, and reproductive system problems; and an overall disruption of ecological cycles on the planet. Pesticide usage is a major public health problem worldwide. Pesticide usage not only leads to disease, but directly destroys the life force of the soil. It reflects a consciousness that is completely out of touch with the laws of nature.

Author's Note: This article does not address the synergistic effect of multiple toxins. For example, as seen in the Gulf War Syndrome, there can be an exponential effect on health when humans are exposed to combinations of toxins.

The Truth About GMOs
by Ellen Simmoneau

Genetically engineered seeds are often referred to as Genetically Modified Organisms (GMOs). They are seeds manufactured by Monsanto Chemical Company and were first introduced commercially in 1996.[15] They now dominate the production of corn, soybeans and cotton in the United States and are now in most of the foods we consume except food that is labeled "organic." They are NOT allowed to sell food that has been manufactured by man and call it "organic" if it isn't.

These man-made seeds are herbicide-tolerant, or the Bt crops, which are known as GMOs. This is an organism that has been changed by injecting it with genetic material from another species. The crops are engineered and produce toxins that will kill certain agricultural insect pests to which nature has produced for the good of us and is part of the food and insect chain as well.

In approximately 30 other countries, including countries in the European Union, they have banned the production of GMOs because they have been proven to be unsafe. The United States will not ban nor will it require any product on the market to label anything that has GMOs. The United States feels there is too much money to be made by not labeling them.

It is important for you to know that 86 percent of corn and 93 percent of soybeans that the United States grows is genetically modified.[16] It is necessary to also be aware of information from the California's Department of Food and Agriculture, that 70 percent of processed foods in American supermarkets now contain GMOs in their ingredients.[17] The USDA has allowed continued planting of GMO sugar beets despite a court order to complete a final Environmental Impact Statement before making any decision on deregulation of genetically engineered sugar beets.[18]

The only way to avoid GMOs is to buy ORGANIC. When planting organic, any nearby farmer who uses herbicides or GMOs must create a buffer zone to prevent contact between organic and non-organic crops.[19] Again, this includes any artificial herbicide-tolerant crops. It is important to insure that any organic crop will have as little as possible contamination from the GMOs from the wind, etc.

The following will give you an idea of just what effects GMOs have:

- They encourage growth of super-weeds. That is similar to taking too many antibiotics when you are ill and building up a resistance to illnesses from the overuse of antibiotics.

- GMOs result in the increased use of toxic and persistent pesticides.[20]

---

[15]http://online.wsj.com/article/SB126862629333762259.html accessed on March 15, 2010.

[16]http://www.ers.usda.gov/data-products/adoption-of-genetically-engineered-crops-in-the-us.aspx accessed on August 29, 2012.

[17]http://www.centerforfoodsafety.org/campaign/genetically-engineered-food/crops/

[18]http://www.reuters.com/article/2011/02/05/us-sugarbeet-usda-idUSTRE7136902011l0205

[19]http://www.rodaleinstitute.org/course/M6/36

[20]http://www.worldwatch.org/node/5950

- In the last 13 years, 383 million pounds of poisonous herbicides have been used on GE crops, in the US alone.[21]

- Increased illness. Female mammals showed signs of liver abnormalities (30.8 percent) and male mammals were more prone to changes in kidney function (43.5 percent) after eating GM seed food.[22]

Now we ask, what are the long-term effects to all of us?

Some of these abnormalities can also be caused by the use of the herbicide "Round-Up" that is sprayed on all GM crops.[23]

It won't be long before you will not be able to buy any seeds that come from nature's plants. They will be manufactured in plants such as Monsanto Chemical and will have no natural insect friends or foes, which are part of the chain for all plants, just like we have for the animal and human chain. In recent conversations, pediatricians have said this would have a catastrophic effect on small children, because their bodies cannot tolerate large amounts of GMOs.[24]

[21]http://www.worldwatch.org/node/5950

[22]http://www.biolsci.org/v05p0706.htm

[23]http://responsibletechnology.org/gmo-dangers/65-health-risks/1notes

[24]http://responsibletechnology.org/docs/BabyFoodCampaignBroch.pdf

Irradiated Food[25]
by Gabriel Cousens

Irradiated food is a biohazard. Irradiating food completely disorganizes the energetic field (this is also true of microwave food). Although it is claimed that irradiation kills all the infecting bacteria, even E. Coli, the bacterium most often cited when arguing for the use of food irradiation, has evolved new forms that are radiation-resistant. In other cases, irradiation does not get rid of the toxins that the bacteria produce. Botulism is one of those cases where the toxin produced is worse than the bacteria itself.

There is no solid evidence to show that eating irradiated food is safe, but there is some evidence to show that it has specific dangers. Food is irradiated with gamma rays. The gamma rays break up the molecular structure of the food and create free radicals. The free radicals react with the food to form new chemical substances called "radiolytic products." Some of these include formaldehyde, benzene, formic acid, and quinines, which are known to be harmful to human health. In one experiment, for example, levels of benzene, a known carcinogen, were seven times higher in irradiated beef than in non-irradiated beef. Some of these radiolytic products are unique to the irradiation process and have not been adequately identified or tested for toxicity.

Irradiating food destroys somewhere between 20 and 80 percent of the vitamins, including A, B2, B3, B6, B12, folic acid, C, E, and K. Amino acids and essential fatty acids are also destroyed. Enzymes, of course, are destroyed, as are the bio-photons.

In addition, food irradiation plants are unsafe. Radioactive accidents have already happened at the few food-irradiation plants that exist in this country and worldwide.

In attempting to determine what to do about food irradiation, the FDA reviewed 441 toxicity studies. The chairperson in charge of new food additives at the FDA, Dr. Marcia van Gemert, testified that all 441 of the studies were flawed. The FDA, however, determined that at least five studies were acceptable under 1980 toxicology standards. The Department of Preventive Medicine and Community Health of the New Jersey Medical School found that two of these studies were methodologically flawed. In one of the five studies, animals eating a diet of irradiated food experienced weight loss and increased miscarriages, possibly due to radiation-induced vitamin E deficiency.

[25] Cousens, M.D., G. (1986). *Spiritual Nutrition*. Berkeley, CA: North Atlantic Books, pg. 507.

The Real Story on Canola Oil ('Can-ugly' Oil)[26]

by Fred Pescatore

In his article, "Canola Oil Real or Imagined," Fred Pescatore, MD, MPH, CCN, author of The Hamptons Diet, explains how canola oil came about, why it is so popular and why we should avoid it. He helps us learn about The Science of Fats, Fatty Acids and Edible Oils.

"Can-ugly Oil" is my pet name for canola oil. Since canola is a completely contrived substance, I thought it should have an equally ridiculous name. Can-ugly oil is derived from the rapeseed, which is a member of the mustard family, which also includes broccoli, kale, cabbage, and mustard greens. Rapeseed oil has been used in traditional Asian and South Asian cooking for many years, without cause for alarm. This is probably because the oil was processed at very low temperatures, usually by hand. A study raised concerns about heart disease and its relationship to one of the fatty acids that was most prevalent in rapeseed oil, erucic acid. Since that was determined, the rapeseed that is used today to make canola oil was bred to eliminate virtually all of the erucic acid so that now instead of 45 percent erucic acid that you get from traditional rapeseed, there is generally less than 25 percent found in common canola oil.

Canola oil is named for a Canadian scientist who developed it, hence, Canadian oil or canola. This new rapeseed was bred to have a fatty acid profile of 57 percent monounsaturated fat, 5 percent saturated fat, 24 percent omega-6 fat and 10 percent omega-3 fatty acids. Because canola oil has a decent level of omega-3 fatty acids, it is not recommended that this oil be heated above 120F or trans fats are formed.

Considering the profile, canola oil looks like a decent product. However, there are some canola oils whose smoke point is 520 F – how did that happen? That is all from manipulation of the chemical structure of the oil through refinement and processing. So, although there is a 2:1 ration of omega-6 to omega-3 fatty acids, unless canola oil is used cold, and even then there is controversy, the levels of trans fats are extremely high at 4.5 percent, more so than margarine.

Traditionally rapeseed oil was probably okay due to its gentle processing technique. However, modern canola oil processing is far from gentle and is what is responsible for making it can-ugly.The oil is removed from the seed by a combination of high temperature mechanical pressing and solvent extraction. As you will recall, traces of the solvent usually remains in the oil. Then the oil is further refined, bleached and degummed, each step requiring exposure to high temperatures and chemicals. Since canola oil has a large amount of omega-3 fatty acids, these easily become rancid and foul smelling during these high-heat processes. It therefore has to undergo another refining process called deodorization. This deodorization process removes a large portion of the omega-3 fatty acids by turning them into trans fats – which can be as high as 4.5 percent.

Now, canola oil is one of the most commonly used oils in processed foods. Since this oil has already been damaged by its refining process, it then undergoes another process that I have already described called hydrogenation, which further increases its trans fatty acid content.

Canola oil is preferred in the processed food industry not only because it is cheap but also because it hydrogenates better than soy or corn oil – an important component for shelf life stability,

---

[26]www.diabetesincontrol.com accessed May 5, 2012.

but not human health.

Canola Oil Mythology

In order to understand how canola oil came from not even existing on the planet to being one of the most commonly consumed oils in the American diet, we really don't have to go back too far – only to the 1980s. At that time, polyunsaturated fats ruled the roost and were the oils that were promoted as heart healthy. Science, however, was beginning to understand that the polyunsaturated stand was unhealthy. The powers that be knew we could also not go back to a position that saturated fats were healthy, after they spent the better part of a decade or longer telling us that the thought of them would kill us. This was the birth of the reign of the monounsaturated fats. But, like most things governmental, the message got distorted by the food processing industry to give us that they can make the most money on. Only now, with the birth of the reign of Mac Nut oil and the success of the Hamptons diet, can monounsaturated fats finally find a good home and be the bearers of the health message that they should.

In the mid-1980, articles on the benefits of olive oil, a natural monounsaturated fat, began to appear in the press. Consumers latched onto this as it seemed natural and the images of the Mediterranean and Tuscany seemed fitting for a healthy lifestyle. However, because of its expense, there had to be a cheaper alternative to use in processed foods; and, because of its relative scarcity, there needed to be an alternative. Another thing to note is that olives do not grow that well in the United States because there are not that many areas of the country that have a Mediterranean-type climate. But, rapeseeds are perfectly suited to growing in the US and thus became the darling of the USDA. So that's when a Canadian scientist developed a rapeseed that was high in oleic acid and low in erucic acid, the poisonous substance – hence, the birth of LEAR (low erucic acid rapeseed), or what is now known as canola oil.

The term "canola oil" did not come into widespread use until the 1990s although it was coined earlier. Since canola oil was a food product that was totally new, and marketers wished to get it into the marketplace right away, it needed to be granted GRAS (generally recognized as safe) status. Otherwise, it would not be allowed into the U.S. food supply, nor sold as food or used in the food processing industry. Without research and testing on the product, which is normally required for many years, this as-yet untested food product was granted GRAS status by the USDA in 1985.

It is interesting to note that stevia, a non-caloric safe and natural sweetener with no friends in the food processing industry, was never granted this same status although it is not a new, man-made contrived substance, nor is it a new food product, having been used for many years without any reported problems by many other countries besides the United States. Unfortunately, Stevia is only allowed to be sold as a nutritional supplement and not as a food. The interest of big business is always at stake, even in our food supply.

Thus, the marketing of canola oil as a health food began in earnest. The marketing genius drew on the fact that canola oil had 10 percent omega-3 fatty acids – which at that time was brand-new to consumers. Canola oil began to be used interchangeably with olive oil, as the lighter alternative with the same healthy characteristics – something that could not have been further from the truth. Unprocessed canola oil, which cannot be found in our food supply, does contain high levels of both monounsaturated fats and omega-3 fatty acids, but not the processed variety, the most common one. That is because a product with that much omega-3 fatty acids is not shelf-stable.

The marketing campaign was very successful and helped push this crop into one of the most widely planted in the world today. It is the oil most commonly used in cholesterol-lowering spreads in place of traditional margarine – a big mistake. And canola oil is the oil of choice in most restaurants.

The Dangers of Can-ugly Oil

There have been many warnings in the health food industry that canola oil is unhealthy and the average health food consumer understands the limitation of this oil. It is interesting to note that canola oil started its meteoric rise in popularity in the health food markets and now is shunned by the healthiest consumers. Several studies in animals have shown that canola oil can decrease the bio-availability of vitamin E, a critical component of cardiovascular health.

Also, canola oil consumption can lead to shortened life spans in other animals. In still another study, growth is retarded and hence the ban on the use of canola oil in infant formulas. If this was so safe, why can't it be fed to human infants? Keep in mind that these studies were all done on animals and it is hard to make that leap into humans. The one thing that is known is that there have never been long term studies in humans as to the health benefits or to the dangers of canola oil – another uncontrolled experiment that only benefits one thing – the food processing industry. That is something to seriously consider when deciding which oil to reach for on the supermarket shelf.

I can't help but wonder if canola oil in and of itself isn't responsible for the dramatic rise in obesity and diabetes that we have experienced since it became fashionable. I guess it is something we will never know.

Agave[27]

Many people seeking a "natural" alternative to dangerous sweeteners like high fructose corn syrup (HFCS) are turning to agave. However, the sticky truth is that agave 'nectar' is often highly processed and not natural by the time it reaches local store shelves.

Just what is agave? Blue agave grows "in the rich volcanic soil of Mexico under a hot tropical sun, boasting a stately flower stem that blooms only once in its lifetime," according to Dr. Joseph Mercola. Agave means "noble," and it's recognized as a superstar of the herbal remedy world, said to relieve indigestion, bowel irregularity, and skin wounds, as stated by Mercola in a 2009 online article, "Agave: A Triumph of Marketing over Truth."

"Agave 'nectar' sellers use agave's royal pedigree to cover the truth that what they're selling is a bottle of high-fructose syrup, so highly processed and refined that it bears NO resemblance to the plant of its namesake," Mercola claims.

Likewise, processed agave nectar's "diabetic-friendly" image is also untrue. Although agave does have a low glycemic index, it has a high fructose content – 90 percent or more, depending on the processing. HFCS averages 55 percent fructose.

Un-naturally Sweet

Agave 'nectar' is not made from the sap of the agave plant, but from the starch of its pineapple-like root bulb, states Dr. Mercola. The bulb consists mainly of starch, similar to corn, and a complex carbohydrate called inulin, which is made up of fructose molecules.

Manufacturers use genetically modified enzymes and a chemically intensive process involving caustic acids, clarifiers, and filtration chemicals to convert agave starch into market-ready syrup, according to Dr. Mercola. This is hardly the natural process many people picture when they see the pretty labels on most prepared agave sweetener.

Fortunately, some organic agave options exist. If you're looking for agave that lives up to those beautiful labels – or at least cuts down the hype – do some research.

---

[27]http://www.articles.mercola.com accessed March 30, 2010.

The Proper Tools and Equipment
Equipment for Healthy Water[28]
by Betsy Bragg and Brian Axelrod

Since we are as much as 70 percent water and our brains are 90 percent water, drinking good water is the most important change you can make for yourself. (See the 21 reasons why.) I'm glad my son persuaded me to buy a water system in the year 2000 as my first piece of equipment for a healthier lifestyle. I bought a Jupiter system to start with, but that didn't last.

I researched water purification systems for several years. **Carbon filter**s, such as Brita, provide a possible 80% purification such as chlorine and organic contaminants, but that isn't enough. **Reverse Osmosis** removes organic and biological contaminants, minerals at about 90 percent which is still not enough. **Distillation** requires four hours to make one gallon of water and provides 99.9% purification, but removes needed minerals which then must be added. **Atmospheric water generators,** like the Atmos used at Hippocrates, extracts water directly from the air and then filters and it's ionized and alkalized and achieves 99.9 percent purification. However, it is very expensive.. I bought and heartily endorse an ionizer, the Kangen System. It tastes better than any other water, greatly minimizes my arthritic pain, energizes me, cleans vegetables, removes stains, softens my skin, cleans and freshens the apartment air I breathe (when used in my humidifier) and is healthier for my plants.

If you would like to taste Kangen Water® and see its effects, come over to my home, fill and take home containers, preferably glass and half gallon mason jars. Bring over some of your water and I will analyze its alkalinity and anti-oxidant qualities. Call me at 781-899-6664 or cell 617-835-2913 for an appointment.

Kangen Water® is alkaline, ionized, anti-oxidant electron rich, restructured, micro-clustered, and active hydrogen-saturated, and it has reduced oxidation. It is essential to drink at least half your weight in water per day. Convert your weight in pounds to ounces and drink at least half of that number. For example, if you weigh 128 pounds, divide that in half, so you should drink 64 ounces or 8 cups (2 quarts)per day. Drink more if you have any health issues. Glass bottles are recommended.

Kangen means "return to the origin" in Japanese. Kangen water dates back to 1931, when world-renowned chemist Dr. Otto Heinrich Warburg won the Nobel Prize for his work in alkalinity and better health. His groundbreaking research showed that all forms of unhealthy cells can be characterized by two basic conditions: high acidity and lack of oxygen. In fact, alkalinity implies higher concentration of oxygen molecules, according to Warburg. He explained that when water molecules split, "if there is an excess of H+, it is acidic; if there is an excess of OH- ions, then it is alkaline."

Lack of oxygen is a very serious and dangerous environment for a cell. If you deprive a cell of 35 percent of its oxygen for just 48 hours, it may become damaged. For better health, Warburg insisted that cells need an alkaline environment. Since unhealthy cells cannot survive in the presence of high levels of oxygen, they cannot survive in an alkaline environment. The first device

---

[28]Lark, S. & Richard, J.*The Chemistry of Success.*

engineered to test Warburg's theory was produced by Russian scientists and was perfected by the Japanese 40 years ago.

To this day, Kangen is the only water that supports Dr. Warburg's findings and is endorsed by the Japanese Association of Preventive Medicine and 6,500 physicians around the world. It is used in over 300 hospitals and more than 3,000 restaurants in Japan, where one in every six families owns an ionizer. There are roughly 400,000 machines owned by restaurants, spas and families in the United States and Canada alone.

Water is the foundation of our cells and working systems in the body. Kangen drinking water, with a pH of 8.5 to 9.5, provides optimal hydration for drinking and healthy cooking. The great taste of Kangen Water®is due to the unique filtration process that does not strip out the natural minerals your body needs. The process of cell hydration is called micro-clustering; this reduces the size of the water molecule cluster by two-thirds and restructures the water into hexagonal clusters, which allows quick absorption as the water enters the cells immediately. Kangen Water®is energetically more powerful than any other water and results can be seen in just three days; people have lost 15 pounds in two weeks, cleared facial acne, stopped getting migraines, stopped excessive mucus production and relieved nasal congestion, just by drinking this water. Take this example: When a fish is sick what do you do? Change its water and the fish comes back to a state of health. Our bodies are the same way. When we consume overly acidic drinks and water, we force our body to work extra hard trying to stay alkaline and not work to heal wounds or act against other ailments. The water does not cure anything, but it allows the body to become more alkaline, and that way the body can heal itself. After all, the body is our powerful healing force.

The most important benefit of drinking Kangen Water®is the Oxidative Reduction Potential (ORP), a measurement of antioxidants. Water with a high negative ORP is of particular value in its ability to neutralize oxygen-free radicals. The water itself contains antioxidants, a huge and booming industry right now because of its anti-aging properties and the defense it gives the immune system. Green tea and Vitamin C contain high amounts of antioxidants; they range at about a -70 to a -30 ORP. Kangen Water®can range from a -350 to a -900 ORP. No other water could ever contain that high of a negative charge mostly because water is supposed to be consumed from the source and within 24 hours. After 48 hours,Kangen Water®starts to lose its high negative ORP due to sunlight, movement and temperature.

Currently the Chief of Surgical Endoscopy at Beth Israel Medical Center in New York, Dr. Hiromi Shinya, a pioneer in colonoscopy techniques, recommends Kangen Water®in his books "The Enzyme Factor" and "The Microbe Factor." He says, "I have a Kangen Water®machine in my New York medical office, and this is the water I drink and give to my patients."

Dr. Gabriel Cousens, in his book "Conscious Eating," says: "Water Ionization could be one of the most important health breakthroughs in our era."

Shan Stratton is a Sports Nutritional Consultant for the NBA (Houston Rockets) and MLB(New York Yankees, Arizona Diamondbacks, and Los Angeles Dodgers), as well as the NFL, PGA, LPGA, NASCAR and the NHL. He states that drinking Kangen Water®is the missing link to overall health and performance for athletes after promoting and counseling the use of high-quality supplements, enzymes, and probiotics for more than 15 years.

Kangen Water®is the standard for water ionization. There are over 105 other water ionizers out there. They all try to match the prestigious Enagic-made model. None of them have won awards like Enagic and they are not guaranteed to last 15-20 years.

21 Reasons why it's important to drink water:

1. It's essential to our survival, we can't live without it. We are 70 percent water
2. It can increase our metabolism
3. Keeping hydrated can help stave off fatigue and help maintain energy levels
4. Flushing our wastes and bacteria from our system and keeping kidneys healthy
5. Adequate hydration reduces the risk of colon, breast, and bladder cancer
6. Helps alleviate headaches
7. Keeps skin moisturized and nourished
8. Aids in digestion, and can help prevent acid stomach and constipation
9. Can lower the risk of a heart attack
10. Keeps muscle cells hydrated when exercising
11. Transports nutrients and oxygen in our blood stream to help keep us healthy
12. Helps with weight loss – ZERO calories, no fat, no sugar, no carbohydrates
13. Acts as an appetite suppressant
14. Helps avoid sunstroke
15. Helps lower blood pressure
16. Makes some medications work faster and more effectively

Additional reasons for using Kangen water:

- Microclustered Kangen water hydrates your cells faster than any other water.
- Kangen enhances flavors and texture of your food, cooks food faster!
- Kangen water's high ORP (Oxygen Reduction Potential) can destroy bad breath and prevent acidic build up after eating.
- Cleaning floors, windows, and eyeglasses, removing stains from clothes with Strong Acidic Kangen water
- Kangen water tastes soft and smooth

Good Knives:

Good Knives are a must, since raw veggies need to be cleaned, cut, chopped or trimmed most of the time. I treasure my Japanese and German knives. Tribest now makes the best – Choisons Precision Knives made of ultra high-quality zirconium carbide ceramic, an extra-sharp lightweight blade which allow you to get difficult slicing and cutting jobs done more quickly and easily than with steel knives. Choisons ceramic blades are sharper than stainless steel knives and retain their edge longer. Ceramic blades don't react with foods, keeping your food looking and tasting fresher longer.

Blenders:

A blender is a kitchen appliance used to mix, puree or emulsify food. It consists of a motor on the bottom and a jar with a blade at the bottom that connects to the motor. You can use the blender to make soups, dressings, dips, smoothies and special sauces.

How to select your blender: The more powerful the motor, the better the blender. You want the jar portion of the blender to be BPA free. You might think the best solution is a glass jar, however, glass can be broken when blending harder items such as nuts.

Good quality blenders are the best choice long term, however, you can get started with any blender. The top-quality blenders listed on Page 59 are followed by other, less expensive choices.

The BEST Juicer, Is There one?[29]
by John Kohler

Often we are asked, "which is the best juicer?" Choosing a juicer is like a choosing an outfit to wear. If you're going swimming, you will wear a bathing suit. If you are going to a formal occasion, you will wear a tuxedo. Choosing a juicer is much the same: You must match the juicer to what you intend to do. There are several "styles" of juicers available on the market today. Some are better suited for juicing certain kinds of produce than others. There is no "perfect" juicer that will perform every juicing operation with equal quality. Evaluate your needs carefully before purchasing an appliance. This article is based on our experience, and is as accurate as possible, but if you have any questions, please visit the frequently asked questions list at http://www.discountjuicers.com/faq.pl.

Before purchasing a juicer, you should ask yourself what considerations are important to you?Some factors you should take into consideration are:

- ease of cleaning
- noise level
- speed of juicing
- length of warranty
- types of produce you will be juicing

One reason why there is no "perfect" juicer is that fruits and vegetables have vastly different properties. The juicing method that is effective for one may not work while juicing the other. Fruits have soft cell walls and therefore require a gentle extraction method. Apples, pears, watermelon, cantaloupe and pineapple are some of the fruits that can be juiced peel and all.*Citrus fruits, such as oranges, grapefruits and tangerines, have a bitter outer rind, and juice from a "whole" orange would be too bitter to drink. It also contains indigestible chemicals.One solution is to grate away the outer rind (the orange coloring on the orange – it is best to leave the white "pith," because valuable nutrients are contained within the white area).The more common method is to slice the fruit in half, and then using a "reamer" style juicer or a citrus press to press out the juice.

* I recommend people purchase organically grown produce whenever possible, especially when juicing produce items skin and all.

Vegetables, on the other hand, have fibrous "tough" cell walls, requiring more aggressive mechanical juicing action than fruit. Due to their low acid content, it is recommended that vegetable juices be consumed within 15 minutes of their preparation, since it has been demonstrated that enzyme activity in juice 30 minutes old is one-half that of freshly made juice. When apple or carrot juice turns brown, it has oxidized.

Juices that are not made fresh, and sold in the store that are bottled or canned will NEVER oxidize. This is because the juice has been heated to deactivate all the enzymes. The enzymes are one of the key reasons why making fresh juice with your juicer can be so beneficial.

I will attempt to explain the various styles of juicers on the market today, how they work, and a brief overview of their advantages and disadvantages.

---

[29]http://www.discountjuicers.com/bestjuicer.html accessed February 1, 2012.

Centrifugal Juicers

The centrifugal juicer design is one of the oldest juicer designs. This juicer uses a grater or shredder disc and a strainer basket with straight sides to hold the pulp in the machine. The shredder disk is at the bottom of the basket, which revolves at a high speed (3600 rpm).The produce is put into the top of the machine, and it pressed through a chute, hits the spinning shredder disc, while the produce is being shredded, juice is released. The basket spins at a high speed, much like a washing machines spin cycle and force pushes the juice through the strainer basket, and comes out of the front of the machine, and the pulp stays inside the machine. Generally this style juicer can make 1-2 quarts before the juicer must be stopped, and the pulp must be removed before further juicing can take place.This is not a continuous juicing appliance. The two centrifugal juicers we sell are the Omega 1000 and Omega 9000. These machines use stainless steel baskets and ball bearing induction type motors. The Omega 1000 offer a 10 year warranty, and the Omega 9000 offers a 15 year warranty. This juicer is good for juicing most fruits and vegetables.

Centrifugal Ejection Juicers

Made popular by the "Juiceman" Infomercial, the centrifugal ejection-style juicer operates much the same way as the centrifugal juicer above operates, except the sides of the basket are slanted. This allows for the basket to be "self-cleaning," so there is no need to stop the juicer and empty it out. The pulp is ejected out of the machine, usually into a collection bin or basket that can be lined with a plastic bag to collect the pulp, and then easily discarded. Due to the short contact time of the pulp in the basket, these juicers must spin faster than the centrifugal juicer, at about 6300 rpm. This style is the noisiest of all the juicers. The Omega 4000(15 year warranty) and Lequip 110.5 (10 year warranty). The latest development in the centrifugal ejection category is the addition of a large feed chute, 3 inches in diameter, which allows the user to juice without cutting the produce.There are benefits and drawbacks to the large chute (visit http://www.discountjuicers.com/widefeed.html for more information).The units we offer with the large feed chute are: Lequip 215XL (10 year warranty) and the Omega BMJ330 Big Mouth Juicer (10 year warranty).Centrifugal ejection juicers are the easiest to use and easy to clean, and are fast. They are good for juicing most fruits and vegetables.

Masticating Juicers

The Champion Juicer, made by Plastaket, combines three operations into one. The Champion Juicer first grates, then masticates or chews the pulp to further break down the cell-wall structure, and then mechanically presses or squeezes the pulp to extract the juice. The Champion uses a powerful slow-turning motor and requires moderate strength to operate. It is definitely not a machine for a physically limited person. It can juice almost every type of vegetable efficiently, including leafy vegetables. By blocking off the juice spout (with the blank or solid plate), the Champion can be used as a homogenizer to make such foods as raw applesauce, tomato sauce and baby food. It can make peanut butter or other nut butters. It also makes wonderful ice cream-like desserts from raw frozen bananas and other fruits. By assembling the Champion without the blank or juicing screen, it can be used as a grater or to make shave ice. The Champion's motor is manufactured by General Electric and its juicing parts are constructed of stainless steel and nylon; it has been manufactured since the 1950's. It is best for juicing most fruits and vegetables. Plastaket also manufacturers a more powerful version of the Champion juicer, its the Champion

Commercial model. The difference is that it has a bit more powerful motor and a stainless steel motor shaft. The look of the machine is the same, as well as all the external parts.

Manual Press Juicers

The press style juicer squeezes the juice out of the produce by pressure. The manual press juicer uses a two-step process: first the produce must be shredded then it is pressed. There are two styles of juice presses. One uses leverage to squeeze the juice while the other type uses hydraulics. The Ito Juice Press is a manual press that uses leverage to extract juice from produce. It is made of all metal and is quite sturdy. The Norwalk is an electric two step juicer that combines grating and pressing operations into one unit, with this machine, the vegetable or fruit was first grated by a revolving cutter into a linen cloth-lined tray, which was then placed into a motor-driven hydraulic press. Extremely high pressure was necessary to extract juice from vegetables (6,000 lbs. PSI), The hydraulic press produced a high- quality juice from both fruit and vegetables, but it was a difficult and time- consuming machine to use and to clean. In addition, the $2000.00 price tag is quite high for the average consumer. A good substitution for the Norwalk juicer, would be to use the Champion Juicer as a grater, and then the Ito Juice Press, Welles press or K&K press, which are operated manually that squeeze the juice out of the produce. Pressing causes the least oxidation of the juicing methods, and produces a pulp free juice, since the juice is strained through cheesecloth. This type of juicer juices fruits (especially soft ones) better than other types of juicers.

Single Auger Juicers

This juicer produces juice by using a single auger that basically crushes the produce into the walls (or screen) of the juicer, and in the process extracts the juice. It runs at a low rpm rate so there is little oxidation. The single auger style juicer has been on the market as a dedicated wheatgrass juicer for many, many years now. A new design allows the single-auger style machine to juice wheatgrass as well as other vegetables and fruits. There are several brands of single-auger juicers. The Samson 9001 (10 year warranty) is a new single-auger machine that juices wheatgrass about as well as a dedicated wheatgrass juicer and does an excellent job juicing leafy greens. It will juice fruits and other vegetables about as well as the twin gear juicers (below).We found that this type of machine was not as effective at juicing carrots, as the twin gear units. The juice made with this machine tend to be really pulpy and it is advised to use the strainer that is included. Fruits and non-leafy vegetables need to be cut into small "cubes" for best results when using this juicer, We find that the single auger juicers, do not produce a high yield when juicing carrots, so if you want to juice a lot of carrots, this is not the juicer for you. For best results when using this machine, the hard and soft produce needs to be "alternated" when feeding into the juicer. As with the twin gear units below, this machine is not the greatest for juicing fruits.

Dual Stage Single Auger Juicers

This juicer works like the single auger style juicer above, but upon the initial crushing of the produce, juice is directed through the stage one juicing screen into the juice cup. The crushed produce continues its way through the machine to the 2nd-stage, where there is a finer holed screen to further obtain more juice. With the single stage auger juicers (above), the juice is only produced in this second stage. In our tests, this style juicer produced more juice and worked better than the single auger juicers. There are two brands that sell the dual stage single auger juicers. Tribest offers the Solo Star and Solo Star II juicer (5 yr warranty) rand Omega offers the 8003 and 8005 model (10 yr warranty). The Omega models are identical except for the color. The 8003 is white, and the 8005 is a chrome color. The new Omega 8004 and 8006 are the upgraded versions of the 8003 and 8005. They include a 15-year warranty, as well as an 8x harder auger. We found that this type of machine was more effective juicing than the single auger style juicer. (read a sample test here). We prefer the Omega 8003/8005 juicer since it is easier to clean than the Solo Star.

Twin Gear Press

These juicers have two gears that basically press out the juice of the produce. The screws turn at a low 90-110 rpm. It is very similar to two gears in a automobile transmission that mesh together. Basically, the produce is pushed (with some force) into the two gears, which first shreds, and then squeezes the produce. These machines are best for juicing vegetables since these machines rely on the fibrous cell wall to push the pulp through the machine. As a bonus, these machines will also juice wheatgrass (Generally a separate wheatgrass juicer is required to juice wheatgrass). The quality of the juice produced with these machines can be compared to the quality of the hydraulic press above. These machines are not for the "faint" or "frail" hearted as some pressure is needed to feed the produce into the machine. Machines in this category are the Green Power Juice Extractor, The Green Star Juice Extractor and the Samson Ultra Juicer. These juicers truly give "the best of both worlds" but there is one drawback: the price. They can be as much as two to three times the price of the Centrifugal or Mastication Juicers. While these juicers are best for juicing vegetables, the Green Power and Green Star machines have a fruit attachment available to help it better juice fruits. (We have successfully juiced hard apples, hard pears, watermelon with rind, and citrus successfully with these twin gear machines). The Green Power, Green Star and Samson Ultra are also able to homogenize as the Champion above, and make raw applesauce, delicious fruit sorbets, nut butters, baby food. Included with the green power and green star is the pasta maker and mochi (Japanese rice cake) attachments. To read a head to head comparison of these style juicers, please see our article, twin gear showdown.

How loud are the juicers?

The noise level of the juicers are all different. A good rule of thumb: The faster a juicer turns (Revolutions Per Minute) or RPM, the louder the machine is. Based on this, the Single Auger and Twin Gear Machines would be the quietest (operating at ~100 rpm) , followed by the Champion (~2700 rpm) ,then the centrifugal machines (~3600 rpm) , with the centrifugal ejection (~7200 rpm) machines being the loudest. I have personally juiced with the Green Power while my roommate was sleeping, and it didn't bother them. I would never try that with any of the other juicers, as they are much louder! Read our article, "How loud is that Juicer in the Window" for the results of our juicer decibel testing.

Blenders

●

Vita-Mix 1300 TurboBlend 4500:

http://www.amazon.com/Vitamix-1300-Vita-Mix-TurboBlend-4500/dp/B0000YRJT6/ref=sr_1_1?s=appliances&ie=UTF8&qid=1328829343&sr=1-1 accessed 02/09/2012

This is the low-end of the champion of blenders.

Euro-Pro Ninja Master Prep Blender and Food Processor

http://www.amazon.com/Euro-Pro-Ninja-Master-Blender-Processor/sim/B002JM2V9K/2 accessed 02/09/2012

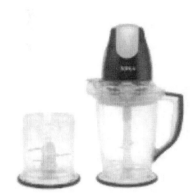

Product Features

● 48-ounce blender and 2-cup food processor with interchangeable power

Advantages

● Price – List price $59.99 on sale $37.27

● Portable / 48oz.

Disadvantages

● 400-watt motor

● Small size makes food prep time consuming

● Grainy liquids

● Time consuming

Magic Bullet MBR-1701 17-Piece Express Mixing Set

http://www.amazon.com/Magic-Bullet-MBR-1701-17-Piece-Express/dp/B001WAKFDY/ref=sr_1_1?ie=UTF8&qid=1328989607&sr=8-1 accessed 02/11/2012

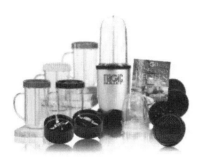

Product Features

- Carafe is size of a coffee cup
- 250 Watts

Advantages

- Price – List price $59.99 on sale $49.99
- Small Blender and Juicer

Disadvantages

- Small size makes food prep time consuming
- Grainy liquids
- Time consuming

Juicers

Green Star Elite Jumbo Twin Gear Juice Extractor (GSE-5000)

http://www.amazon.com/Green-Star-Elite-Extractor-GSE-5000/dp/B002QGXTJK/ref=sr_1_1?s=home-garden&ie=UTF8&qid=1328990503&sr=1-1 accessed 02/11/2012

Product Features

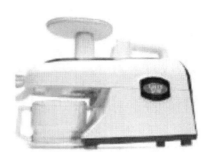

- Juicing Process: Twin gear

- R.P.M. : 110

- Power: 190 W

- Weight: 34 lbs

- Warranty: 5 years

Advantages

- Twin gear extracts more juice (dryer pulp) than single auger

- Easy and quick to clean – 5 parts only

- Fast food prep

- Fine and course screens

- Blank screen makes pate and ices

-

Disadvantage

- Price – List price $629.00 on sale $534.27

New Z-Star Manual Portable Wheatgrass Juicer

http://www.amazon.com/Z-Star-Manual-Portable-Wheatgrass-Juicer/dp/B0007W04AW/ref=sr_1_cc_1?s=aps&ie=UTF8&qid=1328993172&sr=1-1-catcorr accessed 02/11/2012

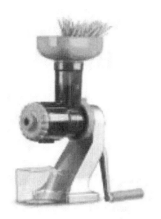

Product Features and Advantages

- Portable

- Affordable

- For wheatgrass only

- Price – Amazon List price $99.00 Optimum Health Solution price $88.00 (profit goes to Real Kids, Real Food)

Disadvantages

- Time consuming

- Requires muscle power

- Hard to clean

Healthy Juicer - Manual Hand Powered Wheatgrass Juicer

http://www.amazon.com/Healthy-Juicer-Manual-Powered-Wheatgrass/dp/B0002LY8PA/ref=sr_1_cc_2?s=aps&ie=UTF8&qid=1328993172&sr=1-2-catcorr **accessed 02/12/2012**

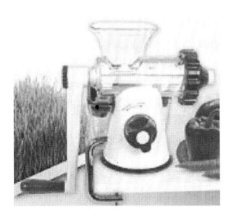

Product Features and Advantages

Portable

Affordable

Handles wheatgrass

Price – Amazon List price $44.95

Disadvantages

Time consuming

Requires muscle power

Hard to clean and leaks

Has to clamp onto counter of correct depth

Cuisinart CCJ-100 Citrus Pro Juicer

http://www.amazon.com/Cuisinart-CCJ-100-Citrus-Pro-Juicer/dp/B00009K3T2/ref=sr_1_1?s=home-garden&ie=UTF8&qid=1328994359&sr=1-1 accessed on 02/11/2012

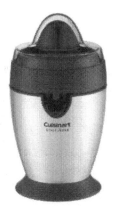

Product Features and Advantages

Squeezes fresh juice quickly and easily; dispenses juice directly into container

Anti-drip spout locks allow for interruption of juice flow

Unique auto-reverse spin feature extracts more juice from pulp

Elegant, brushed stainless steel housing

Includes cord storage and dishwasher-safe parts for easy cleanup

Price – Amazon List price $55.00 on sale $29.95

Food Processors

Cuisinart Prep Plus Food Processor (9cup)

http://www.amazon.com/Cuisinart-DLC-2009CHB-Processor-Brushed-Stainless/dp/B001413A0Q/ref=sr_1_1?s=home-garden&ie=UTF8&qid=1328995030&sr=1-1accessed 02/12/2012 Note: 7-cup too small.

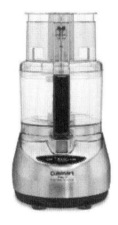

Product Features and Advantages

Lexan work bowl virtually shatterproof, dishwasher-safe

Dishwasher-safe parts

One-piece Supreme wide mouth feed tube holds whole fruits and vegetables

Workhorse, long lasting

Disadvantage

Price – List price $270.00 on sale $135.02

Euro-Pro Ninja Master Prep Blender and Food Processor:

http://www.amazon.com/Euro-Pro-Ninja-Master-Blender-Processor/sim/B002JM2V9K/2 accessed 02/09/2012

For Details see Blenders.

Dehydrators

Excalibur 3900 Deluxe Series 9 Tray Food Dehydrator

http://www.amazon.com/Excalibur-3900-Deluxe-Tray-Dehydrator/dp/B001P2J3K0/ref=sr_1_1?ie=UTF8&qid=132 8996365&sr=8-1 accessed 02/12/2012

Comes in two size: 9 tray and 5 tray

<u>Product Features</u>

Heavy Duty 7" fan

600 watts

Adjustable Thermostat: 85° - 145°F

Built In On/Off Switch

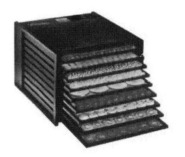

<u>Advantages</u>

Removable trays for casserole

Easy to clean

Teflex sheets available

<u>Disadvantage</u>

Price – List price $260.00 on sale $219.95

Nesco American Harvest FD-37 400 Watt Food Dehydrator

http://www.amazon.com/Nesco-American-Harvest-FD-37-Dehydrator/dp/B003I4F7AS/ref=sr_1_3?s=home-garden&ie=UTF8&qid=1328997042&sr=1-3accessed 02/12/2012

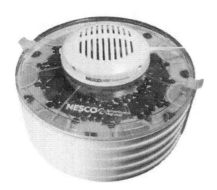

<u>Product Features and Advantages</u>

400-watts of drying power

Expandable to 7 trays

Clear top to monitor the drying process

Fan forced radial air flow means not tray rotation needed

Made in USA

Price – Amazon List price $47.99 on sale $35.99

Kitchen Tools

Spirooli-World Cuisine 48297-99 Tri-Blade Plastic Spiral Vegetable Slicer

http://www.amazon.com/World-Cuisine-48297-99-Tri-Blade-Vegetable/dp/B0007Y9WHQ/ref=sr_1_1?ie=UTF8&qid=1329060157&sr=8-1 accessed 02/12/2012

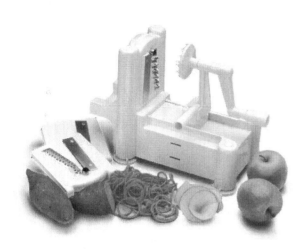

Product Features

3 sets of blades

Handles hard vegetables (yams and beets) and soft vegetables

Price – Amazon List price $49.88 on sale $19.95

Saladacco Spiral Slicer Garnishing Machine – Spirializer

http://www.amazon.com/Saladacco-Spiral-Slicer-Garnishing-Machine/dp/B004IA5X6Y/ref=sr_1_3?ie=UTF8&qid=1329060157&sr=8-3 accessed 02/12/2012

Product Features

Very good for angel hair

Limited use

Only does soft vegetables, e.g., zucchini

Handles only 3 in. pieces

Price – Amazon List price $24.95 on sale $18.95

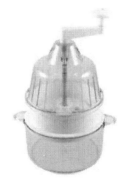

Benriner Cook Helper Slicer

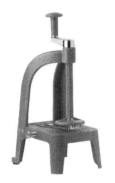

<u>Product Features</u>

fine, medium and course blades

Vertical spiralizer, awkward output location

Price – Amazon List price $59.96 on sale $45.90

OXO Good Grips V-Blade Mandoline Slicer

<u>Product Features</u>

Safety minded with suctions cups

Best for making lasagna

Price – Amazon List price $39.99

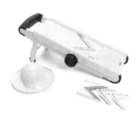

Microplane Premium Zester/Grater

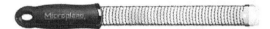

Product Features

Handy tool for mincing ginger and carrots, etc.

Price – Amazon List price $14.95

Norpro 607 Canning Funnel

Product Features

Convenient tool, avoids spilling

Price – Amazon List price $4.30

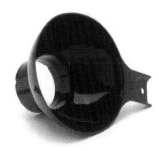

TRIBEST PRICES
www.tribestlife.com
OPTIMUM HEALTH SOLUTION
10 percent DISCOUNT for items over $100
All profits contributed to OHS Kids

Product Description	TRIBEST Sale Price	OHS 10% Discount	MA SH&H	Total
Green Star Elite 5000	$549.00	$494.10	$36.00	$530.10
Green Star 1000	$485.00	$436.50	$36.00	$472.50
Z-Star Manual Juicer	$98.10	$88.29	$15.00	$103.29
Citristar Juicer	$55.95	$50.35	$14.00	$64.36
Personal Blender & Grinder PB 250	$69.95	**	$14.00	$83.95
Freshlife Sprouter	$115.95	**	$16.00	$129.95

** No Sale on Small Items

DVD: Why Kangen Water?

20 minutes

1.   What are the five types of water produced by the LeveLuk and the LeveLuk SD 501?

2.   Is the LeveLuk SD 501 a water cleaner?

3.   What type of water can I use to produce ionized water?

  3a: What if I have well water?

4.   What is active hydrogen?

5.   Is the Kangen water made in Japan effective in the U.S?

6.   What is the problem with bottled water?

7.   Is Kangen water OK for pets?

8.   Is it OK for children to drink Kangen Water?

9.   What advantages does Kangen Water have over reverse osmosis or distillation?

10.   The LeveLuk seems extremely expensive. Is it different from other water cleaners?

11.   Is the LeveLuk electrolyzing tank different from competing models?

12.   How often should the cartridge be changed?

DVD – Food Combining

Proper combining of foods for good digestion. Foods that should never be eaten together. Key information for optimal health.

1. How did our early ancestors eat and why?

2. What is the worst combination of foods?

3. When is the best time to eat protein?

4. How many hours does it take to digest protein in a healthy person?

5. How many hours does it take for starchy carbs to digest?

6. When is the best time to eat starchy carbs?

7. How much fruit should you eat if you are sick and why?

8. What are the 3 categories of fruit? Give 2 examples of each.

9. What are two major rules in buying fruit and why?

10. What two rules in eating fruit?

11. On rare special occasions for an extremely healthy person, which fruits can be combined?

12. What's the rule about fruits and vegetables and give 2 reasons why?

13. What are exceptions to this rule about fruits and vegetables?

14. What is the rule about melons?

15. Where do tomatoes fit into the food chart?

16. When do beans become starchy carbs?

17. How do you feel about powdered and capsulated garlic sold in health food stores?

18. What are complete proteins? Are eggs, dairy and meat included?

Chapter 3
Indoor Sprouting

Overview

This chapter will discuss different techniques of sprouting various legumes, grains, seeds and nuts. Sprouted grains, unlike processed grains, are extremely nutritious and provide a valuable part of any healthy diet. Once sprouted, sprouts have an alkalizing effect on the body. As you learned in chapter 2, one's body needs to be alkaline in order to be in good health. Sprouts, a living food, contain hundreds of molecules of oxygen and are very alkaline.

You will learn:

- Why sprout?
- What to sprout?
- How to sprout?

Sprouting The Easy Way- learned at Hippocrates

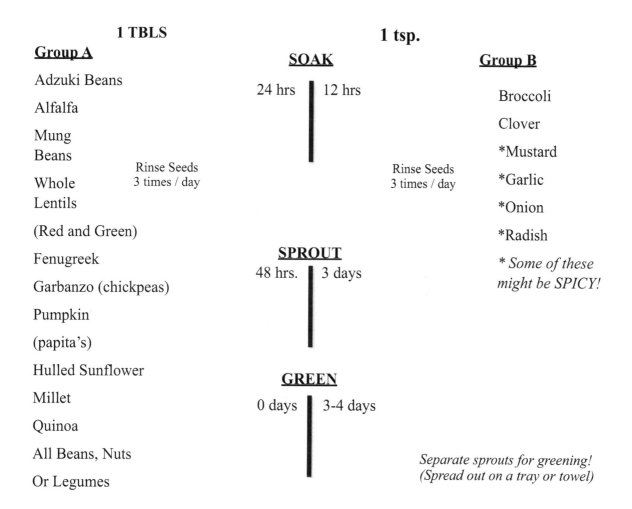

1 TBLS

Group A

Adzuki Beans

Alfalfa

Mung

Beans

Whole

Lentils

(Red and Green)

Fenugreek

Garbanzo (chickpeas)

Pumpkin

(papita's)

Hulled Sunflower

Millet

Quinoa

All Beans, Nuts

Or Legumes

1 tsp.

SOAK

24 hrs. | 12 hrs

Rinse Seeds
3 times / day

SPROUT

48 hrs. | 3 days

GREEN

0 days | 3-4 days

Group B

Broccoli

Clover

*Mustard

*Garlic

*Onion

*Radish

Some of these might be SPICY!

Rinse Seeds
3 times / day

*Separate sprouts for greening!
(Spread out on a tray or towel)*

Both Groups A&B:

- Seed storage: dry and room temperature, DO NOT refrigerate

- Soaking: Fill a glass or stainless steel container 1/3 full with dry seed & fill the container completely with water (it expands).

- Water well 3 times a day and keep in direct sunlight.

- When finished, will last one week in the refrigerator. Rinse well before eating! Enjoy!

The following are extracts from

Sprouts the Miracle Food - The Complete Guide to Sprouting -8th edition, 2010

By Steve Meyerowitz (Reprinted with Permission from Author)

www.Sproutman.com

Why Eat Sprouts?

Seeds are a storehouse of vitamins, minerals, enzymes and essential fatty acids as well as the greatest source of protein in the vegetable kingdom. When sprouting, a seed unfolds and starts to multiply and develop its nutrients in order to provide nourishment for the maturing vegetable. This miracle of nature means that a little sunflower seed has in it the basic formula for nourishing a six-foot plant.

Germination initiates the following changes in the seed:

- Nutrients are broken down and simplified: protein into amino acids, fats into essential fatty acids, starches to sugars and minerals chelate or combine with protein in a way the increases their utilization. These processes all increase nutrition and improve digestion and assimilation. This is the reason sprouts are considered predigested food.

- Proteins, vitamins, enzymes, minerals and trace minerals multiply from 300 to 1200 percent.

- Chlorophyll develops in green plants.

- Certain acids and toxins, which ordinarily would interfere with digestion, are reduced and/or eliminated.

- Size and water content increase dramatically.

Protein: These miniature green vegetables are high in protein when compared to common green leafy vegetables such as spinach and lettuce, but have less protein than bean sprouts such as soybean, lentil and chickpea. Alfalfa and sunflower are richer in protein than spinach or any of the common lettuces and they are free of pesticides and poisons. Alfalfa seed can be as high as 39.8 percent protein although it reduces its concentration as it grows. On the other hand, lettuce and spinach only supply the nutrients developed from one seed, whereas a sprout salad serves up the nutrition from thousands of seeds.

Minerals: Next to sea vegetables, sprouts are the best source of minerals and trace minerals. Most salad sprouts are rich in calcium and magnesium, have more phosphorus than fish, and are excellent sources of hard to find trace minerals such as tritium, selenium, manganese, chromium and others. Because minerals and trace minerals are naturally chelated in the sprout, they are most easily utilized by our bodies. Zinc in alfalfa sprouts increases from 5.8 mg in the seed (per 100 grams), to 18 mg in the sprout (dried weight). One cup (100 mg) of alfalfa sprouts provides twice the US RDA of zinc.

Alfalfa

Alfalfa: One of the most popular, nutritious and delicious of all sprouted seeds with a tasty, sweet, nutlike flavor…

Alfalfa in Arabic means "Alf-al-fa," "father of all foods." In ancient times, alfalfa was used mostly as a remedy to build strength and correct illness. Today researchers are amazed by alfalfa's high vitamin and mineral content. Alfalfa has a rich concentration of vitamin A, B-complex vitamins, vitamin C, vitamin E, vitamin K, calcium, iron, magnesium, potassium, phosphorus and many important trace minerals. It is high in protein, essential amino acids and eight digestive enzymes, and when exposed to light, high in chlorophyll. Alfalfa, as grown in the field, is nutrient-rich because its roots reach down to an average depth of 38 feet and have been known to penetrate as far as 66 feet.

Lowers blood cholesterol… raises HDLs and gets rid of LDLs

Researchers found that fiber in alfalfa pushes cholesterol out of the arteries while its saponins scrub and dissolve it. So impressive was its performance in reducing low density lipoproteins (LDL – the bad kind) that a major research scientist experimented with it on himself. Dr. Rene Manilow, chief of the cardiovascular disease research center at the Oregon Regional Primate Research has studied alfalfa since the late 70's and has unarguably produced the major body of scientific work on it in modern times. He volunteered himself as a human subject and ate large doses of roasted alfalfa seeds for six week periods over 5 months. His blood cholesterol level dropped 30 percent. More alfalfa caused an even greater decline, but there were side effects. He also found that alfalfa replaced the LDLs with the more beneficial high density lipoproteins (HDL- the good kind), increasing the HDL by 40 percent. He also found that steaming the seeds eliminated all potential toxicity.

Remedy for arthritis diabetes, rheumatism, ulcers

Alfalfa tea has been used as a remedy for arthritis, diabetes, rheumatism, ulcers and to promote breast milk in nursing mothers. Doctors in Johannesburg, South Africa were able to lower an 18-year-old diabetic's blood sugar levels from 58 mg per 100ml to 648 mg in 2 hours after drinking alfalfa tea. They attribute the effect to the high levels of manganese in alfalfa.

Estrogenic agent may reduce breast cancer

Alfalfa also delivers much estrogenic-like activity through its abundance of plant hormones. In tests with different female animals in different countries, alfalfa proved itself a formidable estrogenic agenda which may play a role in the reduction of breast cancer. Historically, alfalfa has been described as a "tonic" because of its rich resources of vitamins, minerals and protein. The relevance of other factors such as isoflavones, flavones and fatty acids is now being explored.

Broccoli

Broccoli sprouts for health, vitality and anti-cancer protection…

The cancer-fighting ability of compounds found in plants in the cabbage family has been known for some time. Even so, research scientists were surprised recently to discover that seedlings of broccoli have anywhere from 10 to 100 times more of those compounds (isothiocyanates) than mature plants do. That potentially means that an ounce of fresh broccoli sprouts is as potent as two pounds of head broccoli – and a lot easier to add regularly to your diet. Seeds are quick and simple to sprout on the kitchen counter, and add a sprightly crunch to sandwiches, salads, stir-fries or omelets.

The cabbage family of foods includes...

Chinese cabbage, broccoli, kale, turnip, rutabaga, radish, mustard, rape, cauliflower, collard greens, brussel sprouts and kohlrabi. Of these, the first eight are good for home sprouting. Cabbage is rich in fiber and a good source of minerals, especially potassium, 253 mg per 100 grams, sulfur 1710 mg and vitamins C 47mg, E and A 200 IU. It has a drying and binding faculty that makes it effective for inflammations and hot swellings. Historically, cabbage was used to combat scurvy at sea. Sailors would make sauerkraut from it, which coated their intestinal tract with friendly bacteria and promoted regularity. The fermentation from the kraut remedied the complaints of flatulence that are common with the cabbage family, it is also improved by boiling and draining.

The cabbage family and other cruciferous vegetables are now taken seriously at the National cancer Institute. Recent studies consistently point to lower than average cancer rates for those groups regularly eating dark green leafy vegetables. The crucifers contain compounds called glucosinolates, which block the development of cancer. Turnip greens contain between 39 and 166 milligrams per hundred grams of glucosinolates. When cooked, the concentration drops to a range of 21-94.

Cabbage has the greatest potential in colon and stomach cancer and recent studies demonstrate that people who eat leafy green crucifers have the lowest rate of colon cancer. Other surveys add cancers of prostate, rectum, esophagus, lung and bladder to the list. Isolated chemicals called indoles from cruciferous vegetables are potent antidotes to the development of cancer. Without indoles in a recent study, 91 percent of rats developed tumors. With indoles, only 21 percent succumbed. Dithiolthiones in cabbage cause the body to release glutathiones, a natural body enzyme. Glutathiones neutralize of detoxify carcinogens before they damage DNA. The greater the supply of glutathione, the greater the protection against cancer. Another anti-cancer compound, sulphoraphane, stimulates the cells production of quinone reductase, an enzyme that blocks tumor growth. The consumption of sprouts from the cabbage family is the best source of anti-cancer enzymes.

The author (Betsy Bragg) recommends that everyone read Cabbage: Cures to Cuisine by Judith Hiatt, and in Chapter 10 of this book, read John Duffy's rapid recovery through cabbage juice of many years suffering from ulcers.

Anti-Cancer Broccoli Sprouts

Johns Hopkins recently reported that broccoli sprouts have some 50 times the anti-cancer effect than full broccoli itself. For the last 40 years, broccoli sprouts and others of the cabbage family of sprouts have been part of the Hippocrates' lifestyle. Thousands have been helped to renew their immunity from this simple, yet powerful food.

Anti-Plaque Buckwheat Lettuce Sprouts

Contains the highest concentration of anti-plaque lecithin of any food! It acts to create elasticity in the skin and assists you to have normal digestion and elimination. Beyond this, it is filled with rutin, which promotes healthy circulation

End of Extracts from *Sprouts the Miracle Food* By Steve Meyerowitz

Hippocrates Health Institute regarding the value of Buckwheat Lettuce...

Buckwheat lettuce is very high in bioactive lecithin and helps to eliminate deposits on arterial walls. It is also an excellent source of chlorophyll, and contains good amounts of B-vitamins like riboflavin (the red you see in the stems) and rutin (a brain food).

www.HippocratesInst.org

Pea Greens

Cancer prevention and a great source of fiber

Because peas are legumes, they are rich in protease inhibitors that prevent certain viruses and chemicals that promote cancer. As rich sources of fiber, they are useful in reducing the LDL (bad) cholesterol in the blood.

Great for controlling blood sugar in diabetics

They also help control blood sugar making them a good food for diabetics. Peas have also been linked to a reduction in the occurrence of appendicitis and in a study on dogs, temporarily decreased their blood pressure.

Anti-fertility compounds...

Even a common food like green pea has medicinal benefits. Upon investigation, the anti-fertility compound mzylohydro-quinone was isolated. Although we are not recommending peas as an oral contraceptive, those who are having difficulty conceiving should consider reducing their consumption of peas and pea sprouts. The population of Tibet has remained stationary for about 200 years because of their diet.

Lentil, Mung, Adzuki, China Red Pea, Chickpea

Lots of fiber, lowering cholesterol

Beans have always been said to be "good for the heart." Now we know why. They clear out the dangerous LDL cholesterol in the blood. Simply by eating beans, one man brought down his cholesterol from 274 to 190; another lowered it from 217 to 167. The reason? Primarily soluble fiber. Fiber lowers blood pressure among vegetarians and bean eaters. Sprouting increases bean fiber by 300 percent.

Blood sugar regulators Beans are marvelous regulators of insulin. They make gradual changes in blood sugar and do not draw on the body's natural insulin to keep blood sugar under control. In fact, they provide more receptors for insulin to land, controlling the loss of insulin back into the bloodstream.

Clover

Absorbable calcium and magnesium, a nerve relaxant

Medicinally, clover is known as a tonic, a nutritive and a blood purifier. Jethro Kloss, the renowned herbalist and author of Back to Eden, called it, "One of God's greatest blessings to man." Clover is a wonderful source of volatile oils, carbohydrates, amino acids, flavonoids, minerals, vitamins and saponins. Its profuse and exceedingly absorbable calcium and magnesium relaxes the nervous system and settles the stomach. This accounts for its role as a sedative and an anti-spasmodic.

An expectorant, plaster, compress

A tea made from the blossoms is an expectorant and has been used in the treatment of whooping cough. In the 19th century, clover was a popular ingredient in body plasters. Its lime, silica and other early salts make it an ideal plaster. Plasters were used for sores, boils and cancers. The Shakers used it for cancerous ulcers and burns.

Remedy for eczema, psoriasis and cancerous growths

Plasters and compresses were also used for childhood skin problems such as eczema and psoriasis. The mineral salts also alkalinize the body and promote detoxification. It has a reputation as a remedy for cancerous growths including cancer of the throat and stomach, and was also used for leprosy, pellagra and syphilis.

Promotes fertility and hormonal balance…

The red clover flower is known to promote fertility, probably due to its high mineral content. It includes virtually every trace mineral needed by the gland and helps restore and balance hormonal functions. Its estrogenic activity has been linked to its isoflavone content. It may also balance the acid/alkaline environment of the uterus in favor of conception.

Sprouts of red clover increase energy, purify the blood and improve weak nerves.

The sprouts of red clover share many of the medicinal properties of the other leguminosae (alfalfa, pea, soy, lentil) with an emphasis on blood purification, increasing the energy and improving weak nerves.

Radish

High in Vitamins A, B1, B6, C, folic and panthothenic acid, niacin, potassium, iron and phosphorous. When exposed to light they turn green with chlorophyll. Crisp, slightly hot and tangy, like tiny radishes.

Radish sprouts are definitely expectorants…

Radish belongs to the crucifer family and is a cousin of cabbage, turnip, and mustard. Many of the medicinal properties of the crucifers apply to radish as well. The ribbons of red in the colorful leaves of this sprout alert the unwary gourmet. Radish sprouts actually produce more BTUs of heat than the mature radish bulb. The sprouts are expectorants. They clear mucus from the respiratory tract and are wonderful for colds, sinus congestion, bronchitis and whooping cough, and for the long-term improvement of asthma.

Use as a poultice, plaster, salve or foot bath...

Seeds can be used in plasters like mustard, poultices made from the seeds or ground up sprouts may be placed over various parts of the body with benefit. They relieve chest congestion when placed on the chest in a plaster, poultice, or salve and help rheumatism when placed over the shoulders, wrists and knees. Foot baths made from ground seeds or blended sprouts relieve head congestion.

Intestinal cleansing including expelling worms...

Radish is wonderful for the entire intestinal tract, from the nose to the anus. Its heat-producing action stimulates the elimination of mucus and starts a cleansing process, which can include expelling worms. (Intestinal flora like it).It is anti-putrefactive and antiseptic.

Appetite Stimulant...

Small amounts of radish stimulate appetite. Too much radish, however, will induce vomiting (emetic). Sprouted radish is excellent nourishment during cold weather.

Effective Diuretic and kind to bladder and kidneys...

It is an effective diuretic and restorative for troubles of the urinary tract, bladder and kidneys.

Hippocrates Health Institute regarding sunflower baby greens...

Sunflower greens contain a full spectrum of amino acids (building blocks of all protein) and supply vitamin D without the dairy. These baby greens contain an abundance of the sun's energy and chlorophyll, and are considered "a complete food.

Nutrition of Organic Sunflower Seeds (in Milligrams per 100 grams)

Iron	6.77	Riboflavin	0.25
Vitamin A	50.00USP	Sulfur	87.0
Vitamin E	52.18 USP	Thiamin	2.29
Vitamin D	92.0USP	Magnesium	354.0
Calcium	116.00	Glutamic acid	5.58
Total lipids	49.57	Protein	22.78
Phosphorus	705.0	Aspartic acid	2.45
Linoleic Acid	30.00	Potassium	689.00
Zinc	5.06	Arginine	2.40
Niacin	4.50	Leucine	1.66
Copper	1.75		

Benefits of Mung Bean Sprouts

Mung Beans are a member of the legume family of plants, which. among other things, have the unique capacity to fix atmospheric nitrogen by the nodules on their roots which harbor (in a symbiotic manner) nitrogen fixing bacteria.

In the Ayurvedic approach to health, Mung Beans are one of the most cherished foods because it is believed they balance all three doshas. And according to the American Bean website (http://www.americanbean.org/), research has indicated legumes are the most important dietary predictor of survival among the elderly. A 20gm daily increase in legume intake correlated to a 7-8 percent reduction in the death hazard ratio. In addition, the consumption of 4 or more servings of beans per week decreased heart disease by 22 percent, according to a US study of nearly 10,000 people.

A Nurses Health study indicated the chance of developing colorectal adenomas (the source of most colon cancer) was 35 percent less likely among women who ate four or more servings of legumes a week. Those diagnosed with colorectal adenomas that changed their diets to increase their intake of beans the most, were 65 percent less likely to suffer a reoccurrence of advanced adenomas. The fiber in legumes has the capacity to combine with bile acids. The decrease in bile available for digestion may stimulate the body's conversion of blood cholesterol into bile, resulting in lower levels of blood cholesterol.

Legumes contain a unique phytonutrient, a group of molecules called saponins. See alfalfa and saponins for a more detailed discussion on the health benefits of these molecules.

Unlike most beans, mung beans contain very few oligosaccharides, the sugars responsible for flatulence. This unique biochemistry makes mung beans suitable for children and anyone suffering from delicate digestive systems.

The amazing biochemical process of sprouting transforms this seed, which already has a number of significant health benefits, into a superfood. Most people are aware of the Mung Bean sprouts, where the seed has germinated and is several times bigger than its original size and the white radical or root has emerged. It is often eaten in this form as a snack. At this stage the Mung Bean still resembles a pea in shape.

The sprouting biochemistry has made available minerals, enzymes and vitamins, in a form easily assimilated into the body. The sprouting process makes vitamin C available, which is not found in the seed.

This is the end of the extracts from

Sprouts the Miracle Food - The Complete Guide to Sprouting -8th edition, 2010

By Steve Meyerowitz (Reprinted with Permission from Author)

www.Sproutman.com

Chia Seeds
by Susan Allison

www.thoreaufoods.com - Buy chia seeds locally from Susan.

Chia seeds are an ancient superfood. They are a member of the sage family (Salvia Hispanica). The little black and white seeds were a staple of the Incan, Mayan and Aztec cultures, along with the Native Americans of the Southwest.

"Chia" is actually the Mayan word for strength. The seeds were used by these ancient cultures as mega-energy food, especially for their running messengers, who would carry a small pouch of them with them. Chia has been called "Indian Running Food" and gives an incredibly sustaining surge of energy. Susan goes on to say, "I've definitely noticed for myself the 'running energy' that chia seems to impart. If I eat chia, then run later that day, my endurance and ability to run farther is greatly enhanced — pretty impressive stuff."

The chia from Thoreau Foods is imported from Mexico and is certified organic. In Mexico they say that one tablespoon of chia seeds can sustain a person for 24 hours.

Chia seeds are said to have:

- 2 times the protein of any other seed or grain

- 5 times the calcium of milk, plus boron, a trace mineral that helps transfer calcium into your bones

- 2 times the amount of potassium as bananas

- 3 times the reported antioxidant strength of blueberries

- 3 times more iron than spinach

- Copious amounts of omega-3 and omega-6, which are essential fatty acids

They are also a fabulous source of soluble fiber. Like flax, chia is highly hydrophilic: The seeds absorb water and create a mucilaginous gel. They can hold 9-12 times their weight in water and they absorb it very rapidly - in under 10 minutes.

Chia has high antioxidant content. The seeds stay stable for much longer than flax. Chia seeds can easily be stored dry for 4-5 years without deterioration in flavor, odor or nutritional value. You can substitute chia in any recipe that calls for flax.

The taste of chia is very mild and pleasant. That means you can easily combine it with other foods without changing the taste dramatically. People add chia to their sauces, bread batters, puddings, smoothies and more.

Chia has been called a dieter's dream food because when added to other foods, it bulks them up, displacing calories and fat without diluting the flavor.

Benefits of Eating Chia

Provides energy	Levels blood sugar
Boosts strength	Induces weight loss
Bolsters endurance	Aids intestinal regularity

Chia slows the impact of sugars on the system, if eaten together. Chia gel creates a physical barrier between carbohydrates and the digestive enzymes that break them down, which slows the conversion of carbs into sugar http://www.naturalnews.com/sugar.html. That means the energy from the food is released steadily, resulting in more endurance. This is clearly of great benefit to diabetics in particular. It also means that I can combine chia with super-sweet tastes like apple juice and not get super-spiked.

Due to the exceptional water-absorption quality of chia, it can help you prolong hydration and retain electrolytes, especially during exertion.

Whole, water-soaked chia seeds are easily digested and absorbed. Their tiny dinosaur-egg-like shells break down quickly. They feel light in the body, yet energizing. Their nutrients can be quickly assimilated into the body.

Chia seeds bulk up, then work like an incredible digestive broom, sweeping through your intestinal tract, helping to dislodge and eliminate old accumulated waste in the intestines. Many people find their stools also become more regular once they eat chia.

Chia seed protein contains no gluten. This makes it ideal for anyone with gluten sensitivity or simply wanting a replacement for gluten-containing grains like wheat, barley, rye and oats.

Chia is reported to be beneficial for a vast range of issues, for example:

*weight loss/balance	*diabetes	*acid reflux
*thyroid conditions	*IBS	*lowering cholesterol
*hypoglycemia	*celiac disease	

In the traditional cultures that consumed chia, like the Aztecs, chia was also regarded as a medicine. It was used in myriad ways — from cleaning the eyes to helping heal wounds, topically, to relieving joint pain and so on. It was considered extremely valuable for healing.

One woman we know uses chia therapeutically to manage her acid reflux. Because of the highly absorbent properties of chia, she can swallow a tablespoon of dry seeds with just a little water and they go into her stomach and absorb the excess acid. She makes sure to drink a glass of water a few minutes later, as the seeds are so hydrophilic that if they do not find enough to absorb in the stomach, they will draw from the tissues instead. By allowing the seeds to first absorb the acid, then drinking some more water, our friend is able to very simply, effectively and cheaply handle her condition.

Chia aids rapid development of tissue, due to its incredible nutrient profile and easy assimilation. It can be very beneficial for those healing from injuries, people like bodybuilders who are always re-forming tissues and women who are pregnant or breastfeeding. The most common way to eat chia is to first soak the seeds. They can very rapidly absorb a large amount of liquid, between 9-12 times their volume, in under 10 minutes.

To learn to sprout chia seeds watch http://www.youtube.com/watch?v=xX7RtbB5mBo

Wheatgrass Juice: A Bright-Green Revolution

How to drink it...

Ann Wigmore suggests drinking wheatgrass juice in small amounts throughout the course of the day, always on an empty or nearly empty stomach. In general, two to four ounces every day or every other day is sufficient. Slowly sipping small quantities of the juice gives your body an opportunity to get used to its taste and effect. Taking one to two ounce drinks straight or mixed with other juices (fruit and vegetable) and sipping slowly, will help prevent nausea or stomach upset. On a healing regime, Ann suggests you drink one or two oz. up to 3 or 4 times a day, and to take one day of rest.

The benefits of wheatgrass

Wheatgrass is 70 percent chlorophyll, a key building block for the vast majority of plant life. It traps the sun's energy and transfers it to our bodies. Like all plants that contain chlorophyll, wheatgrass is high in oxygen, which is needed for healthy cell function. Wheatgrass contains more light energy than any other element. Wheatgrass juice is a powerful anti-bacterial agent. Dr. Bernard Jensen, a pioneer in cleansing, says it is speedily digested with minimal energy expended to get that green fuel into the system.

Wheatgrass juice cures acne, removes scars and body odors. It prevents tooth decay and can be gargled for sore throat relief. In addition, it relieves constipation and removes heavy metals from the body.

For scientific references citing the benefits of wheatgrass, refer to *Wheatgrass, Nature's Finest Medicine*, by Steven Meyerowtiz.

also refer to: "Herbal Medicine in the Treatment of Colitis"
http://www.saudijgastro.com/article.asp?issn=1319-3767;year=2012;volume=18;issue=1;spage=3;epage=10;aulast=Ke

How to Grow Wheatgrass as Learned at Hippocrates and from Randy Jacobs, Life Force Growers

1. Soak seeds 8-12 hours (try to use purified water when soaking, tap water is OK)

   a. After soaking, rinse seeds several times thoroughly.

2. Plant seeds on top of soil.

   a. Use three trays. The bottom tray is solid without holes. Place a tray on top of it and fill it half full with soil. The soil that is recommended should be a mix of one part peat moss to three parts soil. (I use Fafard which I buy from Randy Jacobs)

   b. Sprinkle and then mix into the soil a very little Azomite or other rock dust containing natural and trace elements.

   c. Sow seeds so they are touching each other, one layer thick.

   d. Use the third tray to place on top. Tamp it down so the seeds are in the soil.

   e. Remove the tray and spray heavily. Use a gallon sprayer which can be purchased at Home Depot for about $20. Place the top tray back on.

3. Cover seeds during germination period. (first three or four days)

   a. Keep seed covered with an empty planting tray until grass forms and pushes the tray up about 3 or 4 inches.

   b. Spray heavily for the first three days in the morning and evening (do not make mud).

   c. After the grass is 3 or 4 inches high, the sink sprayer can be used. Grasp a handful of grass and pull the mat off the tray turning the mat so that you can spray the bottom of the mat.

4. Let grow in the indirect sunlight until blade of grass splits.

   a. Winter-time 10-14 days, Summer time 7-10 days.

   b. There is no set height the grass should be, just watch for the second shoot.

   c. Air circulation is very important! Ideally...

      i. Open a window near grass.

      ii. Have fan blowing around grass throughout the day.

5. Harvest grass all at once, split grass needs to be cut within a day or two of its jointing stage.

   a. Cut grass will last one week in the refrigerator.

      i. Stored in Deborah Myers bags, grass will last up to 14 days in refrigerator.

6. A second growth will appear and can be used for animals. Please note that the second growth is not as nutritious as the first. It will lose approximately 50-75 percent of its nutritional value.

Lifeforce Growers Price List

Organic Wheatgrass per 1lb. bag or tray	12.00
Organic Sunflower Greens per 1lb. bag	12.00
Organic Buckwheat Greens per 1 lb. bag	12.00
Grow trays each	3.50
Organic Soil 40 lb. bag each	8.00
Organic Glacial Rock Powder per 5 lb. bag	10.00
Organic HRW Wheat seed per lb.	3.50
Organic HRW Wheat seed per 5 lbs. bag	15.00
Organic Blk Oil Sunflower seed per lb.	4.00
Organic Blk Oil Sunflower seed per 5 lbs.	20.00
Organic Buckwheat seed per lb.	2.50
Organic Buckwheat seed per 5 lbs.	10.00
Organic Pea seed per lb.	3.00
Organic Pea seed per 5 lbs.	15.00
Life force grow rack system complete with rack, 3 lights and 6 FS bulbs each	299.00

Randy Jacobs, Director, Lifeforce Growers, Lexington, MA

Cell: 781-492-7624   Fax 781-894-7602
Email:lifeforce1@rcn.com

Visit www.evergreenjuices.com for ordering frozen wheatgrass.Another source for ordering seeds is www.sproutman.com.

Summary Questions

1. What are the benefits of eating sprouts?
2. What are ten benefits of wheatgrass juice?
3. Explain the step-by-step procedure for sprouting Mung beans.
4. Describe the steps in how to plant and harvest wheatgrass.

DVD: Delicate Balance
byAaron Scheibner

1 hour 24 minutes

This movie is produced by the Physicians Committee for Responsible Medicine, a non-profit organization with strong ties to the organization People for the Ethical Treatment of Animals. Thus, this movie has a relative bias against eating animal products and skews some information about the health benefits of an all vegan diet. The film states studies prove certain medical facts without providing adequate evidence to support many of the assertions that the film makes. Take this into account when watching the movie and formulate your own opinions for class discussion.

1. What is an HCA?

2. Describe the China Study and its findings.

3. For optimum health, how much protein do women/men need to eat per day?

4. What is Osteoporosis and what causes it?

5. List some problems with eating fish.

6. How much of the land area of the USA is used to produce food?

7. The human body was made to digest meat. True or False

8. Why is Casein bad for you?

9. What percentage of protein in dairy is casein?

10. What is the best way to absorb calcium?

DVD: Sprouting Seeds and Growing Wheatgrass
by Michael Bergonzi

1 hours 07 min.

1. What 3 things are sprouts good for?

2. What are seeds?

3. How should hulled seeds be kept and for how long?

4. How should unhulled seeds be kept and for how long?

5. What are hulled seeds?

6. What are unhulled seeds?

7. At what temperature should seeds be kept?

8. What is soaking?

9. What is sprouting?

10. Name 3 sources to learn about the nutrients of different sprouts.

11. How do you get enough protein and high energy on the "Living Food" diet?

12. How do you keep your energy up when traveling?

13. How long do you soak the seeds in group A?

14. What is the best type of container for soaking seeds?

15. What can be used for draining seeds?

16. What percent of the jar should be filled with seeds?

17. What kind of water should be used?

18. What do you do after you soak the seeds and how often each day?

19. How long will it usually take for the seeds to sprout before you can eat them?

20. How long will sprouts stay fresh in the refrigerator?

21. Where should the seeds sit in relationship to sunlight?

22. What sprouts fight cancer?

23. How long should you soak Group B seeds and why?

24. How many days does it take to sprout?

25. How often do you rinse the seeds?

26. Explain what is meant by the greening stage?

27. How long will group B's sprouts last in the refrigerator?

28. Should sprouts be rinsed off before you eat them?

29. What kind of bags should they be stored in and why?

30. Give 10 benefits of wheatgrass (see handouts) complete food, detoxer, and chlorophyll

31. At what temperature should wheatgrass be grown?

32. How often should wheatgrass be watered?

33. What other 2 conditions are important to sprouting besides watering and why?

34. What kind of soil to use?

35. How many large and small trays of wheatgrass can you fill with a 30 dry quart bag (the average large size)?

36. What is the difference between hydroponics and soil grown sprouts?

37. What kind of seeds are used to grow wheatgrass?

38. How long does harvested grass stay fresh in the refrigerator?

39. How many cups of dry seed are needed per tray?

40. How long do you soak the seeds?

41. When will the seeds be ready to plant?

42. How much soil do you put in each tray?

43. Why is a third tray needed?

44. How much wheatgrass should you drink a day?

45. How much juice can one get from a large tray?

46. How do you sow the seeds?

47. How should the trays of seeds be watered and how often?

48. After the seeds are sown, what is the next step and why?

49. What do you do for the next 3 days?

50. When is wheatgrass ready to harvest?

51. How do you harvest wheatgrass?

52. What causes wheatgrass to get moldy?

53. What causes wheatgrass to get yellowish in the middle?

54. How do you get rid of bugs?

55. What kind of sunflower seeds should be used and why?

56. How and why should trays of wheatgrass and sunflower seeds be covered?

57. When should sunflower seeds be harvested?

58. How does buckwheat differ from sunflower seeds?

Chapter 4
Internal Awareness - Fasting

By Lorraine Hurley, MD

Overview

Conventional medicine overlooks digestion as a primary source of the disease process. Instead we spend millions on digestive aids that only mask the symptoms and prevent us from being responsible for where illness starts. In order to achieve complete health you must consider all the systems of the body. In this chapter we will study the digestive system and its impact on our health, how to diagnose and treat your own gut for a long life of vitality.

The Hippocrates approach to fasting involves liquid nourishment for deep cleansing. Fasting is the oldest therapeutic method known to man. Even before the emergence of the "medicine man" and the healing arts, humans instinctively stopped eating when feeling ill and abstained from food until health was restored. The Hippocrates approach to fasting is a more modern method for handling a cleanse over a longer period of time. A vegetable juice fast alkalinizes the body faster and speeds up detoxification while providing calories and nutrients to sustain energy.

You will learn:

- The digestive system
- Major glands of the digestive tract
- Fasting on liquid nourishment

Organs of the Digestive System

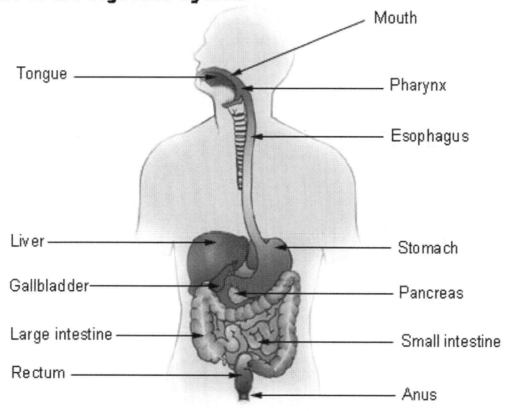

Mouth

Tongue

Pharynx

Esophagus

Liver

Stomach

Gallbladder

Pancreas

Large intestine

Small intestine

Rectum

Anus

The Internal Process of Digestion and Ecology

First, let's review the ideal process of digestion and absorption. This is a simplified explanation, but it is enough for general understanding. First, we will take an idealized scenario, then we will introduce what can go wrong when ideal digestion does not happen.

When you see, smell and taste food, your body is stimulated to prepare for ingestion and digestion. This aspect of digestion is more sensory/emotional than physical. Sensory experience plays a huge role in the enthusiasm of digestion. If we like and desire what we see and smell, this enthusiasm is communicated throughout our gastrointestinal system. Our sensory experience is often linked to whatever emotions eating produced in us as children.

If we have an emotional link to certain foods, often what we learn about healthy eating and what we desire will conflict. For instance, let's take hot dogs. If you have a strong emotional link to eating hot dogs with your dad at a ball game, then it could be really hard to give up hotdogs when we are attempting to eat for health. Even if we are not at a ball game, hot dogs resonate "time with dad."

Make no mistake, our sensory response to food is deeply embedded in our emotional body. It is important to realize this, because it helps you appreciate why changing your diet to affirm health and life force may be so difficult. When we understand that much of our eating is emotional, we can grow our capacity to find other means of recognizing and meeting our emotional needs and surrender eating to a practice that directly impacts life force. In time, we WILL develop discernment, and an enhanced ability to smell, taste and see what is actually before us as food.

So lets discuss the gut, eating, nutrition and digestion in an impersonal way and then expand our comprehension to introduce ourselves to an internal awareness of what happens both functionally and emotionally when we develop a conscious relationship to both food and eating.

Digestion, Absorption and Assimilation

In a general and idealized context, your salivary glands are stimulated in response to sight and smell (hence the term "mouth-watering" to describe the reaction to the sensual experience of food). These enzymes are for the most part alkaline. They break down food so that the enzymes in food itself can be activated. As you chew, your saliva mixes food with several enzymes, but also releases the enzymes present in food (if food is raw and not cooked these enzymes are present in abundance).

Maceration (chewing) plus enzymatic activation (saliva) begin to soften and dissolve the gross structure of your food. This activity (food is coming!) in turn stimulates acid release and peristalsis (movement) in your stomach. There are receptors in your stomach that then stimulate the intestines, gall bladder and pancreas.

Stomach enzymes are very acidic. The stomach also secretes pepsin. This enzyme is critically important in protein digestion. After food is macerated, it proceeds to your stomach where strong acids are ready to further dismantle the information in your food. This interplay of acid/alkaline is the body's way of ensuring that all edible matter is broken down for processing. Food is a complex material, and we are equipped to handle the complexities one step at a time. The stomach initiates a process that has multiple steps.

If the chyme (what leaves the stomach) is appropriately acidic, this stimulates the small intestines, gall bladder and pancreas to secrete their enzymes. The stomach has done a great job of grossly exposing the content of food to your body. But it is a bit like taking off a coat. Underneath the coat is a sweater and underneath that, your shirt, and beneath that, your undergarments. To fully unclothe your food, further digestion is required.

The gallbladder responds to fat content and is highly alkaline (like soap). It requires that chyme be acidic to give out appropriate amounts of bile (a bitter greenish-brown alkaline fluid that sids digestion and is secreted by the liver and stored in the gallbladder). The more fat in your food, the more bile that will be released. The small intestines and pancreas are more specific than the gall bladder and stomach. They secrete several enzymes for the digestion of all the constituents of food. They do require an appropriate "acid signal" to function robustly, but they release several enzymes that function very specifically for carbohydrates, fats and proteins. The stomach and gallbladder are your main acid/alkaline processors. Their job is to see to it that the gross structure of food is broken down so that the intestinal and pancreatic enzymes can process things completely.

The small intestine is where most absorption of nutrients takes place. It has tremendous surface area for this. I was told that if the cells of the gut were laid out as a single "sheet," it would cover an area nearly as large as a football field. This is a pretty astonishing feat of design to put all that absorptive area into a space the size of your abdomen. The small intestines are also where most of the immune cells of the gut reside (referred to as GALT—gut associated lymphoid tissue). The gut is, in fact, your body's largest immune organ. It also has substantial neurological and hormonal function. This has tremendous implications and will be discussed further on.

A rich layer of secretions are produced by the cells of the gut; both specialized cells and immune cells protect the mucosa, or surface of the intestines. Within this layer, the immune cells of your gut keep harmful bacteria from being absorbed along with your food. This part of the intestines absorbs both passively and actively, meaning there are small "holes" in the matrix that allow water and liquefied nutrients to pass into the blood stream. This is passive digestion. There are also areas where nutrient molecules are actively passed – they have to go through an inspection, binding and releasing process. Think of passive absorption as walking through an open door and active absorption as being admitted into a tunnel lined with inspectors. You must pass inspection to be allowed out the other side.

Absorption passes nutrients into a rich, dense micro vascular (blood vessel) bed. Your blood vessels move this nutrient broth up to the portal vein and into the liver. The liver is also lined with immune cells (Kupffer cells - specialized cells in the liver that destroy bacteria, foreign proteins and worn-out blood cells) and is the organ that makes bile for the gallbladder. The liver also does most of our detoxification. All food has active and inactive or waste constituents. What is active we need and what is inactive, or toxic, must be neutralized and eliminated. The liver has two main phases it uses to extract what we need and to neutralize what is left over and other toxins that are present (chemicals in and on food, drugs etc.).

Simply speaking, the body's natural liver detoxification process involves two steps, Phase 1 and Phase 2. A toxin or food initially enters Phase 1 and is reduced to smaller fragments. These fragments are unstable and generally referred to as free radicals. These fragments progress to Phase II where they are bound to several different molecules depending on what the fragment is. Phase II is a very nutrient dependent process. If we are well nourished, phase II can do it's job.

However, not everyone's liver is equal. Phase I can be slow or efficient. Phase II can be slow or efficient. If Phase one is efficient, you have a higher tolerance for toxins. This is where most caffeine, alcohol, drugs and environmental chemicals are processed and "neutralized." In fact, tolerance to caffeine is an indicator of Phase I activity. Studies have shown that it can vary by a factor of 5. People with slow phase I in the 21st century are most likely to develop chronic fatigue, fibromyalgia, multiple chemical sensitivity and cancer.

But, Phase I isn't everything. The substance neutralized by phase I must be bound by a substance in Phase II. If Phase II is adequate, there is a greater binding of free radicals and fewer substances harmful to our bodies released into our blood stream. If Phase II is also slow, then we lose some protection over cellular damage.

There are functional tests of both caffeine clearance and oxidative stress. They can be helpful if you suffer from chronic illness. There are also genetic tests that evaluate individual enzyme abilities in the liver. These are also useful if you suspect that you suffer from a high degree of toxin sensitivity.

See the recommended reading section for web links that provide information in greater detail.

Leaving the liver, we can examine what happens to what is not absorbed. As food is moved out of the small intestines and into the colon, it is still quite liquid. The colon serves three main functions: It absorbs water, eliminates waste and hosts an amazing ecology of microorganisms that are essential to our health and wellbeing. These organisms are also present in our small intestines, though in much smaller concentrations.

Unfortunately, there are many ways in which optimal function and flow of the gut can be compromised. Let's take a look at what commonly goes wrong and how it may affect us.

It is reported that about 20 percent of the US population has some form of functional gastrointestinal disorder. Further, many systemic illnesses and diseases are linked to gastrointestinal dysfunction, particularly autoimmune and neurodegenerative diseases. There are also studies linking cancer, obesity and cardiovascular disease to compromised gut function and ecology. I have included websites in the footnotes to help you investigate specifics on this.

There is a tremendous explosion of research into how gut function and ecology play a pivotal role in whether we are healthy or not. The gut lays the foundation for what is termed our bioterrain. Just as a beautiful and healthy garden or the life of a rainforest require numerous conditions within the soil to thrive, so do we.

Bioterrain

The ecological balance of the organisms living inside our body highlights the truth that we are dependent upon nature. There is a dynamic symbiosis between us and trillions of microbes critically important to our overall health. Together, we participate in some of the most brilliant and intricate of all natural functions.

The GI tract is a hollow, rugate, winding tube that begins with our mouth and ends at our anus. It is as rich in life and process, as the world we think of as outside of us. Most people understand that our GI tract is where digestion, absorption and assimilation of nutrients, and elimination of waste, takes place. But, too few appreciate the eloquence of our relationship to this environment, or how to care for it. When it is healthy, we benefit immensely. When it is compromised, so are we.

The gut also has significant endocrine, nervous system and immunological functions. By current estimates, 50-60 percent of all the immune cells in our body, reside in our gut amid what is referred to as GALT. It is now believed that the microbes of our GI tract assist the body directly with immunological functions and actually train and inform our immune system in necessary and critical ways. They are allies on the front lines of our defense, and they are our generous benefactors in immunological strategic planning.

The GI tract is rich in neurological and hormonal tissue. A full 50 percent of nervous system cells are found throughout the GI tract, rightly earning it the title of "the second brain." There are receptors in the gut for nearly every neurotransmitter and hormone we produce. When we are experiencing a "gut feeling," we are experiencing an intelligence that emanates, in part, from the gut's ability to receive and transmit molecules of intellect and emotion. When we understand how involved the gut is in the whole of human function, it becomes apparent that care of this vital ecology is essential. Almost every problem encountered within medical practice has associations with gut function.

There is a correlation between our environment, both the inner and outer, and disease. Bioterrain refers to the environment that surrounds the cells of our bodies. It contains the fluids, the nutrients, the minerals and trace elements, adjacent cells of all types, and a host of microorganisms both helpful and injurious.

When the bioterrain is healthy, these microbes are primarily symbionts; meaning we need each other to survive and thrive. These organisms colonize our lower GI tract and perform a multitude of brilliant, functional and protective functions on our behalf. Here is the really exciting thing about this ecology–as symbionts, they also participate in genetic regulation and expression of our human genome. The human genome has about 25,000 genes. We are super-organisms; host to a multitude of other organisms in much the way the earth hosts a plethora of life. Our genetic expression is not only dependent on the DNA we inherit from mom and dad, it is dependent upon the organisms we share life with (metabolomics- the study of organisms within us), as well as the environment we live in (epigenetics - regulation of cell function by the environment). Surprised?

What this ecology demonstrates is that at a molecular level (DNA), we depend upon the world of microbes to fully express (or not) our own genetic potential. More amazing, they teach us about a couple of phenomena in nature; specifically the sciences of epigenetics (regulation of cell function by the environment) and pleomorphism (the ability of organisms to change from one to another).

When our bioterrain is overloaded with toxins and pathogens (fungi, molds, viruses, bacteria, etc.), lacks essential minerals and nutrients, is either too acidic or too alkaline, then the vitality of our cells is compromised, or our immune system is overworked.

When the bioterrain is out of balance, our bodies become susceptible to illnesses, fatigue, and a host of other maladies. A healthy, vibrant bioterrain is fundamental to true health, because disease can be easily resisted and cannot establish the conditions that would result in illness.

One of the primary determinants of gut health, and consequently, our bioterrain is the quality of what goes into our mouths. We have already established that living, fresh and organic food is a dynamic exchange of life force and vitally important communication at the molecular level. But, more often than not, what goes into our mouths compromises digestion, absorption, ecology, pH balance, bioterrain and immune system function. It isn't just food quality, but proper food combining that can determine optimal enzyme output from the GI tract.

Let's take a peek at how a typical lifestyle adversely affects us beginning in the gut. We are particularly attracted to certain flavors. This is known and fully manipulated by the food industry. The Monell Institute is given huge funding by major food manufacturers to study the effects of food additives on brain function and satiety. Unhealthy salt, sweet and fat are used heavily in processed foods. This makes them not only palatable, but also addictive. This overrides our sensory processing of food until our preferences are for artificially manufactured substances rather than real food. Processed foods are nutrient deficient and loaded with substances that are frank toxins of absolutely no benefit to us and, in fact, have been shown to have a multitude of adverse consequences on human function and health.

Additionally, most people cook their food. Even if it is fresh to begin with, the process of cooking depletes the food of vital nutrients and enzymes. But, cooked food has a stronger smell and taste. So, we become addicted to the added stimulation of our sensory receptors through cooking. For instance, let's take kale. Kale is a king in pauper's clothing, as far as nutrition goes. It is a leafy green that imparts so much to us when fresh and raw. But, it doesn't smell or taste like much naked and fresh. It may seem very unimpressive, and it may be very hard to chew compared to other foods. Yet, how many people love it when it is sautéed with onions or garlic or doused in a pot of kale soup?

Poor diet can create an entire cascade of dysfunction in the gut. It will dramatically alter the output of enzymes. The use of caffeine, alcohol and drugs (both prescription and non-prescription) further alters digestive enzyme output, but also directly diminishes the mucosal barrier in our intestines.

When Things Go Wrong

Let's take a very common problem associated with GI function, a condition referred to as acid reflux. While marketed as a condition of hyperacidity, this is most often incorrect. It is usually just the opposite. If the stomach has poor acid output, a few different things can happen that affect the overall efficiency of digestion. Low acid means food is insufficiently broken down in the stomach. This creates gas (think about people that burp a lot). Gas creates volume and this relaxes the pyloric sphincter (the muscle between your stomach and esophagus). When the sphincter is open, stomach contents reflux up into the esophagus, causing pain. Why? Because the stomach can tolerate a pH of 1 (highly acidic); its lining is made for that. But, the esophagus will "burn" with a pH as high as 5 or anything less. A pH of 4 or 5 in the stomach is inadequate acidification, but in the esophagus, it burns.

So, reflux is most commonly caused by hypoacidity and not hyperacidity. What causes hypoacidity are diets low in real food and high in synthetic "food stuffs" including caffeine, alcohol, refined carbohydrates and sugar. But, this is only a part of what influences gastric function. Stress (nervous system, gobbling your food and toxicity primarily) directly impact acid output and motility or peristalsis.

What commonly happens is that you are prescribed an antacid. This raises the pH to the point where it no longer burns your esophagus, but you now further confound the balance and efficiency of your entire digestive system.

Another common problem is the use of Non-Steroidal Anti-Inflammatory Drugs (NSAIDS, such as Ibuprofen) for inflammatory conditions. While temporarily alleviating joint pain, they further denude the gut, contributing to a leaky gut, immune excitation and immune complexes in your blood stream that diminish blood flow in small blood vessels and create joint pain.

Traditional medicine is not health care. It is medical care with an emphasis on symptom suppression and not remediation of the cause of illness and disease. Medications more often than not, create a vicious cycle within the body, masking symptoms while promoting the dysfunction that led to illness or disease in the first place.

Let's go back to our symbionts. What this world of microbes teaches us, is that in order to survive, they possess the ability to help us survive. They don't just sit there, and eat, and make nutrients, as bi-products in exchange. They aren't passive like infants waiting to be fed. They possess extraordinary intelligence. They actually communicate with our cells via messenger molecules. They actually stand front and center in our GI tracts and stand down the enemies of the microbial world. Then they go back to our immune cells and tell them how to do this same thing themselves. That is, if they are healthy and able to perform these functions. They also participate in the neurological and hormonal functions of the gut. So, they assist with digestion, absorption, immunological development and defense, hormonal, neurological and genetic regulation. They are essential for human health.

The Human Gut Ecology

What frequently happens, however, is that instead of feeding and caring for this ecology in ways that strengthen it, we rain down sewage upon it. The same foods that make us healthy, make them healthy. When we don't eat right, or expose ourselves to toxins indiscriminately, we begin to stress this delicate ecology. Further, there are energetic constructs in our gut that we can liken to "the atmosphere". If we live in an atmosphere of stress, trauma, hostility and aggression, we translate that information to our department of defense and neighborhood community watch (the microbes of our gut), then what happens? Do they just die and we go on? No, they don't, not on your life. Many will die, but many will utilize a natural phenomenon in nature called "pleomorphism."

In terms of environmental ecology, "pleomorphism" can be thought of as guerilla warfare. Survival at all costs. But, it can also be realized as opportunism. Because our genetic machinery is not static, but morphic (able to respond to environmental queues), we survive. But, we don't thrive when the signal resonating through our bodies is "survive," or our environmental terrain promotes and supports the development and growth of parasites in lieu of symbionts. We adapt, but this is not an optimal state of function. The bodily states of survival and adaptation do not promote creative expansion, but lead to a multitude of disease states.

A good example of what happens in the body when the bioterrain is poisoned can be taken from the work of Ritchie Shoemaker M.D. Dr. Shoemaker was a primary care physician in Maryland when he began to see numerous patients with complaints of serious illness that were "undiagnosable." Many presented with chronic fatigue or fibromyalgia symptoms and many more displayed signs and symptoms of neurodegeneration.

To make a long story short, Dr. Shoemaker, through dedicated and intelligent investigation and research, learned that his patients were suffering from exposure to biotoxins. He traced the exposure to coastal waters near his town. There was a lot of nitrogen runoff into the water (from commercial fertilizers). This caused algae to grow and to consume a food source necessary for the survival of another organism. This organism did not die out: it morphed into a dinoflagellate (a microscopic organism) that did not have to compete for food and that excreted a substance that is toxic to human and animal life. It was not a "new" species, but an existing species that rearranged its DNA and life form to survive hostile conditions. These biotoxins were found in the water and aquatic life that people were consuming. Dr. Shoemaker demonstrated that biotoxins in the environment play a huge role in human illness and disease.

This same process can occur in the body. We have organisms that live harmoniously with us when the bioterrain is healthy. When it is not, they morph into organisms that do substantial damage to us. Dark field microscopy is one method of evaluating our bioterrain for the presence of these morphic species. They generally morph through stages and can be viewed in live blood analysis. There is strong evidence that cancer and other degenerative processes are mediated by pleomorphs–organisms that develop as a result of a toxic bioterrain.

So, if what goes into your mouth injures your ecology, your gut flora change. Promotion of organisms that are opportunistic and do not work for our benefit ensues (called dysbiosis). This imbalanced ecology then begins to secrete toxins that affect the protective layer of the intestines (leaky gut) that in turn stresses and activates the immune system (think auto-immune disease). They also cause a dysregulation of metabolism leading to obesity and other hormonal disturbances.

Because a huge amount of nervous tissue is in the gut, these biotoxins affect our neurological function throughout the body as well. Instead of a properly digested, nutrient-rich soup reaching our liver, a nutrient-deficient, toxic brew, full of poorly digested proteins, microbes and inflammatory chemicals arrive in our liver. Is it any wonder we are a nation of morbidly ill people?

The remedy for auto-toxicity (biotoxins from morphed organisms within the body) and environmental toxicity is to return the body to a balanced pH (through diet and detoxification), to cleanse the body (colon, liver, gallbladder, kidneys) and to optimize nutritional status through living, raw, organic plant based food. There are, of course, probiotics, homeopathic remedies and herbs that can be used to assist with this and these methods are discussed in the following chapter. You can also eat slowly, mindfully and in a relaxed state.

The part of the nervous system that controls digestion and absorption is the autonomic nervous system. The sympathetic branch of this system is your flight or fight mechanism. The parasympathetic is your rest and digest mechanism. If we are excited, irritated, anxious and unfocused, we are running on sympathetic over drive and our parasympathetic function will be suppressed.

One of the most efficacious therapies I know for promoting overall health is colon hydrotherapy. I have witnessed many patients turn the corner on disease and illness after achieving remarkable benefit from colonics. My personal experience with colonics goes beyond the physical, for I have found they enhance creative, emotional and intellectual wellbeing. It is a safe, inexpensive therapy that deserves serious consideration as a key health-promoting lifestyle practice.

There is a tool we can use to powerfully detoxify and de-stress this delicate ecology with amazing results. It is the practice of fasting. Historical records tell us that fasting has been used for health recovery for thousands of years. Hippocrates, Socrates, and Plato all recommended fasting for health recovery. The Bible tells us that Moses and Jesus fasted for 40 days for spiritual renewal. Mahatma Gandhi fasted for 21 days to promote respect and compassion between people with different religions. For much of human history, fasting has been guided by intuition and spiritual purpose. Today, our understanding of human physiology confirms the powerful healing effects of fasting.

The Benefits of Fasting

Fasting is a powerful therapeutic process. It can help people recover from mild to severe health conditions. Fasting provides a period of concentrated physiological rest during which time the body can devote its self-healing mechanisms to repairing and strengthening damaged organs. The process of fasting also allows the body to cleanse cells of accumulated toxins and waste products.

Fasting gives the digestive tract time to completely rest and strengthen its mucosal lining. This expedites the healing of a leaky gut. Fasting also reduces the work of the immune system and liver so they too can heal and find restored balance. As toxins make their way out of your body the growth of healthy flora is promoted and the growth of pleomorphic pathogens is suppressed. A fast that is appropriate for your situation will allow for you to experience some or all of the following:

- More energy
- Healthier skin
- Healthier teeth and gums
- Better quality sleep
- A clean and healthy cardiovascular system
- A decrease in anxiety and tension
- Dramatic reduction or complete elimination of aches and pains in muscles and joints
- Decrease or elimination of headaches
- Stabilization of blood pressure
- Stronger and more efficient digestion
- Stabilization of bowel movements
- Loss of excess weight
- Elimination of stored toxins
- Improvement with a wide variety of chronic degenerative health conditions, including autoimmune disorders.

It is important to understand that the detoxifying and healing processes that occur during a fast are also active when a person is consuming food. But, fasting enables these processes to work more efficiently.

A fast can be helpful for people whose conditions are not improving as quickly as they would like, or for people who have health conditions that require a concentrated period of healing to resolve. It is also crucial to understand that the most important part of a fast is, not only how a person lives after the fast, but also, how a person breaks the fast. Fasting can provide a clean and revitalized foundation upon which you can build and maintain a strong and well-conditioned body by consistently making healthy food and lifestyle choices.

There are several different ways to fast: water fast, fresh juice fast, fruit only fast, etc. If you are very ill, you may not tolerate water only as a fast for more than 24 hours at a time in the beginning. This is because the excretion of toxins from tissues and organs may overwhelm the body's capacity to detoxify. If you are considering fasting for the first time, consult a qualified practitioner to help guide you on the parameters best for you at this time.

The length of a fast can also vary from 24 hours to several days. A very popular and proven reliable method of fasting is to consistently devote one day a week to the practice. Not only will this expedite healing, it has been shown to enhance biological aging and extended lifespan.

What is recommended for liquid nourishment according to the Hippocrates approach, is a drink consisting of sprouts, celery, cucumber and other leafy green vegetables such as kale, bok choy, collard, spinach, dark green lettuces, cabbage, green herbs, etc. Drink at least two quarts of green juice during the day, mostly during the morning hours. Have the last drink at least three hours before bedtime, so you won't have to get up to go to the bathroom during the night. You can drink as much water, lemonade (water, lemon juice and stevia) and herbal teas as you want during the day. The next morning, take an enema followed by a wheatgrass implant as shown in the Hippocrates Health Institute DVD on Internal Awareness. As soon as a half an hour after your first glass of juice, have a light breakfast such as a piece of ripe fruit or sprout salad to give your digestive system a gradual awakening.

If taking responsibility for your lifestyle doesn't sound important to you, consider the following. It is estimated that a full 80 percent of chronic disease and illness and 40 percent of all cancer is preventable. Additionally, the cause of most disease is related to poor lifestyle habits and education. This is stated by the Center for Disease Control (CDC). What the CDC does not acknowledge, but is nevertheless true, is that lifestyle changes that prevent disease and illness can, also, reverse them.

We KNOW how to prevent and reverse most disease and illness, but we don't widely utilize that knowledge in practice. Why? The answer is uncomfortable and inconvenient. As we educate ourselves, we must simultaneously elicit the gut response required to change several beliefs widely held and defended within medicine.

This present medical paradigm, which must be changed, yields four prominent practices in medicine:

1. The focus on a singular, dominant factor (one problem, one disease).

2. The emphasis on homeostasis (treat symptoms to bring parameters, i.e. blood pressure, body temperature, into "normal" range).

3. Inexact risk modification (treat everyone with a blood pressure over 120/80 despite the fact that 30 percent of coronary artery disease happens in people with normal blood pressure).

4. Additive treatments (a doctor and drug for every symptom).

What is the actual result of practicing this way? Nearly 50 percent of our entire population is prescribed at least one drug; 30 percent of the population over 65 is prescribed three or more drugs; and, according to the Journal of American Medical Association (JAMA), medicine practiced this way is the third leading cause of death in our country. Mechanistic, reductionistic science and practice are a disservice to the welfare of living systems, and they fly in the face of the science available to us today.

Quantum theory in physics is, now, confirming what the ancients knew experientially and intuitively. All life is energy and is interconnected through various energy and information fields. Behavior, form and function are the result of complex relationships and both tangible and intangible influences. The parts inform the whole, and the whole, in turn, informs the parts. Life is fluid. Holism, chi, and psychic awareness are no longer "new age" concepts; they are new science frontiers. We don't conquer life; we either participate on her terms or we suffer. What we eat, think, believe, and how we interact with the environment, both within and without, informs our individual template and determines our health status. Growing your comprehension of the wonderful world within you is the first step toward establishing a harmonious and creative relationship with it. As you work with diet and the functions and ecology of your gut, you grow also in competence towards the art and gift of self- healing.

There are numerous scientific and medical academies offering professional education derived from progressive and integrated sciences. The American Academy of Environmental Medicine (AAEM) and The Institute for Functional Medicine (IFM) are two such organizations. Through open-minded inquiry, medical practice can become a vital part of a meaningful solution. Eric Hoffer, an American writer and philosopher, put it succinctly: "Learners will inherit the world, while the learned will find themselves beautifully equipped to deal with a world that no longer exists." May you rise to the challenge of living with affirmation and love for who and what you are, like a phoenix from the ashes. Namaste.

What if...? The Raw Truth
by Lisa Edinberg

What if GMO, artificial sweetener, pesticide-covered vegetables, hydrogenated oil, high fructose corn syrup, dairy from a hormone-filled cow, and all other foods from nutrient-depleted soil produce lack of clarity, a muted heart, your essence from being heard, and a chatter-filled mind? What if the intuitive, all-knowing whisper within, is only heard with a clear mind and an open heart? I argue that the world's authentic guidance system has been silenced by artificial interferences, static that covers up inner truth. Yet, this realization enables hope and possibility for its reversal.

It is hard to know one's truth, one's ultimate purpose when the body is depleted of the nourishment it requires. However, uncover the music, undo the damage, remove the poison that rages within, and the energy you have been lacking comes alive, as if reborn, now engaged in life for the first time. In essence, arrive back to a place from which we came. This renewal changes all that you know to be true; all that you have sensed becomes your potential. The revelation that food matters for all that you are is a truth worth knowing, information worth spreading.

There is a reason that people who go on juice fasts have abundant energy after a couple of days. It seems counterintuitive. Yet our lives have been spent, literally, on digestion, the body's job to breakdown the food and beverage we have consumed, ingested and mechanically sending your whole being energy with which to grow and function. Send nutrient-filled juice and like an injection, the body functions optimally without utilizing energy to digest. Therefore, the surplus of energy is used elsewhere. Want energy? Juice it. Got Energy vs. Got Milk is an excellent slogan for eliminating the treadmill most of us have been running upon.

The body is designed to digest food. Nevertheless, if overworked and underpaid for decades, eventually the workers become restless, weakened, lack spirit, drive themselves into the ground and crave an escape such as alcohol, drugs, and junk food filled with toxins. These foreign entities of the body deteriorate the cells, causing illness ultimately. They begin to form armies, causing a coupe-like reaction against the body. Within this Trojan horse of an exterior shell, they wreak havoc silently for long periods enabling symptoms, until disease is diagnosed, sometimes too late. They ravage cities and towns, the bodily mechanics and systems with capital buildings known as organs, until your surrender, relinquishing all your power. Soon the physical vessel you have called home, which you have been entrusted with in this lifetime, is six-feet under.

We have a choice whether to surrender or even to allow the armies to congregate. Take hold of these militants by sending them peaceful, energetic nutrients that fill their space with a life vs. death option. By sending a living food throughout the system, this physical vessel, all begins to work in harmony. Soon one feels renewed, invigorated, younger, and more like one's authentic self than ever before. ("....more me than I've ever been") The true self shines through, one's essence returns, and like birthing the heart, renews the spirit.

Every decision we make is a choice. When using a toxic-filled mind fueled by the very thing that prevents clear thinking, one understands why change is challenging. Knowing this truth may be the piece of knowledge necessary to transform what has been. The coupe for change must be an overhaul of the good within taking charge, adopting a leadership role. Within, it must pass along the nutrient-based needs of all that is nourishing for itself and bring in the enzymatic pieces of the outside world to harmonize with the inner workings of the body. Together they exhume your being, releasing your essence from captivity it has experienced since the first unrecognizable entity ("edible food-like substances") entered the vessel.

Allowing the healing to take place in the form of life force energy via food, brings the body to optimum health again. This freedom is the destination we strive toward, to enable us to live and breathe our best lives. With this energy and clarity, we can live an openhearted existence. Our life purpose naturally will be lived, while the music of all that we are is played and heard by the world. Living one's authentic life is about retrieving the gifts given, and utilizing them with intention.

The choice is yours for the making. What If...? It's just the raw truth.

Summary questions:

1. What organs comprise the human gastrointestinal system?

2. What is the primary determinant of a healthy gastric ecology?

3. What functions does the GI tract participate in besides digestion and absorption?

4. What conditions within the gut masquerade as systemic diseases?

5. Which organ of the GI tract does most of the detoxifying of our body?

6. Where in the GI tract does most of the absorption of our nutrients take place?

7. Is bile acid or alkaline?

8. In what way does fasting assist our body and promote health?

Recommended Reading and Websites

- "Gut Solutions," by Brenda Watson, ND

- "Desperation Medicine," by Ritchie Shoemaker, MD

- For a thorough review of practical and scientific applications with current understandings, visit
  http://www.scribd.com/doc/24900138/Epigenetics-Role-in-Human-Development.

- http://www.pcori.org/assets/International-Foundation-for-Functional-Gastrointestinal-Disorders-3-12-12.pdf.

- http://www.ranker.com/list/list-of-digestive-system-diseases-and-disorders/diseases and-medications-info.

- http://www.ncbi.nlm.nih.gov/pubmed/22109896

- http://metabolichealing.com/key-integrated-functions-of-your-body/gut/the-role-of-gut-function-in-autoimmune-conditions/

- http://www.annualreviews.org/doi/abs/10.1146/annurev-nutr-072610-145146?journalCode=nutr

- http://www.jci.org/articles/view/58109

- http://www.huffingtonpost.com/leo-galland-md/do-you-have-leaky-gut-syn_b_688951.html

- http://www.everydayhealth.com/digestive-health/what-is-leaky-gut-syndrome.aspx

DVD – Fasting on Liquid Nourishment

Time: 47 mins.

The benefits of fasting on green juice rather than water. A review of the physical, emotional, mental, and spiritual benefits of fasting.

1. What are two similarities of water and juice fasting? What are the differences?

2. How often does Hippocrates recommend fasting and what is its significance?

3. What are our bodies' three areas of energy? Please describe each. What percentage of ourselves should each be and what percentage are they usually?

4. How do we change the imbalance in our lives in these areas?

5. What percent of the brain do most people use according to MRI's?

6. What are the key elements for strengthening the immune system?

7. What is Dr. Kenneth Cooper famous for?

8. Why is weight resistance training important?

9. What are the two major factors why people die?

10. What hours of the day should one fast? When shall one begin and end?

11. Why is it called liquid nourishment instead of fasting?

12. What are the three S's?

13. What are some of the effects of fasting?

14. On a green juice fast, is an enema recommended and can you explain the mechanics?

15. Does fasting reduce the toxic load on the body?

16. What are the results of liquid nourishment for people with dementia?

17. Should you take drugs (medications) on fasting day?

18. Should you exercise or rest on a fasting day?

DVD – Internal Awareness

Time: 38 mins.

The basics of the digestive/eliminative system and how to detoxify. Instructions in the proper way to use enemas and implants.

1. Why is it important to clear the intestinal tract when you are changing your lifestyle?

2. When is it important to do an enema and why?

3. What is the difference between an enema and a colonic?

4. How and what does an enema do in respect to cleaning the intestines?

5. How much water should you take in and why?

6. What is the importance of an implant and what is the procedure in respect to performing an implant?

7. Why is it important to rub the belly when you are performing an enema and what is the procedure of how you should rub your belly in the areas above the intestines?

8. What is the difference between a molecule of hemoglobin and a molecule of chlorophyll?

9. What is the soup like matter called that is created by the small intestines?

10. What happens to the intestinal tract over the years to create a stoppage by not doing its job and what causes the inflammation?

11. What is a villi?

12. What is an hepatic vein?

13. If you don't have wheatgrass for implants, what else can you use?

Chapter 5
Cleansing

Overview

Cleansing prevents decay and periodically revitalizes our physiology. When the body detoxifies it readily cleans the blood of toxins. It does this mainly by removing impurities from the blood in the liver, where toxins are processed for elimination. The body also eliminates toxins through the kidneys, intestines, lungs, lymph and skin. However, when this system is compromised, impurities aren't properly filtered and every cell in the body is adversely affected. Detoxification is very important because of the presence of excessive toxins in our environment. If you are struggling to lose weight, prone to allergies, or have a weakened immune system, then you truly need to detoxify. But you do not need to spend a fortune with the latest detox solutions. All you need to do is to follow the guidelines of the Hippocrates Health Institute and other top experts mentioned in this chapter who have sorted out the best ways to accomplish thorough cleansing.

You will learn:

- How and when to detox
- Why we rest the organs through fasting
- How to stimulate the liver to drive toxins from the body
- How to promote elimination through the liver, intestines, kidneys and skin
- To avoid the dangers in our toxic environment
- To fuel the body with healthy nutrients

Why Detoxification is So Important and How to Achieve It
by Barry Harris

Every day we put potential toxins into our mouths, breathe them into our lungs, and track them into our homes without ever really knowing where they'll end up—or how much damage they'll do when they get there. In fact, if you could peek inside your body you'd find fire-retardant chemicals, heavy metals, pesticides, plastic particles, and dozens of other residues of modern life. It's time to fight back.[30]

What are the best weapons to use for detoxification? The media offers hundreds of options. How do we determine the best methods? Look to what is most natural, with no added ingredients, scientifically validated, and with no hype.

The methods used by Dr. Ann Wigmore have been scientifically validated on numerous occasions. Using these methods, thousands have recovered from life-threatening illnesses since she founded the Hippocrates Health Institute in 1962.

One well-known example is Eydie Mae Hunsberger, who tells about her remarkable recovery in *How I Conquered Cancer Naturally*. In the 1970s she had recurrent axillary lymph node enlargement following lumpectomy for breast cancer. She declined chemotherapy and instead visited Ann Wigmore in Boston where she learned about wheatgrass juice and a live food diet, to which she attributed her recovery and remission from what appeared to be fatal breast cancer. Brenda Cobb, director and founder of The Living Foods Institute in Atlanta, Georgia, attributes her recovery to reading Eydie's book and practicing Eydie's living-food lifestyle.

Another example is Ellie Oster, heir to the Osterizer Fortune, who made a large philanthropic donation to HHI, after recovering from debilitating arthritis. Dr. Ann's wheatgrass treatment cured her when no other methods were effective.

What are Dr. Ann's unique dietary principles? Why have there been such successful outcomes when these principles are faithfully followed, even in terminal or chronic conditions? And the most important question: Why has following these dietary principles resulted in so many more successful outcomes than in following the dietary principles suggested by the nutritional experts in Western medicine?

We gave a clue to Dr. Ann's success when we presented Roy Walford's scientific data in Chapter 1 which showed that rats doubled their lifespan, when fed optimal nutrition with minimal calories. Here is the solution to the mystery. Whereas the Western model of nutrition only looks at the kind and quantity of nutrients the body needs for optimal health, the live-food regimen also looks at how much waste is generated in supplying these nutrients to the body. Minimal waste is an indication that less work was needed to extract the nutrition from the food, which means an expenditure of minimal calories. Dr. Ann used two colorful examples to illustrate.

1) You can determine the health of a meal, by whether you have to do the dishes. A meal that is optimally health producing, is so clean that not only does it leave the body clean, but this is reflected in the ease one has in cleaning the dishes.

---

[30] http://www.health.com/health/article/0,,20411560,00.html

2) In order to produce the required amount of protein building amino acids from a steak, one would leave a room full of dirty beakers. In order to get the same quantity of protein building amino acids from sprouts, one would leave no evidence of chemical processing.

Digestion uses the biggest expenditure of energy of any bodily processes. Because the living food diet expends so little energy in extracting the nutrition from food, all that energy is freed; it can be used not only to release the toxins from the cells which regenerate the body, but also fills us with vitality. Thus, the living food diet uniquely demonstrates the miraculous and unlimited natural healing potential of the body; this is a potential, which has remained hidden to Western medicine.

Follow the live-food dietary regimen and experience for yourself the two steps to miracles. First, cleanse the body with a diet of optimal nutrition and minimal calories. Practices such as colonics, juicing, liver detox and fasting can assist in this cleansing. Then, after detoxification, commit oneself to a diet that won't again accumulate cellular toxins.

How do we know this detoxification, and thus regeneration of our cells, is actually taking place, and we are not just experiencing a placebo effect created by our imagination? Contrary to the thinking of the whole Western medical paradigm, we know we are getting well, by first getting sick. Sickness can be a sign of actual healing, if it occurs after upgrading one's diet to one that is closer to the ideal of optimal nutrition with minimal calories, and if after a few days, one feels better than before the upgrade.

We can thank naturopath and expert in internal cleansing, Dr. Bernard Jensen, for new insight about this process of detoxification/regeneration. Over a million copies of his *Tissue Cleansing Through Bowel Management with the Ultimate Tissue Cleansing System* have been sold. Dr. Jensen suggested that there is much evidence that feeling sick is only a sign that the body is out of equilibrium, and the sickness only lasts until equilibrium is restored. There are two ways the body can lose equilibrium. One way results from upgrading one's diet, and this eventually leads to bodily regeneration. The other way results from downgrading one's diet, thereby going to a lower level of health, resulting in bodily degeneration. Dr. Jensen used the example of the toxic effect of a first cigarette. Our body is brought out of equilibrium by introducing this new poison into our system. But, after a short time, the body restores equilibrium at a lower level of health, and the cigarette's toxins no longer make us sick. Of course, we have the evidence that Dr. Jensen is onto something, from our own personal experience, when we go up or down health levels by our dietary choices. However, Dr. Jensen's model becomes even more credible, and, thus, powerful, when an iridologist sees the evidence in the iris of our eyes. When a person decides to upgrade their diet and start the process of detoxification, there are marked changes in the iris of the eye. When a person downgrades their dietary choices, the iris of the eye becomes blacker and darker, and, eventually, when a section of the iris, corresponding to a particular organ, becomes completely black, tests consistently show that organ has become cancerous. When cleansing, the iris becomes lighter. Some people's eyes change from dark brown to light green or blue by ridding the body of toxins. This does not imply that brown is sick.

Therefore, we should be very grateful for the unpleasant symptoms[31]we experience while detoxifying:

- Headaches
- lethargy
- temporary muscle aches
- mucus or other discharge
- a coated, pasty tongue
- flu-like symptoms
- irritability
- difficulty sleeping
- weakness
- cravings
- nausea
- constipation
- diarrhea
- gas

Experiencing many of the above symptoms means we are doing the cleansing, which will prevent later serious problems.

Keep your focus on the miraculous transformation your body is experiencing, and though these symptoms will still remain unpleasant, they will not be too difficult to endure.

---

[31] http://www.naturaltherapypages.com.au/article/Detox_Symptoms

What is a Healing Crisis?[32]

When a person resolves to eat higher-quality, more natural foods in order to rid his or her body of accumulated toxins, it's important to set realistic expectations. Cleansing is not a fast process, and many people encounter a range of mental and physical symptoms that do not feel like improvements to their health. These symptoms represent a "healing crisis," according to Dr Stanley Bass, N.D. D.C. Ph.D., but this is one crisis that we should welcome.

When a person improves the quality of food he or she eats, and eliminates toxic substances, the body begins to use these better foods to make new and healthier tissue, unimpeded by toxins that previously hindered healthy tissue production. However, instead of making a person generally feel better right away, this process may cause him or her to feel somewhat unhealthy. According to Bass, a "letdown"(healing crisis) can occur as the body eliminates lower-quality foods and toxic stimulants such as caffeine.

Lower-quality processed foods, which dominate supermarket shelves in most places today, include salt, spices and other ingredients that allow these products to sell for longer, but also tend to be more stimulating than natural, less-processed foods. The withdrawal of this stimulation can produce an effect that is similar to when one stops drinking caffeinated beverages—a perceived decrease in energy.

That run-down feeling is actually a good sign: During this crucial cleansing phase, the body is redirecting energies to vital internal organs and starting its reconstruction process. Therefore, you should rest as much as you can if you feel tired during this phase.

This isn't the end of the story, of course. Very often, if a person sticks with his or her decision to consume higher-quality food, additional symptoms begin to appear: headaches, recurring colds / fever, skin breakouts, frequent urination, bowel sluggishness or diarrhea, and feelings of tiredness and weakness are commonly cited during retracing. The person may feel nervous, irritable, or depressed.

If this sounds like a cruel "reward" for attempting to improve your health, it's important to understand what else is going on. During the first phase of the healing crisis, the body begins to remove the garbage that has accumulated in all tissues over the years. Often, people lose weight as wastes are discarded more rapidly and new tissue is made from new and better foods.

The second phase occurs after the excess waste in the tissues has been removed. During this phase weight remains more or less stable because the amount of waste material being discarded daily is equal to the amount of new, healthier tissue being formed. Very often, when symptoms appear, they are not as severe as in the first phase, nor do they last as long.

In the third phase, much of the waste accumulated over a lifetime has been eliminated—waste that otherwise might have eventually caused pain and disease. That doesn't mean you won't encounter additional symptoms in this phase, but they occur less often and generally don't last. The journey toward cleansing—getting your body to be as healthy as it can be—is just that. The symptoms of a healing crisis should be treated as mile markers, not obstacles, during this journey.

---

[32]"What is a Healing Crisis?" http://www.ionizers.org/healing-crisis.html Accessed Dec. 3, 2012

Detox Experience
by Tom Lindsley

For many years, my passion has been nutrition. In college I majored in economics because I enjoyed it, but over time I realized that much of my free time was spent pursuing my passion for nutrition. When I was not working, I immersed myself in reading nutritional books. I called Bastyr University, the best nutritional school in the country, and asked them for a list of all the books they required for their degree. Once they gave me the list, I read every text. For years, I followed the leading journals in the field; I slowly assimilated the "truths" of nutrition, and realized that some of the smartest people who were implementing studies on vitamins and supplements were those who ate whole foods. These smart people realized that the best nutrition comes not from isolated (processed) vitamins, but from the many co-factors and simplest forms of the nutrients themselves - the "living foods." This is what started my journey into greens and superfoods, as well as the foods that are the actual sources of vitamins and minerals. I also sought out the authors of many books to study and learn more. I first began living the truths I had learned back in 1999 using my own body as a laboratory. My purpose was to discover then demonstrate (to myself and others) how ideal foods can have an ideal effect on the body. I hadn't met anyone else who was living this way and did not know it was representative of the Raw Food movement at the time. I have found over the years that different foods are better for different people. However, an overwhelming majority experience success by adopting green living foods and, more importantly, getting rid of accumulated waste in the body. This final factor (cleansing) is the most significant. That's because no matter your illness, or your ayurvedic body type or your meridian - whatever it is that is out of balance, just about everyone is suffering from some kind of internal toxic buildup.

The Role of Cleansing

What led me to cleansing was my profession - I ran a painting company founded in 1984. After 15 years in the business, I developed hypersensitivities and allergies to almost everything chemical; I couldn't even tolerate hair spray. I knew other old timers in the industry who handled paint that had to retire because of this difficulty, yet with my background on studying nutrition I put two and two together and figured that I may have been exposed to something. Sure enough I was diagnosed with above government levels of lead and mercury poisoning—and who knows what else. Working was out of the question. I had to get a truck to carry the paint separately, and I couldn't be around a job for too long, especially if there was drying paint in the vicinity. This was *severely* hindering. The standard therapy recommended is **chelation therapy**, an intravenous treatment designed to bind heavy metals in the body in order to treat heavy metal toxicity. My body even rejected this approach.

Here is an analogy that helped me understand my situation: If your fish is sick, most likely you have a dirty fish tank, and no amount of clean water pushed into that pond is going to make the fish tank clean. You have to pump out the toxic water, take out all the stones and change the air filter. Once everything is clean the fish will thrive. The same is true with all the cells swimming in our body. We each need to focus on the elimination and cleansing process even more than we focus on what we put into our bodies. Almost nobody thinks this way (unless you meet someone older whose health just glows). Few people focus on doing what is necessary to make the body clean. To really shift your body's health paradigm, I discovered (by experience) that what got rid of my hypersensitivities and illnesses in general, was cleaning out all of the organs of the body one by one. Our body is a giant filter, we spend over 50 percent of our energy every day assimilating, digesting and eliminating all of the food that we eat. With half the energy spent digesting and assimilating food, and exercising our bodies and brains, where is the energy left to rid our bodies of the toxins and the things we shouldn't have eaten? Juicing and blenders will free the body of the work digesting so that it has energy to cleanse and get heal.

So I am going to challenge your thinking. Instead of looking what is in your food, ask yourself whether each item of food we eat aids your elimination. How much energy does it take for you to digest and assimilate this food? When I look at when I eat, I look at how young the plant is; a sprout or a plant before it germinates (reproduces) has the most life force. I look at the enzymes and the life in it and what is going to be better for me. Food with more water content and nutrition that is alive will give my body the energy it needs to eliminate the things the elements it doesn't need. This is we lighten our load and get unlimited energy!! Our body is a giant filter. If something that is dead, like a cookie, I know when I eat it, it is going to take a lot of my body's energy and mineral and living water reserves to eliminate, or it's going to stay on my waist or thighs till I start eating foods and doing practices that give my body excess energy to eliminate and rebuild.

An Organ at a Time

The daily routines that are most essential in this lifestyle is deep breathing (see other article), skin brushing, and shaking/rebounding. These big three, and eating live foods, will keep your body cleaning more than toxifying. Once you have the basics down and are also eating a cleansing diet, and are ready for some serious progress and change, then it's time to clean the fish tank!

 I came from a terrible diet, "The Captain-King-Captain meal plan", Captain Crunch for breakfast, Burger King for lunch and Captain Morgan for dinner. OK, not quite that bad, but close. Maybe I had pizza for lunch. When I decided to walk my walk, it was a big change, and physically challenging, and did not happen right away. My food change alone gave me more energy and cleaned up a lot of symptoms. But to completely change my hypersensitivities and most health concerns…involved cleansing, with specific focus on the organs.

With cleansing I recommend starting from the bottom up. The first organ to address in a deep-body cleanse is the colon. I have tried most cleanses, and the best and most difficult cleanse I have tried worked the best for me. It is called the "Arise and Shine" cleanse which includes bentonite, psyllium seed, and other herbs which release toxins from your intestines. The book that I recommend is *Cleanse and Purify Thyself* by Richard Anderson who is also the designer of the cleanse. This book will help change your perspective and open up your eyes to how important it is to cleanse.

As I was doing this month long cleanse and following all the guidelines, about week three of the cleanse - which is the intense phase - I felt a big chunk come off from the inside of my small intestines, and I felt like a part of me left, yet I felt more whole. I remember that I looked at it in the toilet and it looked like a piece of that hard black rubbery stuff, similar to a car tire that you hear about. I couldn't believe that came out of my small intestines. I could see the fine line that the food had to pass through as it went through my small intestines and the food could barely touch the wall of my intestines and get a chance to absorb, before it went inside the rubber gunk again and out the other side. So I realized my food had traveled through caked rubbery walls and barely touched the walls of my intestines where nutrients are supposed to be absorbed.

I firmly believe now that it is our small intestines where most of our health lies. Each part of our small intestines absorbs different nutrients that help different parts of our bodies. For me, one of those parts was obviously my hypersensitivity, and ability to absorb nutrients, because at the end of the cleanse, we are supposed to eat an apple to start getting back to solid food.

Evidence of Change: Apple Example

Now apples was one of the first foods to which I had become allergic. I would just touch it to my lip and it would swell and itch. During this cleanse, I followed everything to the letter, so I was not going to stop now. I cut the apple up, I touched it to my lip and waited a few minutes. And nothing happened! I repeated and no hypersensitive reaction or itching or swelling occurred. I waited and licked the apple, and still no reaction. I decided to bite the apple, and swallow a tiny piece and still I had no reactions and even waited a couple of hours. Then I proceeded to relish my first apple in years - and it was the best apple I have ever tasted. I not only had removed my allergy to apples from doing this cleanse - most of my hypersensitivities were gone! The next thing I knew, I was at the paint store and I had no problems. I had no problems to everything that I was sensitive to before. This amazing recovery lasted about a year before I started getting small little bits of sensitivity back, so I did the colon cleanse again. This next time no symptoms for two years, then some reactions came back again, so I did the colon cleanse again, and no symptoms for four years and then none since. My good health lasted twice as long each time, along with keeping up my good diet. That was the first step and that was the most life-changing thing that I have done. Doing the master cleanse for the whole month and committing to it, even though many people thought I was crazy, was the best thing I have ever done for my health. I did it! I even continued to exercise for the first two weeks. With the amount of burden taken off my body, I felt transformed. Now when I eat something bad, it moves right out of my system, and I don't have to sit around feeling sluggish for three days. I have leeway and my body gets rid of things quickly and assimilates the good things that I do eat. If I eat well for a few days, I need less and less food to function, I can skip a meal or two, and just keep going. My new quote is, "The intestines are to your health, what the spine is to your spirit."

Variety of Method

Of course there are many other intestinal and colon cleanses on the market. There is one called oxyzone, which oxygenates the colon and cleans it out quickly. That seems one of the easiest and still somewhat effective. It basically brings a lot of oxygen to your intestines. Yet it is the 22 feet of small intestine before the colon where the life changing things happen. The psyllium seed and bentonite mixture is tremendously alkaline and draws a lot of the acidic toxins out of your body. The cleanse then alternates the bentonite with the toxin releasing herbs which is a powerful combination. The bentonite pushes the entire waste out and the herbs help to release the toxins from the walls of your intestines. This is a back and forth process of washing your intestines. It worked extremely well for me although I accept it is not for everybody.

You will know when you are doing a deep cleanse because it will start when you see mucus coming out. The mucus comes out white. Mucus protects your intestines from all of the acidic food that we eat, and it hardens over time. It does a good job of protecting our intestines, yet our intestines are supposed to grab all of the healthy nutrients from the food that we should be eating.

126

When you see mucus in the bowel movement you know you are detoxing. It is a good sign and the detoxification will further over time.

Colonics and acidophilus at the same time are recommended. Again, we start at the bottom first because it is not a pleasant experience to have toxic things released further up your system like a gallstone and then getting reabsorbed by slow moving lower intestines. You want the lower intestines to be cleaned and moving first so that as more toxic waste comes out, it doesn't get stopped, and reabsorbed. It is a good idea to have your kidneys moving as well, because if there is a block, you have another way to eliminate waste quickly with urination.

Next Step: Kidneys

The second step when cleansing following the bottom up approach is the kidneys. So before the liver cleanse REMEMBER, you have to cleanse the kidneys. Both cleanses are in another book I recommend *The Amazing Gall Bladder and Liver Cleanse* by Andreas Moritz. Cleansing the kidneys is done with a tea for which I had to gather ingredients. One drinks this tea for about six weeks. For me, I did not notice much difference except for increasing or easing urine flow slightly.

Liver

Step three is cleansing the liver. As mentioned before I highly recommend, *The Amazing Liver Cleanse* by Andreas Moritz. If you have liver stones, kidney stones, or gallstones, you can let your body heal yourself. Why wait and have surgery later? Clean yourself now! Your insides will be so clean you'll feel like whistling Dixie! During the liver cleanse I saw green and white hard matter coming out that is old stones, also some white powder which I understood to be broken up old stones. The idea is to soften the stones for a week by drinking a lot of apple juice, which has malic acid. By following the instructions to the letter, we help prevent cleansing side effects, because the stones that release are very toxic and reabsorbing them in the intestines can make you VERY sick.

Some people may need to do this with the help of a professional. It is set up in a specific way for a reason. Basically the apple juice softens the stones, at the same time giving the liver a break for an entire week. After the week in one night the ports in the gallbladder are widened to release stones by drinking the Epsom salts, then stimulating the liver to work hard by drinking down an olive oil, lemon and grapefruit juice mixture to all of a sudden get your liver contracting, you start seeing everything come out, and surprise, surprise, surprise! I started with about 14 or 15 cleanses once a month until nothing came out. At this time, I simply need to cleanse once a year. What a relief for my system. Each time some stones come out. In the third, fourth, and fifth times, the biggest things came out, but after that it calmed down.

If I did a liver cleanse without a colon cleanse first, I could have been passing one of the most toxic things in my body, and I could've reabsorbed that back into my system, and felt extremely sick. Having a liver cleanse after a colon cleanse is such a gift to your body and health. You don't want this toxicity in your system any more than it should be. If you clean your liver, the last thing you want is to have gallstones sitting in your intestines, even for a day. This would cause you to feel really sick because the toxins are being reabsorbed into the body. The one hallmark principle to remember is that you must cleanse from the bottom up.

Oftentimes, surprising symptoms may arise that pertain to your particular body system. For instance, I had a liver spot, and every time following one of my liver cleanses it would get lighter, yet during the day of the cleanse it would get really dark. Then it would get lighter after more cleansing. I would gauge my cleanses by the liver spot, such that if it became dark, I knew it was time for a cleanse. After a few cleanses it finally went away. This is not mentioned in literature, but if you do these cleanses, these kinds of things do happen. On an emotional note, the liver is where anger is stored. After a few cleanses, my family and I realized a pattern, that I would be irritable and angry the day of the cleanse. My reflections on my emotional nature have told me that I have removed much of my body's stored anger through these liver cleanses. Though humbly I do say I have a long way to go, to rid myself of the emotional patterns and beliefs that caused the anger in the first place. However, that is a subject for another article.

Pancreas / Spleen

After the liver, you clean the pancreas / spleen, which are rebuilt by taking enzymes and probiotics. Eating live foods makes the pancreas better. I had a friend who almost died on the operating table. He lost seven-eighths of his pancreas; he felt like the surgeons removed all the darkness in his life and the one-eighth of his pancreas remaining left him with abundant joy. He had surgically removed the darkness from his system and had an emotional transformation. I believe the pancreas is tied to joy, and that we get joy from fresh green foods that are the color of the heart chakra. We feel more joy as the enzymes in live food give the pancreas a chance to express itself. I am just putting it out there that the pancreas and healthy foods that are alive can actually have an effect on our emotions. A good book on this is *Heal Your Body* by Louise Hay. It lists every ailment, and every emotional connection that has to do with each ailment. For example, when you hear about people with Lyme disease, look at their lifestyle, look at what kind of person they are, look at the similarities between each person with Lyme disease and you will start to notice emotional similarities.

A Lesson in Emotions

I see every challenge in life as an opportunity, to look at ourselves, to look at our emotions, to look at what we face and what is our life lesson. My philosophy is everything is out there to teach us something. This is the way that I look at it, and it has been a tremendous learning experience in emotional health, my psyche, and my patterns. It gets me to face my emotions when I am up against a physical challenge. I suggest trying something different yourselves and experimenting with your own bodies by giving them what you believe is ideal for sustenance, and for living, and removing the burden of what you have done to it.

Lungs and Lymph

Most everyone knows that the largest eliminative organ is the skin. Yet the lungs can eliminate more than any other organ. The organ with the most surface area if you open it up and lay it out (as much as two football fields) are the lungs. After cleansing the pancreas and spleen, the next up are the lungs. You breathe in and out 35 pounds of oxygen and carbon dioxide a day. The lungs are working 24 hours a day. The first thing a runner starts doing is breathing heavy as he builds up lactic acid from his exertion. Deep breathing alone can do more for detoxing the whole body than anything else in the world. The lungs are how we get rid of most of our toxins. As we sleep we go into deep relaxed breathing. Imagine the cleansing done when you breathe as deeply as a runner without the physical exercise. The body quickly cleanses the toxins in the system and then starts on our emotions. I realized that I had blockages in my lungs, because I could not do deep breathing on my own without doing physical exercise. I researched and found the best breath-worker in New England and did over 10 one-on-one sessions where I was coached to stay focused, do deep breathing, and not falsely shut down. What happened was that a lot of emotions came out. A lot of things that I was not willing to face were there, causing me to shut down and have shallow breathing. It took me 13 sessions, and I was more stuck than most. It took me a long time to break through because of my stubborn personality. I even did a breath retreat for three days where I also fasted, but I was finally able to break through these blocks. Now whenever I feel stressed or tense, I do deep breath work and it all just melts away. I highly urge you to do one-on-one coaching sessions. Personally, I feel these are much better than group sessions. If an individual is stuck, you need to be coached through it individually until your body gets rid of the toxin/stored emotion - whether that is emotional or biologically based. One needs to eliminate the blockage.

Skin Brushing

The last cleanse, and an important daily ritual, is skin brushing. A friend of mine came to visit me from the Philippines, but she had to return because her 92-year-old mom became very ill. The only thing that she knew was skin brushing, which was passed down in the family. All she did was skin brush her mother morning, noon and night. This was the only change in lifestyle her mother underwent, and after three months, her mother was out of her wheel chair and walking, and she is still alive at 102 years of age. You work your way up from the bottoms of your feet in strokes toward the heart. One passes over the stomach in a long clockwise motion that covers the large intestines. To finish skin brushing, a few taps/knocks on your chest stimulate the thymus gland. Do it before your shower. Cleaning the lymph and getting the toxins out of the tissues is that important.

Cleansing every day is just as important as what you put into your body. You have to help the body eliminate. It is more important to eliminate than to ingest. Eliminating is the fastest and easiest way to heal. If you do the skin brushing, you will also notice cellulite beginning to disappear. Alternating between a hot and cold shower every 30 seconds is another way of eliminating.

The lymph system is twice as large as the blood system in the human body. It does not have a pump like the blood does with the heart. The lymph system needs movement to function. Every single lymph node in your body is a valve that only eliminates through movement. Another easy way to eliminate is using the rebounder or non-impact shaking up and down from four to 30 minutes. Try it and experience the energy or elimination in your system right afterwards!

With gravity, when you go up and down, every single lymph valve in your whole body opens and closes at once. This effect is similar to that of running, however, it avoids the impact. There is an ashram in Thailand where the people just shake up and down for two hours, three times perday, to clear many stuck emotional patterns. This clearly illustrates how the mind, body, and emotions are intricately connected.

First stage of illness

What are all of the first stages illnesses? All beginning illness or disease in our bodies is where it is stopped up or blocked, and our body starts to eliminate by sweating, crying, boils, fever, vomit, and increased evacuations. The idea is to recognize what our own body needs and unstop the blockages and encourage the elimination of the acidic waste. The second stage of illness or disease is the body does not eliminate the toxins fast enough so it starts to store toxins as fat, or encapsulate the toxins into tumors etc.

A widening circle of change

I have learned that the easiest way to change someone else is by changing yourself, not by pushing being healthy on anyone – they will just resist. Lead yourself, then sooner or later they notice and start to ask questions. My mother saw the changes and saw me get over my issues, and then she knew it was possible to change. The questions started to flow – yet busy as I was at the time, I was not able to answer all of her questions and her desire increased. She went to Hippocrates to fully embrace the lifestyle. My mother got over her debilitating arthritis and food cravings and is now on an upwards spiral.

We clean our physical bodies from what we take in from our mouths. Yet, "the body eats from all its senses," says Mata Amritanandamayi. We have to be careful what poisons/lotions we put on our skin, the type of TV/radio we expose ourselves to and the people we listen to and what we think and say. Having a break from all that assails us through our eyes and ears is invaluable. As my personal saying goes, "Meditate now or medicate later."

A very important point is to not beat yourself or anyone else up. You are doing just as much damage to your psyche if you get angry or really stress yourself out by not giving yourself something you want. You may as well just eat it. I feel we receive more damage by the stress of beating ourselves up, than if you just eat the cookie. I don't force my children to eat or not eat. If your kids are at a birthday party and they want cake, let them have cake. Instead of saying no, just get them thinking. If they don't feel well, ask them what they ate, oh cake? I guess that doesn't agree with you. Or, if they have an upset stomach, I say, "Oh you ate dairy?" I guess we should try something other than that. Get people thinking of alternative positive language instead of saying no.

My daughter, Jane, was raised on green soup. Her mother said to me, "You will never get her to eat that stuff" and the next thing we knew, she was eating the green soup. The first tantrum she had was because she did not have her green soup. We thought it was so funny she was upset because she could not have her spinach! We laughed at her tantrum. This resulted in Jane never throwing a tantrum again!

Why would you spend hard earned money on something that is not good for you, and that will cause you disease? If there is something and it is free, and you are struggling over to have it, it is ok to eat it rather than to stress out over it. For my children, I don't force them to do anything. Examples of what I pack for their lunch are plums, big organic grapes, apples, cherry tomatoes, sunflower sprouts, carrots, and hummus. I try to make a pate every Sunday from nuts and seeds, and it will last for a week. You can put them on crackers or Ezekiel bread.

Levels of Change

Here are four levels of our attitude and how we take care of ourselves:

Level 4:   things that are bad for you, you don't enjoy and hurt you and everyone else, self-mutilation, fighting, alcohol addiction, drug addiction, smoking, etc.

Level 3:   Things that are bad for you but you enjoy them, cigarettes, alcohol, etc.

Level 2: Things that are good for you but you don't enjoy them: colon cleanse, exercise, eating healthy, brushing your teeth, etc.

Level 1: Things that you like to do that are good for you and everyone else: Eating good food, colonics, exercise, brushing your teeth etc.

One might ask - what is the key to a life of joy and wholeness? By changing our attitude, we take our level two experiences and change them to a level one experience.

Detoxing Through Breathwork
by Rosana Gijsen

The most effective mode for the body to detox is through Breathwork. About 70 percent of the body's waste products are eliminated through the lungs, 30 percent through the urine, feces, and skin. Breathwork or conscious breathing is a multiform "healing modality" characterized by specialized breathing. Its purported design is to effect physical, emotional, and spiritual change. Breathwork allegedly: (a) can dissolve "limiting programs" that are "stored" in the mind and body; and (b) increases one's ability to handle "more energy." Anyone can do it with the help of books or with an experienced Breathworker. Most people learn it in ten or more individual breathing sessions. What happens in these ten sessions is magical and amazing for most people. Breathwork is the secret to the health of the soul, as well as the body and the Emotional Mind.

The first goal of Breathwork is to breathe Energy as well as air. The breathing teacher guides the breathing rhythm. After a few minutes of a guided breathing rhythm, the Divine Energy begins to flow in the body. It typically flows stronger and stronger until it peaks, then this flow of Divine Energy recedes naturally until a new balanced Energy Body is achieved and the student feels very peaceful, relaxed, and energized. We usually feel clean inside as well as outside after an Energy cycle in one to two hours. This is a unique combination—relaxed and energized.

In the middle of the session, some people may have many physical sensations and feel fearful. When fear is strong enough, it may cause *tetany*, which is a medical term referring to tightness, or cramps – usually in the extremities, such as hands, lips, feet, and legs. Continued gentle breathing automatically induces relaxation, as tension and tightness disappear. When people experience *tetany* or similar sensations, they should learn to relax and let go and trust life for such symptoms and sensations are always temporary. Once the relaxed connected breathing rhythm is mastered, the symptoms no longer occur. It is important throughout the first 10 sessions to get past the physiological sensations and emotional drama. Breathwork is not about drama or therapy. Rather, it is about learning conscious Energy breathing.

The second goal is to actually notice how we are breathing and to learn how to breathe connectedly, gently, consciously, and intuitively in a way that activates our divine Energy and cleans our Energy body.

The third goal is to have breathing release, which often means reliving the moment of our first breath at birth and releasing the fear and trauma that has been restricting our breathing ability ever since. Releasing this birth trauma memory may or may not occur during the first ten breathing sessions.

The fourth goal, after the first ten guided breathing sessions, is to be able to do the breathing rhythm for an hour without supervision. This goal involves mastering the ability of breathing Energy as well as air. This gives us a new level of spiritual self-sufficiency and a very practical and powerful tool for self-healing. We can use it every day or as often as we like.

Benefits of Breathing
by Rosana Gijsen

Poor Breathing

Inefficient breathing is often marked by tension in one's breathing mechanism. One sign of this may be a contracted belly upon one's inhale. Other signs include forced or inhibited breathing, controlled breathing using neck, head, or back muscles, in a way that is not directly connected to the breathing mechanism of the lungs and diaphragm. There is also tendency under stress to hyperventilate. Hyperventilation involves over-breathing, which reduces the carbon dioxide balance and restricts the arteries to the brain. This causes a shortage of oxygen and signals the sympathetic nervous system to prepare one for flight. Hyperventilation, or improper breathing, can be a response to fear or stress.

Fried (1990) estimates that 60 percent of all the emergency ambulance transport in the United States involves hyperventilation or other breath related disorders. Another study indicates that 10 to 25 percent of the American population suffers from breath related illness every year. Much of this is related to a poorly functioning diaphragm, which will lead to lowered metabolism and decreased vitality and wellbeing. Training of the breath is critical to prevention and recovery of the effects of poor breathing. Other studies indicate that everyone can benefit from breath training, especially people who never had any.

Effects of Poor Breathing

Poor Breathing reduces the efficiency of one's lungs and thus the available oxygen. One must take two to four breaths to compensate. This increases the individual's energy expenditure and heart rate and retards venous flow and discharge of metabolic wastes from the cells to the kidneys and lungs before these wastes can do harm. About 70 percent of the body's waste products are eliminated through the lungs, 30 percent through the urine, feces, and skin. Thus, poor breathing habits contribute to any and all forms of illness.

Good Breathing

Breathing can be trained such that the range the diaphragm contracts can be doubled or tripled thus increasing the capacity of air 250 to 300 milliliter/mm in six to twelve months (Lewis, 1997). With good breathing the chest muscle expands the rib cage out and up slightly and the belly expands during inhale. The increased mobility diaphragm massages the stomach, liver, pancreas, intestines, kidneys, and promotes intestinal movement, blood lymph flow and the absorption of nutrients. Good breathing supports a more consistently healthy Life.

Breathe Training/Sessions

The breath can be trained with "effortless effort," using the proper capacity of our breathing ability. Using direct biofeedback technology, or a good Breathwork teacher, we can be assisted to find our comfort zone. The comfort of inhalation is proportional to our readiness and ability to let go and to trust. Breath training builds energy and endurance, at the same time promoting emotional equilibrium, physical healing and graceful aging. It is also helpful in pain management, mental concentration, and physical performance in sports and has been linked to psycho-spiritual transformation. It raises IQ.

The effect of breath training can be experienced almost immediately and is self-reinforcing. It is pleasurable to learn positive breathing habits and to live greater vitality and balance. It involves simple exercises and completed Energy Cycles.

When we are educated about the significance of our breathing mechanism and decide to breathe properly, we can positively affect our entire health – physically, mentally, and emotionally. The breath is also a key that opens the gateway to the Temple of our spiritual Self.

For information on workshops and individual training sessions please contact:

Rosana Gijsen

Email: soulbreathe@yahoo.com

Mobile: 617-230-9303

What in the World are They Spraying? An Introduction to Chemtrails
by Lorraine Hurley (August 2012)

The official definition for "chemtrails" is given in Section 7, "Definitions" of House Resolution 2977, a bill introduced in the United States' Congress on October 2, 2001 as an "exotic weapons system".

Chemtrails should not be confused with the normal contrails that jets leave behind them as they fly high in the sky. Contrails are simply visible trails of water droplets or ice crystals that disappear rather quickly, whereas chemtrails left by jet airplanes do not disappear. Chemtrails can linger in the sky for many hours. Oftentimes jets crisscross the sky with chemtrails that eventually spread out, creating a haze that can partially block the sun. When this occurs one can observe actual weather changes brought about by chemtrails

Chemtrails have been shown to contain chemical toxins such as aluminum and barium compounds as well as biological materials, such as red blood cells, bacteria, etc. (Visit http://www.carnicom.com/contrails.htm to view evidence.) Some of the symptoms that people often report from chemtrails are a metallic taste, sinus problems, nose bleeds, hacking cough, asthma symptoms, flu-like symptoms, headaches, dizziness, tiredness, memory problems, difficulty thinking, depression, irritability, meningitis-type symptoms, dry skin, rashes, gastrointestinal stress, and diarrhea.[33]

The Guardian, after reporting "potential" geo-engineering projects for a while now, with an entire section devoted to it on their online newspaper last week (2012/8/5) published a map of weather modification programs actually underway. … They report active programs to alter precipitation and regulate solar exposure. This is despite no public debate. Yet Parliament has spoken on the topic, producing policy documents on the regulation of geo-engineering. That document states a "need" for geo-engineering alongside a curious claim that government should not encourage debate on the topic for fear that they would be seen as supporting it, in light of likely public opposition.

Millions of tons of these toxins have been sprayed into our skies since 1995. Each and every one of them does substantial harm to human, animal and plant physiology.

To begin this process of truth discovery for yourself you can simply walk outside and look up. You will one day notice heavy, thick crisscrossing lines emitted from jets that persist, fan out and whiten the sky. Up until recently this was obvious on a daily basis. In the past few months (more than likely due to increasing public awareness) they are spraying more at night and they are using Haarp technology to disperse and move the trails into artificial cloud formations.

Even if at first you don't observe obvious and copious lines from one horizon to the other, you will begin to notice how white our sky has become, how the blue dome of our planet has paled to the faintest of hues and how clouds that are non-descript and unnatural in appearance are the norm. If you do this daily, look up that is, you will eventually see what a growing number of people on this planet see each and every day. There are a multitude of photos and videos avail-

---

[33] http://www.healthfreedom.info/HR%202977.htm

able on line to help you identify what you are seeing, how long this has been happening and the extent of the consequences.

The unofficial official version of this program (both the government and military deny this is on-going publicly but discuss it in documents and articles available to the public—how is that for insanity?) is that it is being done in our own best interests, to mitigate the effects of global warning and to vaccinate the population against biological warfare. Personnel in the armed forces have come forth saying that when they questioned their superiors about the obvious spraying it wasn't denied but was represented as a program of mass vaccination. Further, what too few citizens of the US realize is that it is perfectly legal for our government to spray us with intoxicants and biologicals! (Public Law 105-85 & HR-2977 allow the spraying of chemical and biological agents upon the American populace.)

Geo-engineering is presently being discussed and presented at scientific conferences around the world as a POTENTIAL program for climate control, not as an on-going assault against the planet with out the permission or consent of the people. There are many that have attempted to force a public discussion and acknowledgement from our representative government. Several US governmental officials and representatives deny knowledge of this program when they are confronted on film in the documentary, *What In the World Are They Spraying*? (Available in its entirety on you-tube). And yet Congress has appropriated billions of dollars towards this program and the budget appropriations are available for public viewing!

At the time of this writing there are 27 farming counties in the USA that have been declared disasters due to drought. This will lead to increased food prices and decreased food surplus for an already starving third world. There were 3800 temperature records set this past year. There has been an exponential increase in severe weather and natural disasters such as tornadoes, flooding, hurricanes, earthquakes and tsunamis costing thousands of lives and billions of dollars in damages. This all coincides with the acceleration of geo-engineering that has taken place over the past two decades. We don't hear about this in the mainstream media because the mainstream media is controlled by six multi-national corporations. These multi-national corporations reap grotesque profits from human suffering and sickness.

Consider this; Monsanto has applied for patents for drought resistant seeds, aluminum resistant seeds and now has bullied the organic food industry into accepting GMO's as a fact of life (http://foodfreedom.wordpress.com/2011/01/27/organic-elite-surrenders-to-monsanto/).

To further explore the issues of genetic engineering and for an excellent expose on the full extent of the psychosis that has overrun those in power see http://www.youtube.com/watch?v=pbnTkCTz5VI.

Once you begin to connect dots you will understand the dire necessity of doing all you can to wake up the rest of the world to what is happening and to foster your own locus of personal responsibility in response. You will also then be equipped to take measures to protect yourselves and loved ones from succumbing to the toxic assault falling from our once beautiful blue sky(discussed in an addendum to this article).

Our challenge is to draw out courage from within when standing in truth while simultaneously seeking with all our hearts to grow our awareness of the beauty and joy of living that are abundant at the eye of the storm. We do this through mediation, prayer, breath work and other spiritual work that awakens us to the realization that we are never separated from Source or one another. We are individual cells in the body of life; interconnected, interdependent.

Just as we can choose to accept a disease diagnosis and do nothing to change or we can choose to change the way we live and realize freedom from disease, we can also choose to either accept spiritual sickness in the world or not. Either we believe we are powerless to change our collective condition or we can locate a locus of control within our own lives and, understanding our inter-relatedness, know that we are aiding the planet as we strive to live an empowered personal life.

There's Something in the Air... *But do we want it there?*
by Phyllis Traver, www.yoursafeandsoundhome.com

Did you know the Environmental Protection Agency considers indoor pollution, which is linked to a variety of allergies, ailments, and sleeping disorders, to be among our top five health risks?

New building materials, systems, finishes, and furnishings increasingly contain synthetic and chemical components. As we tighten our buildings to minimize energy costs, these components can pollute indoor climates.

So what can we do to clean the air in our homes? Here are a few suggestions.

Regulate the Humidity

Many airborne organisms, such as bacteria, viruses, mold, and dust mites, are minimized when the humidity level is near 50 percent. During winter our heating systems generate dry air, often with humidity levels less than 30 percent; while summer indoor humidity levels can exceed 70 percent. Exposure to airborne irritants becomes more likely as humidity deviates from the optimal 45-50 percent level.

Use vents in bathroom, kitchens, and laundries to control moisture. Place house plants throughout your home to help balance humidity. Open windows or use humidifiers or mechanical air exchangers to increase humidity during winter months. Dehumidifiers are helpful in summer. Some building materials, such as unsealed wood floors, unglazed tile, and clay plaster walls, naturally regulate humidity by absorbing and releasing moisture.

Reduce AirBorne Particles

Air typically contains millions of particles, most of which you cannot see. Sources include grease, gases, animal dander, pesticides, pollen, carpet fibers, inks, and others. These irritants, some toxic, can be minimized with a few maintenance measures. If you have a forced-air heating or cooling system, use a strong particle filter and replace it regularly. Clean with a HEPA vacuum to minimize exhaust of the unhealthy smaller particles. Avoid wall-to-wall carpet and synthetic and plastic furnishings. They create static electricity that causes irritating particles to remain suspended in the air. If building or remodeling, install vapor-permeable walls to allow natural air filtering.

Minimize Volatile Chemicals

Many common household products, materials, and furnishings contain chemicals that release gas ("VOCs" or volatile organic compounds) at room temperature. Some common VOC sources are synthetic carpets and pads, adhesives, treated fabrics, cleaning supplies, dryer sheets, copiers & printers, paints and solvents, perfumes, air fresheners, and pesticides. Many VOCs are linked to discomforts such as headaches, respiratory ailments, lack of concentration, and dizziness. They also may be associated with chronic serious illnesses. Learn to identify VOCs and minimize their use. Stow questionable products away from living areas. Fully ventilate while cleaning and during renovation periods.

Simply stated, whatever the source of pollution, indoor air typically benefits by an influx of outside air. Consider opening the windows and ventilating your home as much as possible.

Biological Effects of Electromagnetic Radiation
by Phyllis Traver

All life forms are based on electromagnetic energy. Every cell, for example, is electrically charged in a polarized fashion so that nutrients can be delivered across ion channels. There is an all-pervading, fundamental frequency at about 10Hz (a very slow wave) which can be found in humans and in the earth. Our bodies are inseparably linked with the electromagnetic conditions of the outer environment.

Communication in the body is transmitted via electrical current driven by pulsed signals from the heart and brain, and through a semi-conductive, or electronic, fibrous membrane called the cyto-skeleton. Semi-conductors are highly influenced by external electromagnetic fields.

Alternating electric fields created by electrical power lines and internal home wiring, exert forces that result in reversal, or depolarization, and induction of body currents. The body will attempt to become in tune to the higher frequency, which disrupts the body's communication and cell division.

Alternating magnetic fields cause eddy currents and nerve, bone and muscle stimulation. Specific wiring configurations in the home electrical system, and many modern electronic appliances, can create strong magnetic fields.

Higher level frequencies, such as pulsed radio frequencies used in the cellular phone industry, can result in cell membrane dysfunction: cell membranes close to protect the cell, interrupting intercellular communication, nutrient intake, and waste disposal. If membranes are closed for too long, the cell may die, releasing free radicals, or mutate with a closed membrane.

Individuals vary greatly as to their sensitivity to electromagnetic stressors. Plants, animals, and humans that are generally healthy, and/or have a skin connection to the earth, tend to have strong electromagnetic fields of their own, and are less likely to be disturbed. If the extent of the external fields is such that it impairs the central nervous system, endocrine, or immune system, it could subsequently lead to the initiation or promotion of many disorders, especially chronic conditions.

Problems attributed to electromagnetic hypersensitivity are:
1. difficulties in concentration
2. dizziness
3. headaches& nausea
4. aches in muscles and joints
5. cardiac palpitations
6. memory loss
7. coordination problems
8. sleep disorders
9. childhood leukemia
10. Cancer
11. Multiple sclerosis
12. Parkinson's,
13. Alzheimers
14. autism
15. behavioral disorders

16. chronic fatigue

17. fibromyalgia

Most people cannot sense directly the presence of electromagnetic fields, and so it is necessary to measure them with suitable equipment. Remediation may be as easy as distancing oneself from the source or removing the source. It may require the correction of wiring errors, or rerouting of particular circuits. There are many simple solutions that can be employed once the source of the offending field is identified.

Written by Phyllis Traver
Owner, Safe & Sound Home LLC
Sourced from IBE materials

That New Car Smell[34]
by Jeff Plotkin

What's your favorite part about getting a new car? Is it the fact that you have a new toy? Something new to play with? Could it be the change in lifestyle? Or maybe the new car smell? If you answered yes to the last question, then keep reading.

Every new car comes with that smell that we all know and love, as we have deemed it "the new car smell." However, what exactly is that smell and what chemicals go into it? The new car smell contains many volatile chemicals, including benzene, cycohexanone, and styrene which are all possible carcinogens! The plastics and textiles in car's inside are made from a number of dangerous chemicals, including antimony, bromine, chlorine, and lead. Hence, the driver and the passengers are exposed to these dangerous matters by simply inhaling inside the car, but to make matters even worse (no pun intended) the sun's heat can further increase the level of these chemicals which in turn would make them even more dangerous to one's health. According to a CNN article, when driving a new car, you are exposed to harmful chemicals at every square millimeter of your newest purchase. So then you might ask, if the manufacturer knows about this harmful smell, why they spray the car with it. To answer your question, they don't spray anything. The new car smell comes together from a bunch of glues that are used to hold the car together in the first place. The smell can linger for about 6 months after the manufacturing of the car and continue to do damage. It is best to air out the car as best as possible during those first 6 months, especially in the summer time.

---

[34] http://autos.aol.comarticle/toxic-car-interiors/

Cell Phone, Biochips and TriMeters[35]
by Jeff Plotkin

Throughout the past few years, the dangers of cell phone use have been well documented. But, besides the obvious talking and driving or even texting while driving, there is another danger that is less popular to talk about. Did you know that up to 60 percent of the total radiation emitted from a cell phone can go towards the user's head and body? Cell phones often transmit between 800 MHz and 1,990 MHz over a period of a phone call; those numbers closely resemble the frequency transmitted from a working microwave! A cell phone is designed to transmit radio waves in all directions, because a station could be anywhere. Now imagine that these waves are going into your body, but more importantly to your head and brain, where the cells can absorb up to 80 percent of the frequency. The radio waves that are absorbed can cause impairment, damage, and can even kill your DNA, which could then result in cancer. However, as technology is constantly evolving, so is the cell phone. Studies have shown that the newer phones tend to emit less harmful radiation, and they emit the same amount throughout the phone call and day. If you're using an older phone, then you might be out of luck. Reports have proved that the older the phone, the more radiation is emitted throughout a phone call. So, then you might say that you have a blue tooth, which is 10 times better, right? Wrong! A cordless, blue tooth device works by emitting all sorts of radiation which can be up to 6 times stronger than given off by a cell phone! So then, the best hands-free device is one that has a cord, and connects straight to your phone. That way, about 3 times less radiation is emitted to your body. The FDA and FCC have also said that it's just better to use a home phone, which gives off less radiation. However, if you absolutely need to use that cell phone, just to keep the conversation short. So hang up your phone and take a walk and do something healthy!

Concerned about the effects of Cell phone Radiation on your health?[36]
Well, here's good news...

BIOPRO's *Patented* MRET-Shield technology has been proven-—in TEST after test—to neutralize the dangers of EMR (Electromagnetic Radiation) from cell phones & other devices—*Quick Facts* about the revolutionary BIOPRO Cell Chip:

* Neutralizes harmful effects of EMR (electromagnetic radiation)
* Works effectively on cell phones, Bluetooth and PDAs
* Powerful proprietary patented MRET-Shield technology combined with proprietary subtle physics technology (ERT)
* MRET-Shield technology protected by U.S. Patent No.6,369,399 B1
* Substantiated by decades of research and testing in leading labs and universities

Gaussmeter for Measuring EMF Radiation

---

[35] http://www.cancer.gov/cancertopics/factsheet/RISK/cellphones

[36] http://www.cellphone-health.com

The TriField® Meter is as AC gaussmeter, electric field meter, RF field strength meter combined in one electromagnetic instrument. An excellent tool for those concerned about EMF radiation.

The 60 htz TriField Gaussmeter for use in North America and other countries using 60 htz electricity.

The original TriField Meter combines all the features needed for fast, accurate measurements of electromagnetic fields. It independently measures electric field and magnetic field, and is properly scaled to indicate the full magnitude of currents produced by each type of field inside a conductive body. As a result, it "sees" much more than any other electromagnetic pollution meter.

Depending on where the knob is set, the meter detects either frequency- weighted magnetic fields (two separate scales), or frequency-weighted electric fields in the ELF and VLF range. It has significant sensitivity at 100,000 Hz, well past the 17,000 Hz horizontal scan of video displays. The radio/microwave setting can detect up to three billion Hz (3 GHz), which lets you gauge radio wave power, CB and analog cellular phone equipment (most cell phones use digital), and many types of radars.

This meter is the only one that combines magnetic, electric, and radio/microwave detectors in one package, so that the entire non-ionizing electromagnetic spectrum is covered. In addition, the magnetic setting and the electric setting measure true magnitude, a feature found elsewhere only in more expensive meters. If you hold the meter in the center of a room and tip it to various angles, the magnetic reading will stay approximately the same regardless of which way you tip or rotate it. The electric reading is similar, although the presence of your body alters the actual electric field, so readings will vary more. The radio/microwave setting reads the full power of radio waves when the meter is pointed toward the source.

Detox and Elimination
DVD - HHI Lecture 7

The workings of the elimination systems (Lymph, Liver, Lungs, Kidneys, and skin) and your body's reactions to a detoxifying program. 47 minutes

1. What is detox and what is the cycle?

2. What are the filtering organs?

3. Which is the largest?

4. What moves lymph?

5. What does it store?

6. Where are white blood cells made?

7. What is a good total white blood cell count?

8. What is the differential?

9. What are T-cells?

10. What are B-cells?

11. What are the other components of white blood cells and in what percents?

12. What are the different kinds of leucocytes?

13. What happens to the percentages of leucocytes when eating a highly processed diet?

14. Where are lymph nodes?

15. What should you do when you are detoxing (have swollen lymph glands)?

16. What does the lymph do?

17. What are the liver enzymes?

18. How much bile does the liver make and where is it stored?

19. 1 gallon, in the gallbladder.

20. How and where is fat digested?

21. How to clean gallstones naturally?

22. Where are carbohydrates digested?

23. What other healthy foods provide energy?

24. What do the lungs expel and where does it come from?

25. Living food diet is important for the lungs because it's high in what?

26. What are cilia and what do they do?

27. What foods are destructive to cilia?

28. What is asthma?

29. What can dissolve phlegm in the lungs?

30. What do the kidneys get rid of?

31. What are good levels for uric acid?

32. How much should we drink?

33. What causes high uric acid?

34. What are the kidney enzymes?

35. What should the PH of your blood be?

36. Urine and saliva need to be what PH?

37. What is cranberry juice used for?

38. How long is the intestinal tract?

39. How long is the intestinal tract of a carnivore?

40. How often should you fast and cleanse?

41. What is the largest elimination organ in the body?

42. How does the skin eliminate?

43. How do you detox with ginger?

44. What fibers allow your skin to breathe?

What oils can you put on your skin?

45. What emotions are stored in the organs?

46. What harm can coffee cause?

47. How does fruit affect alkalinity?

48. What does garlic do for blood pressure and cholesterol?

Summary Questions:

1. What are the steps you should follow before starting a detox?

2. How long can you live with out air?

3. What are the 6 organs of elimination in the body and how do they eliminate toxins?

Chapter 6
Mind Body Connection

Overview

Because of the results of the latest scientific experiments, we are unexpectedly coming to realize that the mind has the powers to actually create miracles. Miracles will become expected and not seem so miraculous once these experiments prove that consciousness creates perceptual illusion of matter.

Taking care of the mind is just as important as taking care of the body. Being mindful of stress and learning to cope with it effectively is as vital to health as flossing teeth, daily exercise, and eating nutritious foods. Participating in healthy mind-body techniques not only fights stress, but fights disease, too.

You will learn:

- the incredible powers of the mind to transmute matter
- the basics of psychoneuroimmunology
- to train your mind to function positively
- to be mindful
- commitment

The Amazing Powers of the Mind – We are Not Just Physical

by Lorraine Hurley, MD

The Magic Within Us - Epigenetics

Epigenetics is the way the environment around the cell influences the nucleus of the cell and its DNA. This and the power of thought, feeling and intent are great demonstrations of our abilities to create our own bodies. Robert O. Becker[37] whose experiments were later repeated by Dr. Harold Saxton Burr[38] provides amazing evidence of the power of our minds to create our unique body.

Robert O. Becker, Phd, researcher in the field of epigenetics, did an experiment that is phenomenal. Salamanders can re-grow a limb if it is lost. In fact part of their survival arsenal is the ability to detach a limb if they are captured. Frogs, on the other hand, do not demonstrate this ability. UNLESS? Unless the energy field around a lost limb is altered.

The original experiments went something like this. Front legs from both a salamander and a frog were removed. The electrical field of the cells at the open wound was measured. One was found to have a dominant negative polarity and the other a positive polarity. The salamander grew back its limb. The frog's limb was exposed to a magnetic field that flipped the polarity of the cells at the end of the open wound. What do you think happened? The frog grew his leg back. Energy, not biochemistry, induced an alteration of energy field communication to the DNA of his cells so that new growth was enabled. Now, how is it that the frog didn't just grow a blob of new tissue but actually replicated his original limb? How did growth differentiate when the magnetic field was undifferentiated? It happened because of an energy body that I would call the morphogenic field. Other scientists and mystics call it other things, but I use a term coined by Rupert Sheldrake.

A morphogenic field is an energetic replication of your potential. It remains whole even when a limb or organ or other physical part of you is lost. It is an energetic hologram of your highest potential. Again, if it interests you, (and it should ;-) consider doing further reading and study be-

---

[37]Becker, R. et al., The Direct Current System: A Link Between the Environment and the Organism, New York State of Journal of Medicine, vol. 62 (1962), pp. 1169-1176

[38]Dr. Harold Saxton Burr (1889-1973), *Blueprint for immortality: The electric patterns of Life* (London: N. Spearman, 1972) Professor of Anatomy at the Yale University School of Medicine. Dr. Burr discovered "that man – and, in fact, all forms – are ordered and controlled by electro-dynamic fields which can be measured and mapped with precision…the 'fields of life' are of the same nature as the simpler fields known to modern physics and obedient to the same laws. Like the fields of physics, they are pat of the organization of the Universe and are influenced by the vast forces of space. Like the fields of physics, too, they have organizing and directing qualities that have been revealed by many thousands of experiments. Organization and direction, the direct opposite of chance, imply purpose. So the fields of life offer purely electronic, instrumental evidence that man is no accident. On the contrary, he is an integral part of the Cosmos, embedded in its all-powerful fields, subject to its inflexible laws and a participant in the destiny of the Universe" – quoted from E.F. Schumacher's *A guide for the perplexed (*New York: Harper & Row, 1977, pp. 116-17, and used by permission of the Random House Group Ltd.

cause it has extraordinary implications for attaining your highest faculties in life.

This research and knowledge has astonishing implications for healing and it is reasonable to ask why it is not yet widely practiced. It is practiced, but not in the mainstream. There are now centers that use very large magnetic fields to enable those with neurological injuries to re-grow nervous tissue.

Now some might argue that it is still a physical phenomenon. They wouldn't be right because magnetism is a wave function, but here is another example that makes it impossible to argue with energy healing.

What Water Can Teach Us

Masaru Emoto is a brilliant Japanese researcher into the energetic nature and miracle of water. His book is recommended below. He was able to demonstrate how water responded to thought and feeling. Experimenters directed specific thoughts and feelings into water and the water was frozen, sliced and viewed under a special microscope. When words, thoughts and feelings of love were directed at the water, it formed beautiful and unique crystals. When words, thoughts and feelings of hate were directed at the water, there was no crystal formation and the water appeared disorganized and dead.

To demonstrate this on a large scale, several participants were asked to direct loving prayer into a lake in Japan that was "dead" from pollution. I don't recall the exact time frame, but prayer eventually restored the lake to a healthy ecology. Nothing else was done; only consistent and sincere prayers and thoughts of love were directed to the lake.

We are 80 percent or more water at birth. The water content of our bodies diminishes as we age (though this demonstrated in the general population, it is not necessarily "normal").

Water is not just about hydrating us anymore than food is about calories. The microbes of our gut are about a simple exchange of nutrients or our DNA is about a static formula for you. Water is an elixir of life, absorbing and transmitting energy, thoughts and emotions down to a cellular level. Homeopathy is a practice that utilizes this knowledge about water. This amazing quality of water is a great stepping-stone into an appreciation for the fact that thoughts, feelings and beliefs are "things" with real action and real influences on our biochemistry, physiology and quality of life.

Learning to fully uncover our current thoughts, beliefs and feelings so that we may choose and generate new ones that serve us and our planet better, requires that we first unconditionally love and accept what is within us.

Pathway of Awareness

What has helped me tremendously to work with my subconscious feelings and thoughts is a book called "The Presence Process" by Michael Brown. The field of mind/body medicine is expanding rapidly. But, the mind is actually a composite of physical, mental, emotional and vibrational function. When some say the mind, they mean by that, mental or thought. But, the mind is much greater than thought. But, when we are not clear about mind vs. mental, many pursue practices that focus entirely on their thinking and use affirmations and vision boards and other tools in an effort to enact change rather than using the whole mind. These are useful tools, but without a comprehension of the totality of the mind, our tools are not going to do the right job.

Our development as human beings follows a distinct pathway of awareness. When we are in the womb, our experience of life is largely vibrational. We absorb what our mothers think and feel as vibrations as we are without mental faculties yet. These vibrations become part of our sub-conscious mind. When we are born, we now experience life through our emotional body. That is, we are still capable of vibrational communication, but now we can interact with others emotionally. This is our dominant method of communication and growth for the first several years of our lives. Most of us have no conscious memory of our earliest years. But, they are nevertheless present within us as felt-perceptions.

Before further delineating the pathway of awareness, I want to introduce the concept of imprinting and what is commonly referred to as karma (this is bumping into the Akashic field and holographic sciences). Just because we have no conscious recollection of the experiences in the womb or our early childhood, does not mean we cannot recall them non-mentally. The absorption of vibrations in the womb becomes an imprint in our own body. The experiences of our early life are imprinted into our emotional body. The choice of when to be born and to whom is a sacred contract. We come into this world to deliberately work out our needs for continued growth and evolution of consciousness. What we need is given to us through this process of imprinting. It does no good to consider us victims in any capacity. All experiences in our lives are created by both unconscious and later conscious choices we make ourselves. The players are but messengers and mirrors for our own internal landscape of thought and feeling.

In our culture, the development of the emotional body almost stops completely when we enter school. The emphasis is now on developing our mental capacities. In our culture this is more what to think than how to think and it is considered the holy grail of human achievement. Our culture worships the mental body. But, this is the place of ego, limitation and delusion for any who wish to achieve communion with Source or live a vibrantly conscious life. As we approach adolescence, our attention is directed into our physical body reflecting who we "are" and what we "do". By the time we are adults, our world and self-image are largely defined by our work, income potential and pretense about who and what we are.

This means most of us reach adulthood having the emotional capacity of a small child and are completely unconscious about what he or she is doing. What she or he is usually doing is reacting to experiences based on the fear, grief and anger of childhood. The pathway of awareness into the world is more vibrational, emotional, mental than physical. If we want to return to vibrational awareness, we must work backwards. We cannot jump over any aspect of this pathway. The way out is through.

The way "The Presence Process" works is eloquent in its simplicity and dramatic in its effect. Using our breath to draw our attention into our body, so that we are here, NOW and not in the illusions of time (past and future) we develop a capacity to be aware of what we are really thinking. What we think, is an outgrowth of how we feel. Once we are clear on what we are thinking (and come to realize that most of it does not serve us), we are free to allow the emotions beneath these thoughts to emerge. We, then, unconditionally, accept and allow these feelings. We don't sedate, control, judge, deny or interpret them. When we are able to do this, these emotions integrate and no longer fuel unconscious reactions and repetitive trauma and drama in our lives. This is called integration.

What this means is that we grow up emotionally and develop an ability to genuinely feel. While most of what is unconscious is very uncomfortable (otherwise we would not have suppressed it), it is also valid and necessary to be fully alive emotionally. When we learn to integrate our unconscious pain, we open ourselves up to experience ALL emotions fully, freely and responsively. Then and only then are we able to enter into a moment-by-moment relationship with the vibrational. The vibrational is where all limitations, belief in separation, inadequacy and failure dissolve.

Further Wonders

Both the breath and the heart have depth and energetic abilities not defined by their strict physical functions. Breath while drawing air and essential oxygen can be used to draw life force into your body. Practitioners called Breatharians demonstrate this. Breatharians use little to no food but draw life-force from sun and air through specific breathing practices.

The heart while pumping blood and oxygen is also a generator of coherence in the body. Through breath work, meditation, prayer and love we can dissolve the dominance of physicality in our lives and achieve remarkable vitality and well being. Why? Because, coherence strengthens and harmonizes life force. In fact, there is nothing in your body that does not participate in your higher functions. But, you must perceive it to receive it. All experiences in our lives happen that we may grow into the full realization of what we are. When we are sick or stuck or thwarted, we are in actuality being presented with an opportunity to go within and make our way to wholeness and prosperity. We have access to everything we need through our holographic and vibrational "omnipotence".

The Akashic records have been likened to "The DNA of the Universe". Carried within that record is every life, word and deed you have ever had, spoken or carried out. It is an encoded light language. Recent studies have indicated that what has been so arrogantly and ignorantly termed "junk DNA" may actually be that part of us that receives and transmits information into our Akashic record. This research has revealed that DNA emits photons (light) of a very high frequency and that it also changes expression and organization in response to receiving photon energy. Leonard Horowitz termed the expression "our antennae to God". We are endowed with the means to communicate directly with Source. More amazing, is that we are endowed with the means to receive direct communication from Source.

Further, recent research on the pineal gland (metaphorically our "third" eye) shows it is a light receiver and transmitter. We are then ultimately light beings. We are endowed with the means to communicate directly with Source. More amazing, is that we are endowed with the means to receive direct communication from Source.

We've only scratched the surface of this topic. I strongly encourage you to undertake your own program of learning and practice to expand your comprehension and competence with all of your extraordinary "bodies". We live in times where the debts of karma shift and evolve as we do, and we can work with that CONSCIOUSLY. We live in times when accelerated evolution is not only possible but also imperative.

Recommended Reading:
The Presence Process by Michael Brown
The Tao of Physics by Fritjof Capra
DNA: Pirates of the Sacred Spiral by Len Horowitz
Science and the Akashic Field, by Ervin Laszlo
Free Your Breath, Free Your Life by Dennis Lewis
Timeless Secrets of Health and Rejuvenation by Andreas Moritz
The Holographic Universe by Michael Talbot
Gut Solutions by Brenda Watson
Source Field Investigations by David Wilcox

What is The Role of Emotions in The Mind-Body Connection?
by Barry Harris

Has Western medicine made a big mistake with its past focus on manipulating the chemistry of the body as the primary factor in recovering from life-threatening or chronic illness? The results of the latest scientific research brings to mind Christ's powerful metaphor, "They are straining at gnats, while swallowing camels." In this case, it is Western medicine's decision to treat isolated body parts with drugs, which is straining at gnats, while they are swallowing the camel of ignoring the effect of our mind, and, in particular, our emotions, on our body's health and it's recovery from serious illness. In other words, could the dysfunctionality of our present medical system be due in large part to its distraction into the "less important" influences on our health, while ignoring the "most important"

We have been "straining at gnats" ever since Western culture was hypnotized to the illusion of total independence of mind from body, popularized in the model of Renee Descartes in the 16th century. This separation of mind from body was expressed by Descartes in his famous phrase, "Mind must be a different substance than matter, because you can't measure the length of a thought."

Sorry, Descartes, but we now have the theory, provided by modern quantum physics, that strongly suggests not only are mind and matter united as one, but, most probably, mind is creating our perceptual experience of matter, and so, the material world is probably a "perceptual illusion." And we now have the technology to measure the length of a thought, any time we desire, for different thoughts are expressed as different electromagnetic energy waves, and all waves have measurable wave-lengths.

Biochemist, Michael Rull,[1] has taken pictures showing that thoughts of hopelessness express themselves as "hopelessness" molecules, which enter the cells of the immune system, and give instructions to turn off the capacity to fight foreign invaders, such as cancer cells. Modern quantum physics shows that molecules are also electromagnetic energy waves, and thus since thoughts of "hopelessness" are also expressed as electromagnetic energy waves, it is not so surprising that molecules of "hopelessness" have the ability to enter our cells, and have a significant effect on our health.

The latest discoveries are definitely the "Good News," for they reveal a totally new source of empowerment that all of us have over the state of our health. Self-awareness of what our mind, and particularly our emotions, is doing at any one moment, gives us an unexpected control over the unique body that we create. Our body doesn't function as a machine, as was previously believed, but as a creative expression of our minds, and, especially, our emotions.

Unfortunately, so much of that potential for creative expression has become locked up by negative emotional thought patterns we have adopted for protection against childhood pain, and which have been repressed into the unconscious.

Psychologist, David Spiegel's study[39] on women given a terminal diagnosis of breast cancer, and Fawzy Fawzy's study[40] with leukemia and auto-immune disease have proven that emotionally cathartic therapy, in which the individual ends the emotional repression, and, as it's colloquially expressed, "gets it all out," is more important a determinant of life-span and recovery than any miracle drugs.

However, even most psychologists and holistic therapists aren't privy to the secret shared by those in the "living food" community. The committed raw-foodist, by his diet and lifestyle, conserves life force energy, which is then available to detoxify the cells of the body. Negative emotions which have been stored in the cells as neuropeptide molecules, and as disturbed electromagnetic energy patterns are released in the process of regenerating the cells. This is why negative emotional states are often experienced in the first step of detoxification. The hopelessness that Michael Rull observed that turned off the immune system is the kind of negative emotional memory that is released in the process of detoxification/regeneration. Releasing these negative thought forms allows one to truly be born anew.

Perhaps, when Western medicine realizes it's been "straining at gnats, while swallowing camels," there will be a new medical paradigm in which it is recognized that the emotional demoralization and hopelessness that comes from a disfiguring double mastectomy is more harmful than leaving in a few cancer cells, that can easily be eradicated by the immune system of someone who has become a "master of their mind."

 Isn't this prospect worth the discomfort of the self-discipline necessary to be a raw-foodist; after, all, it's your choice to no longer be a victim to your mind and emotions.

"For this is the great error of our day, that the physicians separate the soul from the body."
—*Hippocrates*

Recommended Reading:

Kiecolt-Glaser, J.K., Garner, W, Speicher, C.E., Penn, G., Vlaser, R. "Psycho Social Modifiers of Immunocompetence in Medical Students." *Psychosomatic Medicine 46*, 1984.

http://dir.yahoo.com/social_science/psychology/branches/psychoneuroimmunology

http://www.mnwelldir.org/docs/immune/psychon.htm

---

[39] Dienstfrey, Harris. (1992). *Where the Mind Meets the Body*..New York, New York: Harper Collins.

[40] Ibid.

The Importance of Emotional Detoxification
By Barry Harris

Emotional Detoxification is a new medical paradigm that is replacing the antiquated Cartesian model of the body as a machine. This new paradigm recognizes that the human body can only be understood if one also considers its unity with consciousness. The old paradigm leaves us victims to the universe, and it is truly exciting as we leave the old paradigm behind for a much more encouraging view of reality.

The new paradigm arising from discoveries in quantum physics, energy medicine, neurophysiology, and cellular biology is definitely "good news" for it ends our victimization by restoring the control we have over our body's physiology and thus our state of health.

According to this new paradigm, we do not have a mechanical material body as primary, but we have an energy/information body operating as a messaging system. If the messages for optimal physiological function are effectively transmitted, then there is the possibility for the optimal functioning of the body, and there is even the possibility for the body's miraculous self-repair. Effective transmission of messages requires the production of coherent electromagnetic energy patterns.

What do I mean by coherent electromagnetic energy patterns, and why are they necessary for the body's optimal functioning? The following analogy should bring some clarity. If you have two motor boats making waves as they go through the water, when these waves from the boats collide, the waves will either be dissipated or enlarged depending on whether they superimpose on each other, or cancel each other out. The same is true about electromagnetic energy waves. Waves that cancel each other out are called "incoherent" energy patterns, and waves that superimpose are called "coherent" wave patterns. If the waves cancel each other out, they cannot transmit healing messages throughout the body.

The following quote from biophysicist, Beverly Rubik, gives some of the scientific evidence supporting this new paradigm for understanding health and illness that I have just proposed.

"I'm intrigued by some work done in Germany. In fact, I've gone over there to work with Dr. Fritz Albert Popp. This work involves detecting extremely low-level light that the human body and all organisms emit.... Popp uses very sensitive detectors that can count the photons, the particles of light coming out of the body (i.e. electromagnetic radiation). I think this may be one of the manifestations of the energy dynamics of life. For example, in the Popp laboratory, they have demonstrated that to a large extent the light is coherent like a laser. That means that the light probably has a capacity for carrying information, unlike incoherent light. If that's the case, it's probably not some junk radiation, which is the mainstream opinion. I think that the light, if it's coherent, is maybe involved in both an internal communication system, as well as an external one, that conveys signals between living things......It's interesting that in studying the cancer tissues of patients, they have found losses in the coherence of the light. Perhaps the light has lost informational value, and it cannot communicate with the other cells, and that's why the tissues grow abnormally." (1)

It has been proven that stress causes chaotic electromagnetic energy wave patterns that cancel each other out, and thus under stress, the body cannot transmit healing messages. With stress as the common denominator causing incoherent energy patterns, and thus poor message transmission, we have the foundation for a unified field theory of sickness and health. All sickness is caused by stress, because all sickness is a result of poor message transmission. And this is a unified field theory, because with stress as the common denominator, there are many possible sources of illness, since there are many different kinds of stress. Stress may manifest as dietary stress, stress from environmental toxins, stress from poor relationships, and stress from blocked emotions, just to name a few.

We will be investigating in this article the stress that comes from blocked emotional expression, and the miraculous healing possible just from restoring the energy flow to blocked emotions, and, once again, experiencing an emotional health that may have been absent since childhood traumas caused us to block our emotions and shut our emotions down. This healing of our emotions, that increases our capacity for optimal physical health, is called "emotional detoxification," or "emotional purification."

The work of biochemist, Candace Pert, the discoverer of endorphins, (2), and Bruce Lipton, the cellular biologist who elaborates on Pert's new model of the body/mind (3), gives evidence that the stress of blocked emotions, and the garbled messages that result, actually infiltrate all the cells of the body, and even affect the nucleus of the cell and the DNA. This can explain the study by (??) which proved that individuals with a genetic tendency towards arthritis, were five times less likely to experience arthritis if psychological tests showed they were emotionally healthy. Likewise, Dr. Harold Iker found that women who have suspicious PAP smears were much more likely to have benign tumors if psychological tests showed they were emotionally healthy, and malignant tumors if psychological tests showed they had repressed or blocked emotional expression.

The "good news" is that once the importance of emotional health is recognized, there is a large variety of techniques to get the emotional energy flowing again. Fifty years ago, all that was available were various forms of Reichian bioenergetic bodywork releasing emotions trapped in the body's musculature, as well as modalities like "primal scream." Since then many new techniques have been found to be effective. I can testify from my personal experience to the effectiveness of some of them.

Extended fasts conserve the body's energy and then redirect this energy to cellular detoxification and release blocked emotions from the cells. This toxic, stressful energy of blocked emotions entered the bloodstream, and was responsible for the states of irritability, depression, and foggy thinking that often accompany the first week of an extended fast. If there is any doubt that emotional detoxification is the culprit behind these negative states, the peace and healthy emotional expression experienced at the end of a long vegetable juice fast should reassure any skeptics. This peace is the purified state experienced once all the emotional toxins have been released. It is not a peace that is disturbed by healthy emotional expression, but it is a peace that accompanies healthy emotional expression, even of so-called negative emotions like anger, sadness, and fear. In fact, the effects of fasting taught me how misguided is the human ego's assumption that there are objectively unhealthy negative emotions like anger, fear, or sadness. The truth I discovered was that there is a healthy and unhealthy anger, fear, and sadness, depending on whether the emotion is coming from a state of peace, and thus the emotions flow without blocks, or the emotions are experienced in a stressful blocked state.

From 1985-1992 I worked with live food pioneers, Ann Wigmore (i.e. discoverer of wheatgrass), and Viktoras Kulvinskas (i.e. the first director of Dr. Wigmore's Hippocrates Institute), and while on that diet, even without fasting, emotional detoxification occurred since it is a diet with maximum nutrition.

While involved with the live food community, I was introduced to the work of Dr. John Ray, inventor of "Body Electronics" as a means to optimal emotional detoxification. With this method, large numbers of electrolytes are taken in order to optimize the electrical polarization of the cells, and then acupressure releases many stored blocked emotions, along with the traumatic memories associated with the blockage, and there is often miraculous healing not only in the mental and emotional bodies, but also in the physical body

For the past two years, I have been a participant in an emotional healing group using a technique called "Core Energetics" for emotional detoxification. Emotional detoxification is prime evidence that the health of the body encompasses body/mind and spirit, for as I become healthier emotionally, I see physical symptoms also vanishing.

What kind of miracles are possible when there is optimal emotional detoxification? I have recently been introduced to a process of emotional healing called "The Presence Process." And this process miraculously healed its founder, Michael Brown, of a very painful, neurological disorder, that doctors had assured him would be with him for the rest of his life.

And, finally, most recently, EFT (i.e. the emotional freedom technique) has exploded onto the scene, claiming more and more adherents, because, quite simply, it is found to work miracles, and all it requires is gentle tapping at selected points along the body's meridians.

Perhaps the day will not be far off, that Western medicine recognizes, to paraphrase Christ, "they have been straining at gnats and swallowing camels," which means, our medical paradigm has been focusing on the relatively unimportant (i.e. manipulating the chemistry of the body with drugs), and ignoring the truly important, (i.e. the emotional health of the individual). When that day arrives, finally our medicine will become gentler and kinder as it is accepted that the emotional demoralization that comes from a double mastectomy is more harmful because of its effects on the immune system, than leaving a few cancer cells in the body, knowing that someone who is emotionally healthy has a strong immune system which can neutralize the problem.

Research on Mind-Body Connection
Shows We are More than We Think We Are
by Barry Harris

Who are we really? Is it possible that we are not who and what we thought we were? Is it possible that we have experienced ourselves as powerless machines, only because we have been hypnotized by an inaccurate, misguided paradigm of the body as machine, and the mind as part of this machine?

Modern science, and particularly modern quantum physics, and holographic theory as a part of this modern physics, are strongly suggesting, that who we are is part of universal consciousness, that creates the illusion of a body, and then uses this body to carry out its creative projects.

This new view of who we are gives us new eyes to see that, perhaps, the mental state of one's mind is the most important factor in our health, even more important than one's diet. If this is true, then the statement by Brian Clement from his article in Hippocrates News would seem to logically follow: "You can't be doing all the right things, and thinking all the wrong things, and still expect a positive outcome."[41]

The results of the latest scientific research has ended the past machine paradigm, and is responsible for this new paradigm, which takes the influence of mind and our emotions, out of the shadows, and makes them front and center. It is the scientific research that is proving emotional turmoil, depression, remorse, resentment, and other negative mental conditions have measurable, negative physical effects on our body's physiology. Therefore, as biochemist Candace Pert, the discoverer of endorphins, emphasizes in her groundbreaking book, "Molecules of Emotion," the medicine of the future will be based on our awareness of what our mind, and, thus, our body is doing moment to moment.

---

[41]Clement, Brian. "The Mind-Body Connection." Hippocrates News, Volume 6, Number 2, Hippocrates Health Institute.

Centering the Mind Comes First[42]

Why Meditate

Meditation is the art of silencing the mind. When the mind is silent, concentration is increased and we experience inner peace in the midst of worldly turmoil. This elusive inner peace is what attracts so many people to meditation and is the key to health.

Meditation reduces stress levels and alleviates anxiety. If we can reduce stress, health will follow.

Numerous scientific studies have shown that meditation alleviates stress and the physical and emotional problems stress can lead to. Meditating can help with chronic pain, heart disease, migraines, anxiety, depression, high blood pressure and many other ailments.

Practicing meditation slows breathing rate, blood pressure and heart rate; and some studies even show that a meditator's brain may be more "fit" than the next guy's. If you're suffering with a health condition or making lifestyle changes to prevent illness, check out some guided meditations for specific health conditions.

While many of us do think of meditation as a solution to a problem — a way to rid ourselves of worry, stress or anxiety — there's much more to this picture.

For example, researchers have shown that meditation can increase compassion, love and forgiveness. Visualization, a practice closely linked with meditation, is being used by more and more people to help heal physical or emotional illness. And some have found that practicing meditation over time can help them access deeper, more expansive effects from meditation. You may begin feeling more spiritually fulfilled, experience a profound therapeutic effect or gain greater sense of happiness and peace in your life.

Some suggestions that I've found helpful:

- Practice everyday at the same time
    - Early morning between 2 am and 8 am is recommended – follow nature - this is when flowers bloom and all is still
    - I've found once you meditate for 21 days, your body will be trained to expect to center at this time. It becomes a habit.
- Practice on an empty stomach so your body/energy is not focused on digestion.

---

[42] http://life.gaiam.com/guides/meditation-answers-solutions-go-guide

- Sit erect in a hard-backed chair (not leaning back on chair). Place your feet flat on the ground in front of you (if the chair is too high, use a footstool). Place hands on your knees with palms up with your pointer finger touching your thumb that for me creates a circuit). Touch your palette just behind your front teeth with your tongue which will keep you awake.

- Lower your eyes –half closed while focusing on a spot on the floor in front of you

- Focus on breathing out and breathing in. Just be. Use any technique you find helpful.

- Be gentle with yourself. Don't take it on as a task but a state of mind to be achieved. When it's new, it's special. Then it becomes routine and nothing special. It's O.K. to be nothing special. An analogy is flying in an airplane. At first, it's exciting buckling up and hearing the rev of the engines and rising above the clouds. At some point when you are up there, you forget that you're up there flying high. It's no longer special. However, you now see each moment clearly with no attachment, no stress and no anxiety.

To attain life force energy, the body needs to be clean. Like a car, it needs good gas and oil and a clean engine.

The Grace That Flows From Commitment

by Valarie Spain
Mindfulness Educator & Coach
Mindful Eating & Diabetes Lifestyle Change

Everyone struggles to change habits that lead to making poor health choices. My struggle to understand the legacy of an eating disorder became especially urgent when I was diagnosed with Type 1 diabetes. Now, after years of mindfulness meditation practice, attention to diet and physical activity, more often than not, I experience the benefits of that attention. There were many ah-ha moments and little epiphanies, but no single event or experience brought change, rather, it was simply the persistent doing that bore fruit after many years. Mindfulness meditation, basically a daily sitting practice, was essential, but so were my creative practices of making art and writing poetry.

Persistence in practicing any good thing results in beneficial states of body and mind, like open-heartedness, joy, compassion for oneself and others, physical and emotional wellbeing, including better reactions to stress and anxiety. In the beginning, one has to have faith in the inherent goodness of these activities, even when benefits seem elusive. Commit to doing them routinely, whether daily, weekly or monthly. Don't strive for perfection, but at least hold the intention to practice, because intention will eventually spur action, which, in turn, will bring the benefits you seek.

Remember that we can't change alone. Reach out to a supportive circle of friends, colleagues–find a support group. Even a few people who have your best interests at heart can make a great difference.

Practices for deep and lasting change include mindfulness meditation and nonviolent (NVC) communication. You can use them as "techniques" but I encourage taking them on as practices. Choose something and make it an integral part of your life. Both meditation, especially metta practice, and NVC, nurture empathy for oneself and others; they help practitioners become aware of actions that trigger or induce fear, because fear is a key component that causes us to act in familiar, predictable, and often unhelpful, ways. Meditation and NVC ground practitioners in the present moment, helping them act skillfully in the face of challenging events and people–even that challenging person we know as us! They create healthy new habits to replace old destructive ones.

An NVC practice that dovetails nicely with meditation practice is called Breath, Body, and Needs, where each word is a prompt to remember an action. Breath says, become aware of your breathing–just breathe. Body says, become aware of your body: feel your feet on the ground, your breath moving in and out; feel where you actually are in this moment. Needs are universal to all sentient beings: the need for warmth, shelter, respect, meaning etc. What do you need in the moment? Do you know? If not, then it's time to find out!

The grace of commitment is available to everyone. In a world that desires quick fixes, such practices may seem like too much effort. Yes, effort is required, but it's never too late to begin. What I've learned in hindsight is that grace begins as soon as we do, often we're just too preoccupied to notice. Practice wakes us up and makes us notice.

Mindful Eating

by Kate Kilmurray

Food is a celebration, a daily opportunity for nourishment, sensuality, community and environmentalism all rolled into one. There is simply nothing like eating good, wholesome food that sustains our bodies while awakening our spirits and helping to preserve the planet at the same time.

The following are suggested guidelines for mindful eating:

- Sit down to eat your meals slowly and without distraction.

- Eat in an orderly, calm manner.

- Chew each mouthful completely: digestion begins in the mouth.

- Avoid mixing foods in the same mouthful.

- Keep your meal times regular.

- Eat only the quantity you need.

- Occasionally, eat in silence. This experience enhances your ability to fully taste, smell and appreciate your food while remaining connected to your appetite. When fully focused and present, food nourishes deeply.

Kate Kilmurray, a longtime yoga and meditation practitioner, mentors others on the path of awakening and mindful living. www.katekilmurray.com

Love, Pray – Nutrition and Polarity Therapy
by Karen Woeller

h we travel many roads, one of those being nutrition. We know that by
to what we choose to feed our body we affect how our physical body
and repairs itself, thus increasing our Life Force Energy. Another road we travel has to do with our energetic systems or more to the point, "what we think". What we think and act upon also affects our physical body and our Life Force. And as we travel these roads we discover who we really are in this world and being our true self brings us joy and manifestation.

Polarity Therapy is about taking care of our energetic systems. It's about choosing to feed ourselves with nourishing thoughts and feelings, cleansing away those that no longer support us, and learning how to repair these systems when needed. As we do this we gain Life Force Energy so we can manifest that which we truly desire.

Polarity Therapy was developed by Doctor Randolph Stone, D.C., D.O. who believed diet, nutrition, stretching, exercise, manipulation and the role of lifestyle and individual thought patterns are all important in creating a healthy body. He directed his attention to the "energy anatomy" of the human body which seeks to release and balance the energy that is blocked and causing pain and disease. To maintain health energy must flow freely through its fields, to and from its source.

How Polarity Therapy is done:

A session with a polarity therapist takes approximately one hour. You remain clothed and lay on a massage table. The therapist does some gentle body work using specific points and pathways to move the energy in your body to clear and balance the areas where energy has gotten dense or blocked because of trauma, stress, or emotional issues and works to create flow in your life force. Polarity activates the parasympathetic nervous system (the rest and relax part) that creates deep relaxation. You may experience a tasmic or alpha state of being which is like falling asleep but yet still fully aware. This state allows us to tune into our inner self either consciously or subconsciously. Polarity also clears the energy of old traumas and issues so we are free to move on and discover our true selves. Releasing blocks and allowing the body to fully relax boosts the healing ability of the body.

After a polarity session you will feel refreshed and deeply relaxed and may have new insight into the issues and questions you may have. Over time as energy is released and balanced you will also feel physically better and especially if you are also making lifestyle changes such as diet, exercise and practicing relaxation techniques.

Summary questions:

1. What are the amazing implications of the salamander – frog experiment?

2. What does psychoneuroimmunology mean?

3. What are the magic properties of water?

4. What has modern quantum physics discovered which helps us understand miracles?

5. What are ways recommended to help you meditate?

6. Why are emotions more important to our health than reason?

7. Why is it more harmful to do a double mastectomy, then to leave a few cancer cells in the body?

Chapter 7
Enzymes and Vitamins

Overview

The nutrient content of food has fascinated people for a long time.

The idea that what one eats makes a difference in improving one's health is often the subject of numerous magazines and TV shows. It has its roots in serious research from peer-reviewed articles, available on the Internet.

While some details vary as to what is emphasized in the nutrient content, it is consistent that plant-based food has rich health-building properties. Actually, they may have nutrients that have not yet been discovered!

The organic choices are always the best in order to ingest high quality plant nutrients, and thus to avoid consuming artificial chemicals.

We have been conditioned to pay attention to vitamins, minerals and protein, as the top content in food, but none of these have any effect on us without enzymes. Enzymes are the catalyst for nearly all biochemical reactions in our body; they hold our life force.

This chapter briefly discusses enzymes, the benefits of plant-based food, herbs and supplements. It includes charts reprinted with Brian Clement's permission from his book Life Force, that references scientific studies backing its claims. Furthermore, it contains Susan Comeau's Life Force Energy class presentation on the medicinal value of herbs.

You will learn:

- the value of enzymes

- the whole food sources of vitamins and minerals

- why supplementation is necessary

- the difference between plant-based and synthetic supplements

- the health benefits of plant-based food

- the therapeutic value of herbs

Enzymes[43]

The great raw-food pioneer and co-founder of the Hippocrates Health Institute, Viktoras Kulvinskas, wrote in his book *Survival in the 21st Century*, *"There is an evolutionary step beyond periodic internal cleansing which I call 'youthing'. It's the actual reversal of aging. To be able to become physiologically younger even as you chronologically get older, you'll need to increase your level of enzyme supplementation as well as the quantity of enzyme –rich superfoods you eat."*

The word, 'enzyme', he writes, comes from Greek and means to 'ferment' or 'cause a change'. *The medical dictionary defines an enzyme as "a protein produced in a cell capable of greatly accelerating, by its catalytic action, the chemical reaction of a substance (the substrate) for which it is specific."*

Scientists have found over 3,000 different enzymes in the human body, all which play a specific role. The enzymes in white blood cells digest foreign substances. Enzymes are responsible for cleaning the blood, digesting food, transporting nutrients to organs, building protein into muscle, and balancing hormones and cholesterol in the body.

There are three types of enzymes: food enzymes, digestive enzymes and metabolic enzymes. Food enzymes are found in raw foods, which are foods in their natural state or foods cooked below 118 degrees. Once a food is cooked above this temperature, enzymes can no longer survive or carry out its functions. Food enzymes work together with other nutrients to boost the immune system and cleanse the body. Digestive enzymes come from organs that aid in breaking down food. The main types of digestive enzymes are amylase which break down carbohydrates, protease which break down proteins, and lipase which break down fats. Metabolic enzymes are created by the body's cells to deliver nutrients, clean and transport blood to organs and tissues.

Although raw foods have the enzymes necessary to break down food, providing supplemental enzymes can help to break down and clean up toxic substances that are in the blood. Many leading cancer experts such as the Gershwin Institute and Dr. Nicholas Gonzalez use proteolytic enzymes as a successful cancer treatment. Cancer, bacteria and viruses, being made up of proteins, can be successfully treated with protein digesting enzymes.

Advocates of enzyme therapy regard enzyme bankruptcy as a health catastrophe that can cause many bodily functions to cease prematurely. They suggest that even when eating on the best nutritional plan and supplementing with vitamins, that supplemental enzymes can aid with vitamin absorption into the system.

Do we really need plant enzymes?

While some medical authorities deny the importance of enzymes as supplements, proposing the body makes its own enzymes, Victoras Kulvinskas writes, *"Everyone would benefit from extra enzymes. The studies on longevity show that cultures that were noted for low infant mortality, low disease patterns and outstanding longevity, had in common only one dietary factor, consuming enzymatic beverages that were being created by friendly bacteria action. There are over 3,500 enzyme complexes that play key roles in digestion, immune action and metabolism.*

---

[43]Kulvinskas, V. (1982)*Survival in the 21st Century*. Hot Springs, AZ: 21st Century Publications.

When you eat cooked food or breathe in pollutants, the enzymes are used by the immune system to clean up the internal pollution. The human body is an incredibly resilient organism using enzymes to control every known biochemical process. Every cell in the body produces enzymes, which are used to power physical movement, regulate organ function, and power the immune system. Even thinking and breathing are processes that depend on enzymatic activity. Digestion of food is also dependent on enzymes. In fact, an enzyme is the only known compound capable of the hydrolysis of food. Digestion of foodstuffs in the absence of naturally occurring enzymes negates the process of pre-digestion forcing the body to produce pancreatic enzymes to digest 100% of the nutritional factors of that food."

Dr. Edward Howell, father of enzyme nutrition and therapy, stated that enzymes are the very substances that make life possible. After working with enzymes under an electron microscope, Brian Clement, from the Hippocrates Health Institute, states that in every case when an enzyme was split open, an actual electrical charge was observed. From this he concluded that enzymes are the most important nutrient that our bioelectrical bodies require.

Further Reading:

- Dr. Edward Howell, *Food Enzymes for Health & Longevity,* 2nd edition
- D.A. Lopez, M.D., R. M. Williams, M.D, K Miehlke, M.D., *Enzymes, the Foutain of Life*
- Tom Bohager, *Everything You Need to Know about Enzymes*
- Dr. Anthony J. Cichoke, *The Complete Book of Enzyme Therapy*

My Personal Experience with Enzymes

I studied live blood analysis with Anna Maria Clement while I was attending the Hippocrates Health Institute as a Health Educator student. At the time I was tested, and Anna Maria took a sample of my blood, I was going through a detox. Therefore, some of the signs of toxicity of blood sample included: my plasma appeared almost black; the red corpuscles were stacked like pancakes; the white blood cells looked like packmen as they ate up the candida. Anna Maria gave me ten digestive enzymes to take. Fifteen minutes later she took another blood sample. Amazingly, the plasma was clear and the red corpuscles were calmly floating around. Now, I take digestive enzymes with each meal, systemic (metabolic) ones at the beginning of the day and eat a sprout, leafy green plant-based diet most of the time. And, as a result, I'm "youthing".

Further Reading:

- Viktoras H. Kulvinskas, *Survival in the 21st Century*
- Dr. Edward Howell, *Food Enzymes for Health & Longevity,* 2nd edition
- D.A. Lopez, M.D., R. M. Williams, M.D, K Miehlke, M.D., *Enzymes, the Foutain of Life*
- Tom Bohager, *Everything You Need to Know about Enzymes*
- Dr. Anthony J. Cichoke, *The Complete Book of Enzyme Therapy*

Summary Of Syndromes Common To Enzyme Deficiency

Amylase Deficiency

Breaking out of the skin – rash

Hypoglycemia

Depression

Mood swings

Allergies

PMS

Hot flashes

Fatigue

Cold hands and feet

Neck and shoulder aches

Inflammation

Protease Deficiency

Back weakness

Fungal forms

Constipation

High Blood Pressure

Insomnia

Gum disorders

Gingivitis

Acne

Gall bladder stones

Gallstones

Hay fever

Prostate problems

Psoriasis

Urinary weakness

Constipation

Diarrhea

Heart problems

Combination Deficiency

Chronic allergies

Common colds

Diverticulitis

Irritable Bowel

Chronic fatigue

Sinus Infection

Immune depressed conditions

Lipase Deficiency

Aching feet

Arthritis

Bladder problems

Cystitis

Hippocrates Health Institute Supplements[44]

If you want to fight disease and achieve maximum life span, you can't do it with diet alone. You need the extra nutritional boost that only supplements can provide. The nutrients in our soil have been depleted from years of pesticides and pollution.

"During the 20th century, according to this report, about 85 percent of all nutrients have been depleted from crop soils from North America. Asia and South America lost 76 percent of soil nutrients. Africa lost 74 percent and Europe experienced 72 percent decline. These nutrients were stripped from the soil by fertilizers, pesticides, herbicides, farming practices and other human induced causes. At least 90 of these depleted nutrients are considered essential to human health including 60 minerals and 16 vitamins that are crucial to proper immune system functioning..." [3]

Additionally, the packaged and processed foods that are so common in our culture are not only nutrient void; they actually rob our bodies of vital nutrients. Consequently, even a person whose primary concern is optimal nutrition may still be lacking in some of the most basic nutrients.

The following were prescribed for me and also for most participants of the Hippocrates program by Dr. Brian Clement, director of Hippocrates Health Institute.

- Apple Cider Vinegar or lemon juice in water on arising & retiring (Put 3 T in 1 qt water). This health procedure takes fat deposits out between muscles.

- Lifegive Systemic Enzymes 3 Capsules during the day before meals – formulated with proteolytic enzymes vitamin C and select botanical antioxidants that were specifically chosen for their ability to combat oxidative stress, support healthy circulation, support muscle and joint recovery after exercise and it also provides other systemic benefits.

- Lifegive Biotic Guard– 2 capsules twice daily with beverage at least 30 minutes before a meal or, 2 tablespoons of fermented vegetables such as sauerkraut with your lunch and dinner. BioticGuard contains life supporting, healthy bacteria, which populate the digestive tract and in particular the small and large intestines. This superior and powerful probiotic is a soil-based organism formula comprised of a matrix of pure food-derived probiotics and healthy bacteria from organic soil. BioticGuard repopulates intestinal flora at the highest levels, helping to revitalize digestive and eliminative function, thereby creating greater immune cell development. The primary ingredients are minerals, amino acids, FOS (derived from chicory), as well as chlorophyll and its naturally occurring antioxidants. BioticGuard is the most advanced intestinal ecological supplement available today and is a safeguard supplement for all of us living in a modern, stressful and toxic world.

- Lifegive HHI Zyme (digestive enzymes) for maximum benefit 20 during day – take at least 3. Digestive enzymes provide essential nutrients, vitamins, minerals and enzymes to enhance digestion of foods. They may help increase the electromagnetic frequency around the cell and fight off free radical damage, which is the cause of disease and aging. Contains amylase, protease, glucoamylase, invertase, malt diastase, protease, cerecalase, cellulose, lipade peptidase.

- LifeGive Chlorella – 10 (can take 3 x daily) makes blood stronger; takes away sugar cravings –Excellent source of protein that is easily digested. Also helps the body to get

---

[44]LifeGive Supplement Guide, Hippocrates Health Institute.

more out of vitamins and minerals. Helps with blood sugar regulation glycemic episodes. Detoxifies the body of Heavy Metals, Also may be helpful before and after Chemotherapy. Contains sodium, vitamin C, calcium iron, Vitamin E, Thiamine, riboflavin, niacin, vitamin B6, folate, vitamin B12, Biotin, Pantothenic acid, phosphorus, iodine, magnesium, zinc, copper, potassium, chlorophyll, RNA and the essential amino acid

- Ocean Energy B12 Probiotic 3 capsules in morning – nutrients enhance energy and endurance, increases Hemoglobin (iron levels in the blood, a blend of kelp and blue green algae, kamut (green algae)

- Phyto Turmeric 3 capsules daily, 30 min before meal at least – take with green drink – whole food turmeric with its active "curcuminoids" contains a symphony of disease inhibiting elements such as vitamins, minerals and enzymes. Each caplet contains 800 mg of pure naturally occurring standard (NOS) curcuminoids, which have been scientifically shown to enhance brain function and pack anti-cancer effects along with pro-digestive and anti-inflammatory properties.

- Sea Vegetables provide necessary minerals. Dulse kelp, arame, hijicki are 4 most common of the seventeen hundred different species. Use in everything you eat -salad dressings, salads, soups, crackers.

Vitamin B-12 Replication Suggestions[45]

This vitamin is the most controversial with some indicating that it cannot be acquired without meat sources. It is produced by bacteria so we consume it when we consume plants or animals with bacteria on them. For this reason, unwashed organic produce may contain B-12. We have B-12 producing bacteria in our bodies, but most individuals have incapacitated their system's ability to produce B-12 by modern lifestyle. The sources named below are thought by some to have small amounts of B-12.

Food Sources

- Bean sprouts
- Other sprouts (especially alfalfa, clover, sunflower and buckwheat
- Seaweed (especially kelp, dulse and nori)
- Raw sauerkraut
- Wheatgrass and barley grass
- Bee pollen
- Capsicum
- Chickweed
- Comfrey
- Dandelion
- Fenugreek
- Ginger
- Ginseng
- Hops
- Licorice
- Miso
- Peas
- Almonds
- Tempeh

These sources contain B-12 in its natural bacterial state yet much does not convert to useable B-12, so supplementation is critical.

---

[45]Ibid.

Supplement:

- Lifegive Ocean Energy (preferred since it contains B-12 grown on a food source and blue green algae)

Function:

Vitamin B-12 is needed to form blood and immune cells and support a healthy nervous system. A series of closely related compounds known collectively as *coalmines* are converted into active coenzymatic forms *methylcobalaminor 5-deoxyadenasylcobalamin.*

Sun - D, The Sunshine Vitamin[46]

Sun-D offers you a daily pure and powerful plant source of life-supporting and living Vitamin D for general health, prevents nutrient deficiencies and development of threatening health conditions, thereby enhancing optimum health. Most of us know Vitamin D as the "Sunshine Vitamin" since it is well documented that exposure of our skin (the body's largest organ) to sunlight is one of our best sources of Vitamin D. This helps our skin to synthesize Vitamin D.

A good source of vegetable Vitamin D comes from Shitake mushrooms. This may seem unintuitive since we know that many mushrooms do not get much sunlight, but some do and Shitake mushrooms do get sunlight both directly and indirectly.

Vitamin D is currently known as a pro-hormone involved in mineral metabolism and bone growth. It's most dramatic effect is to facilitate intestinal absorption of calcium, although it also stimulates absorption of phosphate and magnesium. In the absence of Vitamin D, dietary calcium is not absorbed efficiently. Vitamin D stimulates the expression of a number of proteins involved in transporting calcium for the lumen of the intestine across the epithelial cells and into the blood. So, Vitamin D is essential for the absorption and use of calcium in our bodies and for maintenance of strong bones, immune strengthening and anti-cancer support and is now known as the most important nutrient in preventing osteoporosis and in reversing depression. It is a fat-soluble vitamin that is stored in the body fat and released as required.

There are several sources of Vitamin D mainly divided into synthetic sources made chemically in labs and natural sources found naturally occurring in foods. All main forms of Vitamin D can be found naturally and synthetically. Vitamin D3 is widely accepted as the best source of naturally occurring Vitamin D. This form, known as Cholecalciferol, is the most potent for general health and specific health conditions. Studies have indicated that Vitamin D may play a role in the prevention and/or mitigation of various health conditions including the following: atherosclerosis; breast, colon & ovarian cancer; depression; epilepsy; hypertension; IBS (inflammatory bowel disease); kidney disease; liver disease; multiple sclerosis; osteoporosis; periodontal disease; preeclampsia; psoriasis; tinnitus and ulcerative colitis.

Synthetic Vitamin D like other synthetic vitamins is drug-like and is an isolated chemical which does not contain "life" or the naturally occurring supportive nutrient factors known and unknown as found in naturally occurring plant sources.

Naturally occurring Vitamin D in foods is scarce. Fresh-water algae, sea vegetables, shitake mushrooms, and edible weeds are the vegetable sources highest in naturally occurring Vitamin D.

Adequate Vitamin D is necessary for health, but consuming large quantities of synthetic Vitamin D is dangerous. According to Dr. Brian Clement, a single dose of synthetic Vitamin D of 50 mg or greater is toxic for adults. The immediate effect of an overdose of vitamin D is abdominal cramps, nausea, and vomiting. Toxic doses of Vitamin D taken with time may result in a buildup of irreversible deposits of calcium crystals in the soft tissues of the body that damage the hearts, lungs, and kidneys.

---

[46] Ibid..

Health Benefits of Plant-Based Food[47]
by Brian Clement, PhD

4.Therapeutic Sprout Juices	
•SPROUTED SEED JUICE	•BENEFITS
Alfalfa	Strengthens blood, which in turn builds strong tissue, reduces edema, and strengthens muscle and bone
Anise	Good for the respiratory and cardiovascular systems. Also enhances the development of T cells associated with the immune system.
Broccoli	High in phytonutrients. Reduces the potential for mutagenic growths, including cancer. Facilitates healthy and consistent elimination.
Cabbage	Helps to combat an irritated or inflamed digestive tract, ulcers, cancer, osteoarthritis, and osteoporosis.
Cantaloupe	Increases sperm and egg production. Regulates blood sugar, whether low or high.
Cayenne	Countervails heart attack, stroke, and deficient circulation, and benefits those who have had these conditions. Strengthens the cardio vascular and circulatory systems.
Cress	Builds blood by multiplying red blood cells, decreases toxins in the respiratory system, prevents fibroids an cysts, and acts as an anticarcinogen.
Fennel	Builds white and red blood cells, Increases digestive enzymes.

1.   [47]Clement, Brian R., PhD. Hippocrates Health Institute Lesson III-8.

4. Therapeutic Sprout Juices

Fenugreek	Fights gastrointestinal disorders. Neutralizes body odor. Normalizes blood sugar by helping to regulate both hypoglycemia and diabetes.
Garlic	Fights cancer, ulcers, and parasites. Improves the protein levels of blood cells.
Jamaica ginger	Harvested as a small, sprouted plant and then juiced. It helps to regulate the internal thermometer—including slightly elevated temperatures—to combat microbes and mutagens. It also assists in the prevention of motion sickness.
Kale	Rich in calcium and sulfur. It builds bone and acts as a digestive aid and pain reducer.
Mango	Rich in enzymes. It promotes healthy digestion and elimination. Helps build a reserve of vitamins and minerals to create healthy and stable organs.
Mustard	Relieves hemorrhoids, eliminates mucus from the respiratory system, and reduces the term of colds and flu.
Onion	Antimutagenic and anticarcinogenic. Purifies the liver, gallbladder, spleen, small intestine, and large intestine. Builds immune cells and red blood cells.
Orange	Provides powerful phytonutrients to combat viral and bacterial disease. Assists the neuronal functions of the brain.
Papaya	The high enzyme content encourages gastric, digestive, and pancreatic juices to build blood platelets and reduce external and internal scar tissue.

178

4. Therapeutic Sprout Juices

Quinoa	Harvest and juice these sprouts on the fifth day of sprouting. High protein content and low glycemic properties make this juice a super-fuel that energizes all bodily functions. Increases stamina, strength, and muscle development.
Radish	Increases digestive capability. Reduces fibroid and fibroid cystic growths. Is a powerful antimutagen and anticancer agent.
Red pepper	This juice is a powerhouse of vitamin C and effectively reduces and event prevents viral infections. Helps to prevent blood clots and strokes.
Sweet potato (sprouted leaves)	Builds healthy tissue, compensates for various nutritional deficiencies, and creates elasticity of ligaments.
Tomato	Increases metabolism and reduces excess weight. Reduces fluid in edema. Lycopene and other phytonutrients attack cancers of the prostate, breast, and colon. Combats hepatitis A, B, and C.
Uva-ursi (bearberry)	Eliminates excess mucus and resists microbial infections. It is a diuretic, astringent, mucilage, antiseptic, and disinfectant.
Xanthium (cocklebur)	This antiviral juice helps those with hepatitis A., B and C, HIV, colds, flu, SARS, and other microbial infections.
Yam (sprouted leaves)	Balances hormones and minimizes the effects of PMS, menopause, mood swings, and low sex drive.
Yucca root (sprouted leaves)	Elevates endurance and energy levels and stimulates the immune function of glycosides to combat all forms of disease.

Therapeutic Vegetable Juices

VEGETABLE JUICE	BENEFITS
Asparagus	Assists renal function, neutralizes kidney stones and bladder stones, and regulates urinary flow.
Artichoke	Enhances the functioning of digestive, immune, and renal systems.
Beet	Consumed in small quantities, it is a blood purifier and blood strengthener. Reduces varicose veins and cleanses arteries and the cardiovascular system.
Brussels Sprouts	Contains a protein that helps generate insulin, thereby improving pancreatic function and combating digestive disorders.
Cauliflower	Improves the functioning of skeletal, digestive, and elimination systems.
Celery	Facilitates dermal detoxification and circulation. Reduces uric acid. Improves electrolyte function. Detoxifies the system of the effects of nicotine and caffeine. Promotes dermal flexibility. Provides organic sodium.
Cucumber	Benefits respiratory, renal, joint, and ligament functioning. Increases dermal elasticity/
Daikon radish	Acts as a blood thinner. Maintains electromagnetic functioning of the solar plexus.
Dandelion	Creates red blood cells. Strengthens gums and teeth. Assists healthy bone development (skeletal and dental).
Endive	Improves vision and reduces the potential for and the severity of cataracts. Creates strong ventricular tissue.

Therapeutic Vegetable Juices

Horseradish	Consumed in small amounts, removes excess mucus. Diuretic. Helps to counteract colds and flu.
Iris flower	Builds ligaments, tendons, and cartilage. Strengthens joints and improves membrane development.
Jerusalem artichoke	Stabilizes blood sugar disorders. Generate energy.
Leek	Anticarcinogenic and antimutagenic. Prevents ulcers and inhibits parasites.
Lettuce	A subtle aphrodisiac and mood enhancer. Helps restore hair and skin.
Lily flower	Builds capillaries. Strengthens vision and hearing. Assists the H cell development of the immune system.
Nasturtium	Builds the immune system, fighter cells, and eosinophils. Purifies the lymphatic system and the bloodstream.
Parsley	Minimizes the pain of menstrual cramps. Fights coronary disease, cataracts, conjunctivitis, and glaucoma. Improves vision, cardiovascular functioning, and blood count.
Pepper (ripe red, yellow, purple)	Reduces bloating, flatulence, colitis, and colic. Rich in vitamin C. Strengthens metabolism, specifically of the heart, and reduces the risk of microbial infection.
Potato (white)	High mineral content, especially potassium, assists renal and cardiovascular function. Effective against arthritic and osteoporotic conditions.

Therapeutic Vegetable Juices

Sauerkraut (raw)	Improves dermal elasticity and appearance. Cleanses and builds the digestive organs. Enhances the probiotics in the gastrointestinal tract, which in turn strengthen immune cells.
Sorrel	Enhances healthy skeletal and dermal development. Creates greater bone density in the lower extremities.
Spinach	Prevents anemia, convulsions, neuronal disorders, and adrenal dysfunction. Builds red blood cells to cleanse the liver, thereby improving immune function.
String bean (green, purple, yellow)	Regulates blood sugar (in both diabetes and hypoglycemia) by insulin stimulation. Develops proteinase (protein-digesting enzymes).
Tomato	Contains minimal amounts of lycopene. Although it is effective in the reduction of prostrate breast, and colon cancers, and in combating hepatitis A, B, and C, it is less effective than tomato seed sprout juice. Detoxifies the liver and gallbladder
Turnip greens	Consumed in small quantities, builds bones, facilitates digestion, and prevents colon polyps and hemorrhoids.
Violet flower	Consumed in small quantities, stimulates the spleen and assists in the production of healthy red blood cells, fingernails, and toenails.
Watercress	Consumed in small amounts, increases hemoglobin to prevent anemia and chronic low blood pressure. Strengthens joints, cartilage, tendons, and ligaments. Helps to reduce tumors by improving circulation.

Therapeutic Vegetable Juices

Yellow squash	Packed with bone-building minerals. Acts as a diuretic and relieves constipation.

Sprouts and Their Health Benefits

TYPE OF SPROUT	1.HEALTH BENEFITS
Apple and Apricot	Apple and apricot seeds contain high levels of abscisic acid, a plant hormone and anticancer agent. Scientific evidence indicates that sprouted apple and apricot seeds assist in recover from all forms of cancer.
Broccoli	Cruciferous vegetables contain a phytonutrient that inhibits the development of cancer. Sprouted broccoli seeds are several dozen times more effective in combating cancer than other vegetables in this family.
Butternut squash	Dried butternut squash seeds germinated in soil produce a succulent green plant (similar to sunflower sprouts) containing nutrients that build the blood an help balance the heart. Cardiovascular problems may be neutralized by the consumption of butternut squash sprouts and sprouts from other members of the winter squash family in conjunction with a health-supporting lifestyle.
Cabbage	Cabbage sprouts contain anticancer phytochemicals and help battle ulcers and digestive disorders.
Carrot	Carrot tops and sprouted carrot greens are excellent sources of beta-carotene, which benefits vision, healthy pigmentation, and blood purification.

Sprouts and Their Health Benefits

Daikon	The sprouts of the Asian daikon radish yield benefits, unique to the radish family, which include purifying blood, improving circulation, and deterring the development of tumors.
Dill	The consumption of sprouted dill seeds alleviates menstrual problems and helps stabilize blood pressure.
Eucalyptus	Eucalyptus sprouts are very powerful and help combat respiratory and pigment-related disorders.
Fennel	Fennel's ability to build red blood cells and purify the body help to combat clotting problems and breathing disorders.
Fenugreek	Fenugreek sprouts, the heartiest of all sprouts, yield a medicinal gel that helps combat diabetes, digestive disorders and even body odor.
Garlic	Garlic, a member of the lily family, produces the most antimutagenic, antifungal, and antimicrobial sprout. Its mutagen-fighting capacity is equaled only by that of onions.
Gourds	Conventionally used as seasonal decorations, gourds contain seeds that, when sprouted, produce powerful and positive effects on the body's nervous system and skeletal structure.
Hops	Sprouted hops have a calming effect; they also facilitate the neuron activity of the brain.
Impatiens	The seed of this edible flower produce sprouts that benefit hair and improve vision.

Sprouts and Their Health Benefits

Jamaica ginger	When this root is planted in organically fertilized soil and watered daily, it sprouts a stalk, which should be consumed before it reaches two inches in height It helps regulate our internal body temperature to combat microbes and mutagens. It also assists in the prevention of motion sickness.
Jojoba	The sprouted sees of the fruit of this relatively rare member of the cactus family provide fatty acids for brain tissue development and optimal cardiovascular function; they also help stimulate the immune system's T cells.
Kale	Kale is part of the cruciferous family of vegetables; its significant sulfur and phytonutrient content facilitate cellular function, skeletal repair, and the prevention of cancer.
Kava	Kava seed sprouts help relieve depression without any harmful effect on the liver.
Leeks	Sprouted leeks, which are part of the onion family, benefit the body's respiration, hearing, and glands.
Lima beans	Lima bean sprouts help sustain maximum functioning of the pancreas and kidneys; they also assist in warming the body as necessary.
Mango	The seed within the mango can be dried, placed into soil, and watered twice daily to start the birth of a mango tree. However, to be used as a beneficial sprout, it should be cut and consumed before it reaches two inches in height. The extraordinary enzyme activity in this tropical seed assists weight regulation and cholesterol reduction and inhibits gallbladder malfunction.

Sprouts and Their Health Benefits

Mung beans	Mung bean sprouts (Chinese bean sprouts) are the most easily digestible food; there potent content of zinc, other minerals, and digestible proteins can help prevent prostate problems, glandular dysfunction, and breast cancer, as well as premature balding and graying.
Nettle	The seed of the stinging nettle develops by midsummer, and it can be easily found throughout much of the world. Sprouted mettle seeds are among the finest blood purifiers and blood builders in the world of germinated foods.
Nuts	All raw nuts can be sprouted, although you should not sprout or consume peanuts or cashews because they are toxic. For walnuts and pecans, after a lengthy soaking, place the nuts in soil and water them regularly. East the shoots before thy reach two inches in height. Almonds, hazelnuts, macadamias, pine nuts, and pistachios require overnight soaking. Afterward, place them on an unbleached paper towel, and spray them with pure water at least twice daily. They will be ready to harvest and eat around the third day. All these sprouted nuts, which are rich in protein and essential fatty acids, strengthen the cells, build muscle structure, and sustain the heart.
Onion	Like garlic sprouts, onion sprouts area among the best anticancer foods; they also remove and emulsify pollutants in the organs and circulatory systems,

Sprouts and Their Health Benefits

Orange	When dried and sprouted for three days, orange seed sprouts function as an astringent, assisting the removal of bacteria while simultaneously helping white blood cells to cleanse debris from the bloodstream.
Oregano	When sprouted, oregano seeds are among the most effective antifungal and antiyeast foods available.
Peas	Pea sprouts, which should be grown on soil for five days, help to build muscle, strengthen teeth, and stimulant H cells.
Poppy seeds	Poppy seeds should be soaked for six hours, then placed on unbleached paper towels and sprayed with pure water at least three times a day. Harvest and eat them on the fourth or fifth day. They are a powerful relaxant and a mood-enhancing food
Quinoa	The prominent protein content and low glycemic properties of quinoa sprouts make them a super-fuel that energizes all bodily functions, increasing stamina and strength. Quinoa sprouts should be harvested in two days.
Radish	Radish sprouts—which are different from daikon sprouts—facilitate digestion, elimination and blood cleansing, and they are antimutagenic.
Rye	Rye seed sprouts are beneficial in several ways: they strengthen the liver and gallbladder, boost energy, and increase sexual potency.
Sesame	Sesame seeds maintain excellent hair, teeth, and bone. These powerful seeds should be soaked for six hours, placed on an unbleached paper towel, sprayed with pure water at least three times per day, and harvested on the fourth day.

Sprouts and Their Health Benefits

Spruce cone	Spruce cone sprouts are created by placing the cone into rich soil, watering it twice a day with warm water, and waiting for the arrival of the baby sprout of the spruce tree. Harvest the sprouts before they are three inches long. Spruce cone sprouts are unique in their ability to strengthen the lungs and enhance brain function.
Sunflower seeds	Sunflower sprouts may be grown on soil or hydroponically in nutritionally enriched pure water for seven days. These sprouts are essential to the Hippocrates Program. They are considered the most balanced of all of the sources of essential amino acids, and they are a perfect source of complete protein. They activate every cell in the immune system, and they build the skeletal, muscular, and neurological systems.
Teff	Teff is a staple of the Ethiopian diet. The sprouts benefit the ventricular, endocrine, and cardiovascular systems.
Tomato	Tomato seed sprouts are remarkable because of their significant phytochemical content. They combat glandular disorders, prostate problems and breast-related concerns, including cancers.
Uva-ursi (bearberry)	This fascinating plant, a small evergreen shrub, is often called the "upland cranberry." Its seed, dried and then sprouted for three days, is a diuretic, astringent, mucilage, antiseptic, and disinfectant.
Valerian	Valerian sprouts should be consumed in small amounts, as they fuel the nervous system. They can benefit those who suffer from insomnia and should only be consumed before rest or sleep.

Sprouts and Their Health Benefits	
Violet flower	Easting violet flower seed sprouts benefits the cardiovascular system and vision, and facilitates neuron activity in the brain.
Water chestnut	Water chestnut is a root-like herb. Planted in soil and watered twice a day, it produces a plant that should be harvested when the attached sprout extending from it is no more than one inch long. It should then be washed and either juiced or sliced into a raw salad. Its ability to strengthen the lungs and kidneys makes it a desirable and delicious part of the diet.
Wild yam	Yam—also known as "China root and rheumatism root"—can be planted in soil and watered twice daily to create a sprouted vine. Clip and eat once inch of this sprout. It improves hormone balance and is especially useful for regulating progesterone, estrogen, and DHA. It also eases the functioning of the stomach and bowels, especially when they are inflamed.
Xanthium (cocklebur)	Xanthium is an herb that grows in china, Japan, Korea, Taiwan, and various parts of Europe. Its roots, stems, hairy leaves, and fruits are used in traditional Asian medicine to combat the common cold, headaches, German measles, and other diseases and illnesses. Use the dried seed and sprout it for three days.

Sprouts and Their Health Benefits

Yucca root	Yucca is a starchy root vegetable that should be planted in rich soil and watered twice a day. It will then sprout a green plant that should be harvested before it is three inches tall. The sprouts help elevate endurance and energy levels and stimulate leukocytes (white blood cells), which is an important immune function in the battle against all forms of disease.

• Whole Food Sources of Vitamins

• CHOLINE

BEST SOURCES: broccoli sprouts, cauliflower, grapes, onion sprouts, ripe tomatoes

MAJOR SYMPTOMS OR DEFICIENCY	MAJOR SYMPTOMS OF TOXICITY
impaired lung functioning	enlargement of the liver and spleen, anemia, increasing physical and mental degeneration

• FOLATE Folic acid

BEST SOURCES: beet root greens, broccoli sprouts, lettuce (all kinds), sprouted black-eyed peas, sprouted chickpeas

MAJOR SYMPTOMS OR DEFICIENCY	MAJOR SYMPTOMS OF TOXICITY
miscarriage, complications of pregnancy, birth defects, neurological malfunction, heart disease	renal toxicity causing kidney enlargement and possible kidney failure

•VITAMIN A beta-carotene; retinol

BEST SOURCES: chia sprouts, cruciferous vegetables, green leafy vegetables, sea vegetables, sunflower green sprouts (Supplemental vitamin A should be consumed as beta-carotene, which is a precursor of vitamin A.)

MAJOR SYMPTOMS OR DEFICIENCY	MAJOR SYMPTOMS OF TOXICITY
night blindness, dryness of various parts of the eye, blindness	liver damage, irritability, weakness, diminished menstrual bleeding, psychiatric disorders

• Whole Food Sources of Vitamins

VITAMIN B_1 thiamin; thiamine

BEST SOURCES: wheatgrass, raw sauerkraut, sprouted corn, sprouted sweet potatoes, sprouted peas

MAJOR SYMPTOMS OR DEFICIENCY	MAJOR SYMPTOMS OF TOXICITY
beriberi, headaches, irritability, fatigue, lethargy, neurological diseases	allergic reactions

VITAMIN B_2 riboflavin (formerly cited as vitamin G)

BEST SOURCES: buckwheat green sprouts, cabbage sprouts, corn sprouts, kamut grass

MAJOR SYMPTOMS OR DEFICIENCY	MAJOR SYMPTOMS OF TOXICITY
soreness of the mouth and tongue, skin and genital rashes, neuropathy, anemia	possible increase of tumor growth and related complications

VITAMIN B_3 niacin; nicotinamide; nicotinic acid

BEST SOURCES: dulse, kelp, spelt and kamut grasses, sprouted wheat

MAJOR SYMPTOMS OR DEFICIENCY	MAJOR SYMPTOMS OF TOXICITY
circulatory and cardiovascular disease	burning, itching, headache, nausea, vomiting, duodenal ulcers, liver failure

VITAMIN B_5 pantothenic acid; calcium pantothenate

BEST SOURCES: avocado, apricot seeds, organic apples, pecans, sprouted sesame seeds

MAJOR SYMPTOMS OR DEFICIENCY	MAJOR SYMPTOMS OF TOXICITY
Respiratory infection, fatigue, cardiac irregularities, gastrointestinal complications, rashes, staggering, muscle cramps, disorientation	Diarrhea, water retention

VITAMIN B_6 pyridoxine; pyridoxal; pyridoxamine

BEST SOURCES: brussel sprouts, cabbage sprouts, sprouted mango seed, sprouted sweet potatoes, wheatgrass

MAJOR SYMPTOMS OR DEFICIENCY	MAJOR SYMPTOMS OF TOXICITY

• Whole Food Sources of Vitamins

rashes, seizures, carpal tunnel syndrome, anemia	Unsteadiness, muscle weakness, systemic weakness

VITAMIN B₁₂ (considered a probiotic) cobalamin; cyanocobalamin; hydroxocobalmin

BEST SOURCES: there are no reliable food sources of vitamin B_{12}; supplementation is necessary

MAJOR SYMPTOMS OR DEFICIENCY	MAJOR SYMPTOMS OF TOXICITY
pernicious anemia (which sometimes causes unpleasant internal electrical impulses permeating the lips, nose, and extremities), susceptibility to colds and other infections, bruising, impaired blood clotting	allergic reactions; rashes

VITAMIN C

BEST SOURCES: black currants, broccoli, cauliflower, kiwifruit, sprouted papaya seed

MAJOR SYMPTOMS OR DEFICIENCY	MAJOR SYMPTOMS OF TOXICITY
scurvy and its symptoms (primarily spontaneous bleeding), edema and wounds that do not heal, cardiovascular disease, cancer	excessive urination, kidney stones

VITAMIN D

BEST SOURCES: arame, blue-green algae, clover sprouts, olives, sprouted pinto beans

MAJOR SYMPTOMS OR DEFICIENCY	MAJOR SYMPTOMS OF TOXICITY
impaired vision, dermal impairment (causing blotches, lack of tautness, and weakness of the skin, hair, and nails)	Anemia, weakness, loss of appetite, vomiting, diarrhea, kidney failure, death

VITAMIN E

BEST SOURCES: avocado, sprouted almonds, sprouted hazelnuts, sprouted pine nuts, sunflower green sprouts

MAJOR SYMPTOMS OR DEFICIENCY	MAJOR SYMPTOMS OF TOXICITY

• Whole Food Sources of Vitamins

anemia, degeneration of the spinal cord and peripheral nerves, weakness	nausea, flatulence, diarrhea, allergic contact dermatitis

VITAMIN H biotin

BEST SOURCES: hemp seeds, raw sesame tahini, sprouted almonds, sprouted hazelnuts, walnuts

MAJOR SYMPTOMS OR DEFICIENCY	MAJOR SYMPTOMS OF TOXICITY
disorientation, tremors, loss of memory, speech impairment, unsteady gain, restless legs syndrome	Cartilage erosion

VITAMIN K

BEST SOURCES: alfalfa sprouts, broccoli sprouts, cabbage sprouts, kale, sea kelp

MAJOR SYMPTOMS OR DEFICIENCY	MAJOR SYMPTOMS OF TOXICITY
blood dilution	blood clotting

•Selected List of Medicinal Herbs

1. MEDICINAL HERBS	P.. BEST SOURCES	1. ATTRIBUTED MEDICINAL RELIEF
Angelica	fresh root, leaf	respiratory, bronchial, antiviral
Basil	fresh leaf	mild sedative, antiseptic, relieves nausea
Catnip	fresh leaf	colds, catarrh, bronchitis
Dandelion	fresh root, leaf	liver maintenance, diuretic, laxative, juice combats warts
Elder	root, stem, leaf	coughs, catarrh, rheumatism, sciatica, combats cysts
Feverfew	complete plant	headaches, migraines, natural insect repellant
Geranium	plant or flower	cardiovascular benefits

·Selected List of Medicinal Herbs

Horseradish	root	benefits lungs and circulation, blood cleanser
Iris	fresh flower	ligaments, tendons, joints, cartilage, membrane development
Juniper	berry, leaf	digestion, renal function, blood cleanser
Kohlrabi	root, stem, leaf	antimutagenic, ulcers, digestion
Lavender	flower, leaf	antiseptic, equilibrium, rheumatism, relaxant
Marigold	stem, flower	heals wounds, conjunctivitis, bee and wasp stings
Nettle	root, stem, leaf	arthritis, internal bleeding, skin conditions, detoxification
Orris	root, leaf	throat infection, bladder problems
Pennyroyal	stem, leaf, flower	flatulence, nausea, headaches
Quinoa	root, plant	builds red blood cells, strengthens neurological system
Rue	seed, root, leaf, stem, flower	epilepsy, eczema, psoriasis, ointment for eyes and throat
Sorrel	stem, leaf	diuretic, kidney tonic
Tarragon	stem, leaf	toothache, antimutagenic
Uva-ursi (bearberry)	root, leaf	backache, bladder congestion, renal congestion, prostate, gonorrhea, syphilis
Valerian	root, stem, leaf	sedative, tranquilizer, insomnia, nerve disorders

Selected List of Medicinal Herbs

Wallflower	stem, leaf	cardiovascular functioning, arterial elasticity
Xanthium (cocklebur)	seed	hepatitis, colds, flu, SARS, other microbial infections
Yarrow	stem, leaf flower	diarrhea, dysentery, astringent
Zingiber	root	combats microbes and mutagens, controls elevated temperature, prevents motion sickness

Herbal Life Force Energy Class Presentation[48]
by Susan Comeau

WHAT IS AN HERB?

Medicinally, an herb is any plant part or plant used for its therapeutic value. Yet, many of the world's herbal traditions also include mineral and animal substances as "herbal medicines"? An herb used for medicinal value has several levels of interaction. First, an herb is known for its action, or its affect on the body. Examples are, stimulates increase energy. Many herbs have multiple actions and act differently when combined with other herbs. This is one of the basic levels to learn about an herb use. There are many other levels of an herb to learn, starting with the energetic or vibration properties, the spiritual impacts as well as magical qualities of the herb.

HOW ARE HERBS DIFFERENT FROM PHARMACEUTICALS?

Most pharmaceutical drugs are single chemical entities that are highly refined and purified and are often synthesized. In 1987 about 85 percent of modern drugs were originally derived from plants. Currently, only about 15 percent of drugs are derived from plants. In contrast, herbal medicines are prepared from living or dried plants and contain hundreds to thousands of interrelated compounds. Science is beginning to demonstrate that the safety and effectiveness of herbs is often related to the synergy of its many constituents.

HOW IS HERBAL MEDICINE DIFFERENT FROM CONVENTIONAL MEDICINE?

The primary focus of the herbalist is to treat people as individuals regardless of the disease or condition they have and to stimulate their innate healing power through the use of such interventions as herbs, diet and lifestyle. The primary focus of conventional physicians is to attack diseases using strong chemicals that are difficult for the body to process, or through the removal of organs. Not only does this ignore the unique makeup of the individual, but many patients under conventional care suffer from side effects that are as bad as the condition being treated. The philosophical difference between herbalists and conventional physicians has profound significance. Herbalist look at healing holistically, they look at the whole person and combined experiences, to find the trigger for the symptoms that are presented where as conventional medicine treat the symptoms of the disease.

WHAT IS AN HERBALIST?

Herbalists are people who dedicate their lives to working with medicinal plants. They include native healers, scientists, naturopaths, holistic medical doctors, researchers, writers, herbal pharmacists, medicine makers, wild crafters, harvesters and herbal farmers to name a few. While herbalists are quite varied, the common love and respect for life, especially the relationship between plants and humans, unites them. Persons specializing in the therapeutic use of plants may be medical herbalists, traditional herbalists, acupuncturists, midwives, naturopathic physicians, or even one's own grandmother.

---

[48]Comeau, Sue F. Herbal Life Force Energy Class Presentation.October, 2011.

HOW CAN HERBS AND HERBAL MEDICINE HELP ME?

Herbs can offer you a wide range of safe and effective therapeutic agents that you can use as an integral part of your own health care program. They can be used in three essential ways:

1) To prevent disease

2) To treat disease

3) To maximize one's health potential.

Herbs are also used for the symptomatic relief of minor ailments.

HOW CAN I KNOW IF A PARTICULAR HERB WILL WORK FOR ME?

Medicine is an art, not just a science. No one can predict which herb will work best for every individual in all situations. This can only come with educated self-experimentation and experience or by seeking the assistance of those who are knowledgeable in clinical herbal medicine. The simpler the condition, the easier it is to find a solution. The more complicated the condition, the greater the need there is to seek expert advice.

HOW LONG DOES IT TAKE FOR HERBS TO BE EFFECTIVE?

The success of herbal treatment always depends upon a variety of factors including how long the condition has existed, the severity of the condition, the dosage and mode of administration of the herb(s) and how diligently treatment plans are followed. It can be as short as 60 seconds when using a spoonful of herbal bitters for gas and bloating after a heavy meal; 20 minutes when soaking in a bath with rosemary tea for a headache; days when using tonics to build energy; or months to correct long-standing gynecological imbalances. Difficult chronic conditions can often take years to reverse.

HOW SAFE ARE HERBS?

It depends on the herbs. Most herbs sold as dietary supplements are very safe. When used appropriately, the majority of herbs used by practitioners have no adverse side effects. A review of the traditional and scientific literature worldwide demonstrates that serious side effects from the use of herbal medicines are rare. In fact, of all classes of substances reported to cause toxicities of sufficient magnitude to be reported in the United States, plants are the least problematic."?

HOW IS THE HERBAL INDUSTRY REGULATED?

The Federal Trade Commission (FTC) primarily regulates the marketing and advertising of products. The Food and Drug Administration (FDA) primarily regulates the manufacture and labeling of herbal products and has legal authority over assuring that products are manufactured correctly and are truthfully labeled with respect to ingredients and claims. Additionally, there are a number of trade associations that require member companies to adhere to specific codes of ethics and conduct their own testing programs.

HOW DO HERBALISTS PRACTICE?

Herbalists can practice either as primary health care providers or adjunctive health care consultants. Most visits to an herbalist begin with a consultation about your past and current health history, your dietary and lifestyle practices, or other factors related to your health issue. The herbalist, with your involvement, should develop an integrated herbal program that addresses your specific health needs and concerns. You should be treated as a whole person, not as a disease.

ARE THERE DIFFERENT APPROACHES TO USING HERBS?

Various herbal traditions have developed worldwide. In the West there are a number of different traditions which include folkloric herbal practices, clinical western herbal medicine, naturopathic medicine, practitioners of Ayurveda or Chinese medicine and numerous Native American herbal traditions. Some practitioners use highly developed systems of diagnosis and treatment while others base their treatments on individual knowledge and experience. Every person must find the herbal practitioner that is most appropriate for them.

Types of Medicines used by Herbalists

1. Tinctures - Alcoholic extracts of herbs such as Echinacea extract. Usually obtained by combining 100 percent pure ethanol (or a mixture of 100 percent ethanol with water) with the herb. A completed tincture has an ethanol percentage of at least 25 percent (sometimes up to 90 percent). The term tincture is sometimes applied to preparations using other solvents than ethanol.

2. Herbal wine and elixirs - These are alcoholic extract of herbs; usually with an ethanol percentage of 12-38 percent .Herbal wine is a maceration of herbs in wine, while an elixir is a maceration of herbs in spirits (e.g., vodka, grappa, etc.)

3. Tisanes - Hot water extracts of herb, such as chamomile.

4. Decoctions - Long-term boiled extract of usually roots or bark.

5. Macerates - Cold infusion of plants with high mucilage-content as sage, thyme, etc. Plants are chopped and added to cold water. They are then left to stand for 7 to 12 hours (depending on herb used). For most macerates 10 hours is used.[68]

6. Vinegars - Prepared at the same way as tinctures, except using a solution of acetic acid as the solvent.

7. Capsules-Powered herbs encapsulated for ease of administration

8. Topical:

- Essential oils - Application of essential oil extracts, usually diluted in a carrier oil (many essential oils can burn the skin or are simply too high dose used straight – diluting in olive oil or another food grade oil such as almond oil can allow these to be used safely as a topical).[69]

- Salves, oils, balms, cream and lotions - Most topical applications are oil extractions of herbs. Taking a food grade oil and soaking herbs in it for anywhere from weeks to months allows certain photochemical to be extracted into the oil. This oil can then be made into salves, creams, lotions, or simply used as oil for topical application. Any massage oils, antibacterial salves and wound healing compounds are made this way.

- Poultices and compresses - One can also make a poultice or compress using whole herb (or the appropriate part of the plant) usually crushed or dried and re-hydrated with a small amount of water and then applied directly in a bandage, cloth or just as is.

1. Whole herb consumption - This can occur in either dried form (herbal powder), or fresh juice, (fresh leaves and other plant parts

2. Syrups - Extracts of herbs made with syrup or honey. Sixty five parts of sugar are mixed with 35 parts of water and herb. The whole is then boiled and macerated for three weeks.

3. Extracts - Include liquid extracts, and dry extracts. Liquid extracts are liquids with a lower ethanol percentage than tinctures. They can (and are usually) made by vacuum distilling tincture.

Some Kitchen Herbs Used by Class Members

Basil

(Octimum basilicum)

Common Names: Common basil, St Josephwort, sweet basil

Medicinal Part: The herb, leaves and stems

Description: Basil is an annual plant found wild in the tropical and sub-tropical regions of the world: elsewhere it is cultivated as a kitchen herb. Its thin, branching root produces busy stems growing one to two feet high and bearing opposite, ovate, entire toothed leaves which are often purplish, hued.

Properties and Uses: Antispasmodic, stomachic, carminative, and galactagogue. Basil's usefulness is generally associated with the stomach and its related organs. It can be used for stomach cramps, vomiting, and constipation. As an antispasmodic, it has sometimes been used for whooping cough. Basil has also been recommended for headache.

Preparation and Dosage: Steep 1 tsp. dried herb in ½ cup water, for 10 minutes. Take 1 to 1 ½ cups a day, a mouthful at a time. Can be sweetened with honey for cough

Bay Leaf

(Laurus nobilis)

Common Names: Sweet Bay, Victors' Laurel

Medicinal Part: Leaves, berries, seed

Properties and Uses: Antiseptic, Antifungal, gastric tonic, stomachic, nutritive, mild sedative. Bay Leaf oil is anti-dandruff, carminative, cholagogue and vermifuge. Used for weak digestion, poor appetite, hot and soothing to a cold stomach, use for urinary infections, decocted, for chest infections, use berries, use seeds for rheumatic pains (only externally)

Preparation and Dosage: Decoction –1 ounce of crushed leaves to one pint of water simmered down to three-quarters of its volume. Dosage is a half cup three times a day.

Bay Bath-place crushed leaves in a small muslin bag, and put in 2 quarts of water and bring to boil, simmer for 15-20 minutes and add to bath.

Diet-taken as a culinary herb with potatoes, salads, soups, stews, etc.

Cardamom

(Elettaria cardamomum)

Common Names: Bastard cardamom, cardamom seeds, Malabar cardamom

Medicinal Part: Seed

Description: Cardamom is a perennial plant found commonly in southern India but also cultivated in other tropical areas. The simple, erect stems grow to a height of 6-10 feet. The leaves are lanceolate, dark green and glabrous above, lighter and silky beneath. The small, yellowish flowers grow in loose racemes on prostate flower stems. The fruit is a three-celled capsule holding up to 18 seeds.

Properties and Uses: Appetizer (loss of appetite), stomachic, carminative, stimulant, warm and soothing to stomach, colic and flatulence. Cardamom seeds are useful for flatulence, but they are usually used as adjuvants with other remedies. They are also used as a spice in cooking and as a flavoring in other medicines.

Preparation and Dosage: As a tea, crush seeds in a pestle and mortar. 1 tsp to one cup of water; bring to boil; remove from heat when it boils, infuse for 10-15 minutes. Dose-1/2 to 1 cup. As a tincture, ½ tsp, or 3-4 drops in honey after meals promotes digestion, and removes odors of garlic, onions

Cayenne

(capsicum frutescens)

Common Names: American pepper, chili pepper, Spanish pepper

Medicinal Part: Fruit

Description: Cayenne is a perennial plant in its native tropical America but is an annual when cultivated outside tropical zones. Growing to a height of three feet or more, it stem is woody at the bottom and branched near the top. The drooping white to yellow flowers grows alone or in pairs between April and September. The ripe fruit or pepper is a many seed pod with a leathery outside in various shades of red or yellow.

Properties and Uses: Appetizer, digestive, irritant, Sialagogue, stimulant and tonic. In powder form cayenne is used as a stimulant to build up resistance at the beginning of a cold. It can also be taken as an infusion for stomach and bowel pains or cramps. The fresh fruit stimulates appetite. For external use, cayenne is made into plasters or liniment or the tincture and applied to increase blood flow to areas of rheumatism, and arthritis.

Preparation and Dosage: Use ½ to 1 tsp. pepper per cup of boiling water. Take warm, 1 tablespoon as a time. Take in powder form for acute conditions, take 2-3 capsules, for chronic conditions, 1-3 capsules.

Chives

(Allium schoenoprasum)

Medicinal Part: Leaves

Description: Chive is a widespread perennial plant, both cultivated and wild. It grows to a height of 8-12 inches. The leaves are hollow, cylindrical, closed at the top and dilated to surround the stem at the bottom. It flowers in June and July, with purple global flowers.

Properties and Uses: Appetizer, digestive. Chives help to stimulate appetite and to promote the digestive processes.

Preparation and Dosage: Always use fresh, and avoid heating. The common method is to cut and sprinkle over your food just prior to serving

Coriander

(Coriandrum sativum)

Medicinal Part: Seed

Description: Coriander is a small annual plant that has been cultivated for thousands of years and is still grown in North and South America, Europe and the Mediterranean area. From June to August the white to reddish flowers appear. The brownish, globes seeds have a disagreeable smell until they ripen, when they take on a spicy aroma.

Properties and Uses: Antispasmodic, appetizer, aromatic, carminative, stomachic. Coriander can also be applied externally for rheumatism and painful joints. Coriander also improves the flavor of other medicinal preparations.

Preparation and Dosage: Steep 2 tsp. dried seeds in 1 cup of water. Take 1 cup a day. Powder take ¼ to ½ tsp at a time.

Dill

(Anethum graveolens)

Common Names: Dilly, and garden dill

Medicinal Part: Fruit

Description: Dill is an annual plant widely cultivated as a spice but also found growing in North and South America and in Europe.

Properties and Uses: Antispasmodic, calmative, diuretic, galactagogue, stomachic. Dill tea, made with water or white wine, is a popular remedy for upset stomach. Dill also helps to stimulate appetite, and decoction of the seed may be helpful for insomnia as well as for pains due to flatulence. Nursing mothers can use dill to promote the flow of milk, particularly in combination with anise, coriander, fennel and caraway. Try chewing the seeds for bad breath.

Preparation and Dosage: Steep 2 tsp, seed in 1 cup of water for 10-15 minutes. Take ½ cup at a time, 1-2 cups a day.

Mint

(Mentha spicata)

Common Names: Spearmint, lamb mint

Medicinal Part: The herb

Description: Spearmint is a perennial plant found in wet and moist soil in temperate climates. The plant grows 2-3 feet high, with aromatic leaves.

Properties and Uses: Antispasmodic, carminative, diuretic, stimulant and stomachic. Spearmint shares many of the uses described under peppermint

Sage

(Salvia officinalis)

Common Names: Garden sage

Medicinal Part: Leaves

Description: Sage is a shrubby perennial plant which grows wild in southern Europe and the Mediterranean countries and is commonly cultivated elsewhere as a kitchen spice. A strongly branched root system produces square, finely hairy stems which are woody at the base and bear opposite, downy, oblong leaves. Purple, blue, or white two-tipped flowers grow in whorls. Flowering time is June and July.

Properties and Uses: Antihydrotic, antispasmodic, astringent. Sage is best known effect is the reduction of perspiration, which usually begins about two hours after taking sage tea or tincture and may last for several days. This property makes it useful for night sweats, such as those common with tuberculosis. A nursing mother whose child has been weaned can take sage tea for a few days to help stop the flow of milk. The tea has also been prescribed for nervous conditions, trembling, depression, and vertigo. As an astringent, it can be used for diarrhea, and gastritis. As a gargle, the tea can be used for sore throat, laryngitis and tonsillitis. It also helps to eliminate mucous congestion in the respiratory passages and the stomach. Finally crushed fresh sage leaves can be used as a first aid for insect bites.

Preparation and Dosage: Use leaves collected before flowering, more medicinal live force in leaves before flowering, life force of plant moves to flowers then seeds. Steep 1 tsp. leaves in ½ cup water for 30 minutes. Take 1 cup a day, a tablespoon at a time. Tincture, take 15-40 drops 3-4 times a day.

Summary Questions:

1. What is an enzyme?

2. Why are enzymes important?

3. Why are supplements necessary?

4. How do phytochemicals contribute to our health?

5. What is the major difference between synthetic vitamins and plant-based vitamins?

6. What are some examples of the health benefits of plant-based foods?

7. What are some examples of the health benefits of using herbs?

We are deeply saddened by the sudden accidental death of Sue Comeau in January 2012; Sue was much loved by me and her fellow classmates and as an intern of the September 2011 Life Force Energy class. She is greatly missed. Her husband gives permission to reprint her article.

DVD - Hippocrates "Supplements" Q & A

1. Who was Dr. Lee and why was he important?

2. What does bio-active mean?

3. What does "HOPE" stand for?

4. What brought about the birth of chemical supplements?

5. What problems arose with the birth of chemical supplements?

6. What affect did bio-active supplements have in the Hippocrates study of an ill population?

7. What are the four legs of the table of health?

8. Why take whole food supplements even if well?

9. What was the result of the 2-year Hippocrates study on use of taking bio-active supplements with both the well and the ill population?

10. What supplement should everyone take? Name 2 kinds of this supplement.

11. How does it protect our DNA?

Chapter 8
Holistic Medicine

Overview

More and more people are taking responsibility for their health, and, therefore, are turning to alternative forms of treatment. These treatments are used in conjunction with traditional medicine. In this chapter we will examine the role living food nutrition takes in the healing process.

Holistic medicine encompasses a number of therapies, all basically using the same principles, promoting not only physical health, but also mental, emotional, and spiritual health. Quality nutrition is also a high priority. Processed foods found in the standard American diet contain chemical additives and preservatives, are high in fat, cholesterol, and sugars, and promote disease. Alternative nutritionists recommend natural organic fruits and vegetables whenever possible while minimizing animal products including dairy and eggs. In fact, it is common for many alternative practitioners to promote vegetarianism to detoxify the body.

The goal of holistic medicine is to harmonize all the areas in an individual's life. Self-responsibility, obviously, is key. The practice of holistic medicine does not rule out the practice of allopathic medicine; the two can complement each other.

The optimal holistic health regimen can safely and often completely eliminate even acute health conditions. Relying on holistic health is often superior because it is not an invasive procedure nor does it employ pharmaceuticals. Also, it treats the source of the illness rather than the symptoms; it's preventative.

Here are some of the major holistic therapies:

- Functional medicine
- Tong Ren
- Herbal medicine
- Naturopathic medicine
- Ayurvedic medicine
- Chiropractic
- Psychotherapy

- Energy medicine
- Quantum Touch
- Homeopathy
- Traditional Chinese medicine
- Nutritional therapies
- Stress reduction
- Massage

Holistic medicine, using a multi-faceted approach, often takes advantage of a team of experts treating the whole person as compared to focusing on an isolated symptom.

You will learn:

- The unexpected healing power found in these therapies
- Alternatives to allopathic medicine
- A number of non-invasive approaches for restoring the body to optimum health
- A new experience of personal empowerment when applying these therapies

Functional Medicine and Beyond -

The Real Future of Healthcare, Self-Care, and Longevity

Dr. Tel-Oren, Adiel, MD (Europe), CCN, DABFM, DACBN, LN, DC(ret), DABOM, FABDA

http://www.ecopolitan.com/doctor-t

Dr. Tel-Oren does not necessarily agree with some of the statements or concepts or principles included in this book, or espoused by the Hippocrates Health Institute.

For more information please contact office@ecopolitan.com" as well as his bio.

Practice Focus

- Nutritional, Environmental, & Functional Medicine

- President & Founder, Ecopolitan Eco-Health Network (www.ecopolitan.com)

- President Emeritus & Professor of Nutrition and Functional Medicine, University of Natural Medicine

What is Functional Medicine?

The term "functional medicine" was first coined about 20 years ago in order to define the comprehensive, multi-specialty, integrated medicine of the future. Functional medicine combines scientific research with innovative tools for accurate diagnosis and safe and efficient medical treatment of complex and chronic conditions. The emphasis is to elucidate how different aspects of an individual's life - the physical and emotional environment, general lifestyle, as well as genetic factors - can all lead to deviation from health and manifest in disease over time. This is highly relevant today, since the vast majority of chronic conditions seen in clinical practice are attributable to these lifestyle and genetic factors.

Many degenerative or chronic conditions are caused by various combinations of disease triggers and promoters, such as nutritional deficiencies, toxin accumulation, allergenic exposures, emotional stressors, metabolic imbalance, and infectious load in food, water, and air. Additionally, digestive disturbances may cause nutrient mal-absorption and exposure to toxic compounds, as in the prevalent "leaky gut" syndrome. … They utilize advanced, scientific functional laboratory tests and other diagnostic procedures—including comprehensive medical and socio-emotional history - to uncover tacit illness or the initial deviation from health even in the absence of overt or significant symptoms. The goal is to effectively and sustainably address the triggers, promoters, and biochemical imbalances in order to stop the progression of symptoms, reverse them whenever possible, and prevent the appearance of new conditions, while increasing overall wellness and improving the body's resistance towards disease.

How does Functional Medicine Differ from Allopathic Medicine?

The common approach of allopathic (orthodox) medicine focuses mainly on suppressing the symptoms using artificial substances, which pharmacology and toxicology experts agree are toxic and poisonous for the body, as their central or primary effect. Paradoxically, the occasional alleviation of symptoms is in fact the "side effect." For example, the allopathic approach would recommend a pill to lower temperature for high fever, prescribe a synthetic pill to elevate mood in treating depression, or a pharmacological anti-inflammatory drugs for simple immune reactions.

Functional medicine, on the other hand - rather than simply "chasing symptoms" while ignoring the causes - searches for and addresses environmental factors, nutritional deficiencies, genetic tendencies, biochemical dysfunctions and emotional and social stressors that can together cause the development of symptoms. …

The causes continue to accumulate until there is a perceived "need" to use even more poisonous drugs, in ever-increasing doses, which inevitably cause new illnesses. This leads to gradual (sometimes rapid) deterioration of the patient's health, which the orthodox allopath assumes is "the normal progression of disease" - when in fact it is the toxic intervention (and the neglect of causes) that created this deterioration. Consequently, a "statistic" is born, allowing the practitioner to "predict" the unfortunate outcome of treatment, thereby creating a self-fulfilling prophecy. The chronic orthodox disregard for environmental or nutritional causes is the reason for the ever-present "idiopathic diseases"—which is the medical textbook's description for syndromes or conditions that allegedly have "no known cause." Therefore, pharmacological symptom suppression, despite its toxicity and futility in addressing chronic disease, becomes justified as the only viable therapy by "conventional" medical training centers (benefiting the Medical Industrial Complex and big Pharma). By diagnosing and treating the underlying causes (or just a few of them) in a scientific manner, functional medicine practitioners can promote improvement or healing of many health conditions considered chronic or incurable by allopathic doctors.

Functional medicine is characterized by a personalized approach to each patient, since similar symptoms or dis-eases can derive from different causes. The patient is approached as a whole being of integrated body, mind, and spirit.

The clinical application of functional medicine is based upon a profound knowledge of the following:

- Physiological and biochemical function of the body, from the cellular level to the organ and system level.

- The biochemical uniqueness of each individual, based on personal and family history, environmental and nutritional exposure, life style, genetics, and emotional factors.

- The appropriate clinical interventions for beneficial alteration of gene expression.

- The basic biological processes in all the body systems and their mutual interactions, requiring integration of all areas of medical specialization.

- The influences of nutritional, environmental, social, emotional, and physical factors on human function.

- Scientific diagnostic tests (functional lab tests) designed to expose non-linear diversity of causes for any health complaint: Each symptom may have several factors acting simultaneously, therefore the treatment has to be multifaceted, relying on scientific diagnosis of multiple elements of health.

What Do Functional Medicine Practitioners Treat?

Functional Medicine does not revolve around specific sets of diseases and syndromes - it concerns itself with an extremely wide variety of health disturbances. Although many of these "disturbances" seem to differ a lot in symptomatic appearance - including diverse conditions such as fibromyalgia, irritable bowel syndrome, heart disease, diabetes, mood and cognitive disorders, various autoimmune disorders, PMS, TMJ, chronic pelvic pain, interstitial cystitis, chronic low back pain, chemical and food sensitivities, allergies, asthma, and cancer - they all seem to share common courses of formation.

The common denominator for these disturbances appears to be chronic stress, which may typically be thought of as deriving from mental or emotional origin, although many other factors can stress the body, like unhealthy food, nutritional deficiencies, environmental toxins, insufficient rest, infections, physical strain, and injury. All these factors contribute to the body's level of "total stress"—causing it to cross a previously invisible threshold where chronic health disturbances can manifest. The current global epidemic of chronic diseases is especially marked within industrialized nations, where the inhabitants experience relatively high levels of "total stress." While some acute stress factors may help us survive and even thrive, chronic stress factors that seem unpleasant, undesirable, or painful can lead to unhealthy changes in our immune system and in other body systems.

Recent findings indicate that these common stress factors—whether nutritional, environmental, physical, or psychological—can in fact alter, from day to day, the expression of genes in the cells. These alterations can lead to significant changes in physical symptoms and general health. Functional Medicine researchers are now convinced that syndromes of functional nature such as fibromyalgia, chronic headaches, and irritable bowel syndrome are likely to be initiated by different stress factors that can change the expression of DNA and lead to symptoms of chronic disease. Accordingly, when a person is suffering from chronic or aggravated symptoms, assessing and addressing all or most of the stress factors involved can be the key to recovery.

Further Reading:

http://www.ecopolitan.com/health-services/eco-healing/functional-medicine/330-functional-medicine-and-beyond-the-real-future-of-health-care-self-care-and-longevity

"Textbook of Functional Medicine" / Institute for Functional Medicine (IFM), David S. Jones, MD, Editor in Chief "Immunotics" / Robert Roundtree, MD

"Genetic Nutritioneering" / Jeffery S. Bland, PhD

"Functional Nutrition" / Institute for Functional Medicine (IFM)

Tam Healing System -
Healing is Balance, Removing Resistance and
Encouraging Natural Abundance
by Joseph Lucier, LMT, NANP

Nature thrives on homeostasis and balance. Balance is the normal state of our bodies, minds and spiritual being. In healing, as in life, the goal is simple; remove resistance and blockages interfering with this process, and support and nourish ourselves so we thrive and support our physical bodies as well as our entire human community.

As Ann Wigmore stated, there are two main causes of disease or disharmony:

1. Toxicity - Poison and Inflammation

2. Deficiency - Malnutrition and Negativity

Toxicity

Toxicity is poison and this can be physical as well as emotional. The environment can influence us by pollution, our mind can influence us by toxic or negative thoughts and above all, we can receive toxins from our food. Remember, we make food decisions about 1,000 times a year so we have a lot of control over this one. As for negative thoughts, our control over this is self-awareness, compassion, self-reflection and transformation. In my opinion, a toxic mind is equally harmful as a poor diet and polluted environment. Working on the positive aspects of our mind is greatly enhanced by our spiritual practices and by our community. Working on our food choices greatly enhances our physical body. Additionally, a healthy body supports a healthy mind and spirit.

Our bodies, when we are out of balance, have many mechanisms for self-healing and self-preservation. Inflammation is one of those things, and in low levels, this is a healing mechanism such as a fever. When inflammation continues for prolonged periods of time, the body reacts to rectify this such as in the cases of artery inflammation and patching and eventual arterial plaque buildup. Cancer cells in the body are normal, but, when the body is in a diseased, acidic, inflamed or toxic state, oxygen starved (anaerobic) state, cancer cells thrive.

Deficiency

Our body needs resources to regenerate and maintain ones self. This is simply done with the quantity of food, as well as with the quality of food. The United States has more available resources than just about any country in the world. Surprisingly, we have some of the highest disease rates, obesity rates (even in children) and malnourishment rates in the world as well. Some people are overweight, but malnourished because they eat lots of food overall, but it is not nourishing food and the body is still deficient and oftentimes craves even more food since it is starving for the vital nutrients it needs to survive. Poor food is simply stored as fat (the body surrounds the toxins with fat in order to survive), as the body tries to manage this onslaught of non-food. Eating 15 pounds of junk food is not going to satisfy the body as much as one or two pounds of fresh fruit or vegetables. Likewise, spiritual and emotional deficiency is also harmful and negatively impacts the body, mind and spirit. A regular spiritual practice and connecting with nature nourish us tremendously.

Healing

With that said, when we are out of balance, when we are sick and have disease, how do we recover? Remember, so much of the influences of disease are choices we make. So many illnesses are simply caused by a blockage from long-term toxicity or deficiency. The blockage is the core element that must be removed. In many healing systems, they focus on these blockages. Allopathic medicine in general, focuses on the symptom instead of the cause. For long-term healing, I see it in two steps:

1. Remove the blockage causing bioelectrical (neural), biochemical, or vascular resistance (blood, hormone and oxygen delivery). These are the communication and distribution methods of our bodies. Long-term poor health, trauma, or even accidents create these blockages and when removed, homeostasis is possible again. The body is amazing in its ability to heal and regenerate.

2. Remove, manage or resolve the underlying cause of illness and eventual blockage such as emotional trauma, poor diet, pollution, inflammation, lack of exercise, accidents or even structural damage or anomalies.

Remove the Blockage - Tam Healing System

There are many ways to remove a blockage and as a healer, I have followed the Tom Tam Healing System. It focuses more directly on blockages than any other system I have ever seen. It is very effective in the areas of cancer and many other diseases. Our primary focus is on blockages in the Central Nervous System. Opening blockages in these areas revive bioelectrical transmission of signals to organs and other functional areas. In the cases of cancer, if there is a nerve blockage, the energy signal is impeded and the targeted areas and cells of the organs is reduced. Basically, the cells do not get enough energy to perform properly and can mutate. A blockage in our system is very specific, and removing the blockage improves our success rate for our three techniques of healing; Medical Massage Therapy, Acupuncture or Tong Ren Distance Healing.

Summary - Remove Underlying Causes of Blockage And Disharmony

Balance is the key. When eating, eat a wide variety of fresh fruits, vegetables, nuts and seeds and drink plenty of water, and then we will thrive. By doing this along with regular exercise, we can achieve balance and homeostasis. What a radical concept, eat healthy natural unprocessed foods, drink water, and exercise. How's that for a crazy idea!

Doing this gives us plenty of nutrition and health. For the long term, this will prevent toxicity, deficiency, and allow for optimal mental functioning, and the eventual clarity that results from mindfulness supports spiritual growth and balance as well. We have choices and do not need to be disempowered by advertising, marketing, negative thoughts, or uncreative health practitioners. We must take responsibility and take charge of our lives and do our research and never give up hope. Hope, like faith, is the true healer. It removes a blockage that eliminates us from a connection to our true selves and nature or the Dao itself as healthy physical, mental and spiritual beings. Connecting with nature is what we are and this is what can heal us and ultimately, give us clarity, humility, appreciation and respect for the beauty and sacredness of our own existence as well as the entire planet and all the wonderful sentient beings that share our beautiful world.

Joseph Lucier, LMT, NANP, is a licensed medical massage therapist, student of herbalism, software engineer and a long time student of Asian culture. He is also an advocate for plant based nutrition and veganism, a Vegan Chef, health educator and lecturer, spreading the benefits and amazing healing and spiritual opportunities of plant based nutrition and the vegan lifestyle. He has a degree in Chinese Studies from Boston College, Boston MA USA. After college, he moved to Asia and lived there for 15 years. He then returned to the US, worked as a software engineer while also focusing on Medical Massage Therapy. In 2001, he learned the Tam Healing System, inspired by the self-less dedication of Tom Tam to remove suffering and help people. He also balances out his practice of Tui Na hands-on work with Tong Ren Distance Healing and has patients worldwide including both people and animals with a wide ailments ranging from cancer to the common cold.

Check out his websites http://www.TongRenHealer.com and http://www.LiveFoodCuisine.com.

Further Reading:

Joseph Lucier LMR, NANP Tam Healing System Volume 1 - Illustrated Anatomy Point Location - Tong Ren

Joseph Lucier LMT NANP Tam Healing System Volume 2 - Illustrated Anatomy Point Location- Cancer Strategies

Tong Ren Definition

Developed by Tom Tam, and an integral part of the Tom Tam Healing System, Tong Ren is a form of energy therapy for restoring health and vitality. Tong Ren is based on the belief that disease is related to interruptions, or blockages, in the body's natural flow of chi, neural bioelectricity, blood, or hormones. Blockages are very commonly found physically, rather than energetically, commonly along the spine inhibiting the natural circulation of the body's central nervous system. Tong Ren Therapy utilizes the concept of the collective unconsciousness to remove these blockages, restoring the body's natural ability to heal itself, even when illnesses are chronic, debilitating, or otherwise untreatable.

Tong Ren combines western knowledge of anatomy and physiology with the ancient principle of "chi," or life force energy, to create what many consider to be a powerful new healing modality. Drawing on the Jungian theory of the "collective unconscious," Tong Ren is believed to access energy from this universal source and direct it to the patient. Because no physical contact is involved or necessary, Tong Ren is often practiced as distance healing.

In a typical therapy session, the Tong Ren practitioner uses a small human anatomical model as an energetic representation of the patient, tapping on targeted points on the model with a lightweight magnetic hammer. The practitioner directs chi to blockage points corresponding to the patient's condition, breaking down resistance at these points. As blood flow, neural transmission, and hormone reception are restored, the body is then able to heal.

See www.tongrenhealer.com for Joe Lucier's outstanding book, *Tam Healing System,* for understanding the Tom Tam Healing System theory. Also recommend Rick Kuethe's book, *Tongren Therapy.*

www.tongrenstation.com - The groundbreaking new energy therapy for healing cancer, osteoporosis, arthritis and more .Safe and Natural. Supported by Dana Farber and Spaulding Rehab. Available live 24 hours a day. You can call in with your challenges and be worked on.

Importance of Coherent Energy Patterns for Physical Health

A new model for illness and health: Understanding the need for coherent energy patterns to transmit healing messages to the body.

by Barry Harris

"Over the last few decades scientists have developed more than adequate measurable and logical connections between biological energy fields and generally accepted scientific knowledge. Methods have been developed to measure subtle but important energy fields within and around the human body. A few decades ago these fields were considered non-existent by academic medicine. Not only are we documenting the presence of such fields, but researchers are understanding how fields are generated and how they are altered by disease and disorder." (1a)

"Energy Medicine: The Scientific Basis" by Dr. James Oschman, Phd; Harcourt Publishers, Ltd..

What is electro-magnetic energy?

Electro-magnetic energy, also called electro-magnetic radiation (often abbreviated E-M radiation or EMR) is a phenomenon that takes the form of self-propagating waves as in the ocean, radio waves or light waves. For example, if you have two motor boats making waves as they go through the water, when these waves from the two boats collide, they will either be dissipated or enlarged depending on whether they superimpose upon each other or cancel each other out. The same is true about electro-magnetic energy waves. Waves that cancel each other out are called incoherent energy patterns. If the waves cancel each other out, they cannot transmit healing messages through the body. There is now new technology that proves that the mind transmits messages throughout the body using electro-magnetic energy waves. It's also been proven that stress causes chaotic electro-magnetic energy patterns in which the waves cancel each other out and thus, cannot transmit healing messages. With stress as the common denominator causing incoherent energy patterns, and thus poor message transmission, we have the possibility for a new unified field theory of medicine. All sickness is caused by stress, and there are many forms this stress can take: dietary stress, stress from environmental toxins; stress from blocked emotions; stress from body losing its muscle tone; etc.

As the above passage indicates, recent discoveries have proven that the messages needed for the body to optimally function and heal, are carried by coherent electromagnetic energy waves. This discovery has initiated a whole new model of illness and health. This model is truly good news for it's proven to be both non-invasive and more powerful than the present allopathic model. The past medical paradigm has been handicapped by a focus on the material aspect of the body. The new paradigm focuses on the electro-magnetic energy transmission occurring in the body. This new paradigm ends our hypnosis that the human body is primarily a material body minimally affected by our thoughts and emotions; a paradigm that has been with us ever since the model of reality given to us by Rene Descartes in 16th century. The main assumption of Descartes' philosophy is that mind had minimal effect on the material body because mind and matter are such totally different substances. In Descartes' famous phrase, "You can not measure the length of a thought". Because of the latest technology, such as the SQUID machine, we measure the length of a thought all the time now. The importance of this discovery , made by the new technology showing mind (ie mental processes such as thoughts, emotions, and images) expresses itself as electromagnetic energy waves, combined with quantum physics showing that matter also expresses itself as electromagnetic energy waves, give us the common denominator -electromagnetic energy waves - for how mind can affect the body, and the body can affect mind. Descartes was just flat out wrong. There are new technologies, such as the QXCI machine, which actually diagnose health conditions by transforming the material molecules in the body into their electromagnetic energy wave pattern equivalents.. When it has been discovered which organ systems are exhibiting incoherent electromagnetic wave patterns, the QXCI then finds the appropriate electromagnetic energy wave patterns to add to the diseased organ system, in order to bring it back into coherence, and thus balance. This is one example that when the body is seen as an electromagnetic energy system, new possibilities arise both for understanding how our body functions and for new very powerful non-invasive treatments.

 Summarizing. The new model of the body sees the body not as a material machine, but as an electromagnetic energy wave messaging system. Our body has incredible powers to heal if the messages can be sent with great clarity. This requires coherent electromagnetic energy wave patterns that reinforce each other rather than incoherent electromagnetic which cancel out and prevent transmission of healing messages. Stress in any form creates incoherent electromagnetic energy wave patterns that cannot carry either the messages for the body to optimally function before it becomes sick, or to heal, after it becomes sick.

Biophysicist, Beverly Rubik, explains this new approach in the quote below, which best illustrates the point I'm trying to make.

"I'm intrigued by some work done in Germany. In fact, I've gone over there to work with Dr.. Fritz Albert Popp. This work involves detecting extremely low level light that the human body, and all organisms emit…Popp uses very sensitive detectors that can count the photons, the particles of light coming out of the body (ie. Electromagnetic radiation). I think that this may be one of the manifestations of the energy dynamics of life. For example, in the Popp laboratory, they have demonstrated that to a large extent the light is coherent like a laser. That means that the light probably has a capacity for carrying information, unlike incoherent light. If that's the case, it's probably not some junk radiation, which is the mainstream opinion. I think that the light, if it's coherent, is maybe involved in both an internal communication system, as well as an external one, that conveys signals between living things.….It's interesting that in studying the cancer tissues of patients, they have found losses of coherence in the light. Perhaps the light has lost informational value, and it cannot communicate with the other cells, and that's why the tissues grow abnormally."

"Towards A New World View," by Russell DiCarlo, pages 52-53. Published by Epic Publishing, P.O. Box427, Erie, PA 16507

Bio of Barry Harris. Barry worked at the Hippocrates Health Institute in Boston, editing health booklets for Dr. Ann Wigmore, the founder of the live food movement. Hippocrates Health Institute was a healing center with a powerful spiritual focus and extreme dietary regimen which often attracted those who Western medicine had labeled as "terminally ill." While working there, Barry witnessed many miracles. It was clear to Barry that those who experienced miracles were uniquely empowered people who had been so changed by their illness, they actually saw their terminal diagnosis as a gift. This inspired Barry to undertake a 22 year study in quantum physics, energy medicine, and cellular biology, among other disciplines, in order to discover both the secret to miracles, and the nature of the spiritual transformation of those who experienced them.

For the last five years, Barry has been presenting a course in either a 14 evening or two weekend format on his findings, and, in addition, will soon see his book "Beggars At God's Banquet: Miracles Are Our Birthright" published by XLibris press. Barry also teaches "Voice As A Spiritual Path," and explains in his instruction the relationship of the ego to breath patterns, and to surrender to a higher power, and uses this information in his course.

Further Reading:

Dr. Oschman, J, PhD. "Energy Medicine: The Scientific Basis." Harcourt Publishers,

Ltd. DiCarlo, R. "Towards A New World View," pages 52-53. Published by Epic Publishing, P.O. Box 427, Erie, PA 16507

The Shift in Consciousness – My Quantum Leap[6]
by Marlene Campbell

"There is a thought in your mind right now. The longer you hold on to it, the more you dwell upon it, the more life you give to that thought. Give it enough life, and it will become real. So make sure the thought is indeed a great one."   *Ralph Marston*

- Did you know that thoughts are real energy?

- Did you know thoughts and emotions affect all life?

- Did you know they affect the environment?

In the late 1990's I found myself desiring to make changes in my professional life. I had been teaching grammar school for many years and loved what I did. But there was a part of me that had been speaking to me for a while saying that there is more for you to learn and do. Now that inner voice was getting louder. I found that I could no longer ignore that voice.

At the same time, there was an issue in my life that needed resolution. The issue was affecting my health- physically and emotionally. A friend suggested that I try some energy work and recommended a therapist. That decision was made with ease. It was that decision that made all the difference in my world.

I had no idea what energy healing was. Yet I listened. I trusted my intuition. I made an appointment, and entered a wonderful world of energy, holistic healing, and higher vibration. It has opened up a world of so many wonders in the amazing realm of natural healing. This world of *Holistic Healing* is truly healing of body, mind, and spirit.

When I made that decision to experience energy healing, I had no idea where it would lead. That first experience instilled in me a desire to have more sessions. I was seeing colors. I was remembering long forgotten events. I was releasing energy physically from my body. I was "hearing" my inner voice, and I wanted to act upon what I heard. I experienced changes physically, emotionally and mentally. And at the same time, I had to learn what these experiences were all about - experiences that affected my body, mind and spirit. What was really happening to me?

It was then that I made a decision to begin my formal training in energy and healing. And because my love is teaching, all of it eventually led to sharing and teaching others that which I have learned.

In 1998 I studied Reiki Jin Kei Do with Patricia Warren, attaining Levels I and II and Ennersense Levels I and II. Next I enrolled and completed the Holistic Massage Program, the Advanced Polarity Program, and the RYSE Practitioner / Instructor Program at Spa Tech Institute, in Westborough and Ipswich, MA. In 2005 I studied with author, composer, and internationally known peacemaker James Twyman for 2 years. I, also, studied with Betsy Bragg at the Optimum Health Solution's Course, a course filled with a vast amount of knowledge in the field of holistic health, nutrition, and life force energy

I continued to take many other courses and seminars. I found that as I read more, studied more, and met new people, I had a strong desire to learn more. I just could not get enough! This was, and is, the Law of Attraction, the principle of resonance that like attracts like. I was filling a deep desire that had been dormant for a long time.

One day my friend Sue introduced me to Quantum-Touch®. As I explored the book and DVD set, *Quantum Touch, The Power to Heal*, by Richard Gordon, I knew that this was what I had been searching for. I knew I wanted to incorporate this into my private practice with clients. And because I am a teacher by profession, I knew I wanted to teach Quantum Touch, sharing with others this amazing simple method. As G. Norman Shealy, M.D., Ph.D., founding president of the American Holistic Medical Association, states, *"Quantum-Touch appears to be the first technique that may truly allow all to become healers."*

Quantum Touch is a healing modality that works with the life force energy - chi - that flow of energy that sustains all living beings, to promote wellness. Quantum-Touch teaches how to focus, amplify, and direct this energy, for a wide range of benefits with surprising and often extraordinary results. It is based on the concept of vibrations—love being the universal vibration that allows people to transfer healing to another. It allows this transfer to animals, plants, situations, the world at large. It can be done in the presence of the other or at a distance! We have all heard that *love heals all*. This gave a whole new meaning to that expression.

Consciousness affects matter. Mankind's consciousness affects matter at a subatomic level, at a quantum level. It is at this level that healing, balance, comfort and structural alignment – healing- take place. It helps maximize the body's own extraordinary capacity to heal itself by addressing the root cause of disease; all healing is self-healing.

When your thoughts are charged with emotion, either positively or negatively, there is a great electromagnetic field created within and around you. The Law of Attraction states that like energy attracts like energy. You attract more of what your electromagnetic energy field is vibrating.

Research conducted at the Institute of Heartmath in Colorado has shown that the heart is a powerful generator of energy. The heart produces an electromagnetic field that is 5,000 times greater in strength that that of the brain. This heart energy affects every cell in your body and extends outward in all directions from you, affecting living beings in close proximity and at greater distances. This is another confirmation of the statement that *love healsall*. Quantum-Touch teaches that "Our love has impact. Our love matters." I believe that can be stated as our *love materializes*.

In The Intention Experiment, Lynne McTaggart writes: "A sizable body of research exploring the nature of consciousness carried on for more than 30 years in prestigious scientific institutions around the world, shows that thoughts are capable of affecting everything from the simplest machines to the most complex living beings. This evidence suggests that human thoughts and intentions are an actual physical "something" with the astonishing power to change our world. Every thought is a tangible energy with the power to transform. A thought is not only a thing; a thought is a thing that influences other things

We are energy. Everything is energy. With this awareness comes an understanding of the energetic impact that your thoughts, words and emotions have on your body, all living beings, and your reality. Awareness is the key to all change, to letting go of fear and living in greater peace and joy.

We are living at a critical time. When there is a deliberate change in consciousness—in our thoughts, words, and emotions — things change. We can individually and collectively use this power. It is this Great Shift in human consciousness that brings creative and constructive solutions to personal and global problems.

It is imperative to use this knowledge and to bring this message to adults and to children, for children are the future.

Marlene Campbell is a Certified Quantum-Touch Practitioner and Instructor, Levels 1 and 2, and Self Created Health. She brings years of experience and training as a teacher and facilitator of healing, intuitive arts, and personal empowerment techniques, for adults, children, and groups of all sizes.

marlenecampbell@townisp.com

www.rippleeffectworkshops.com

Beverly Paoli Reviews Kevin Gianni's online audio event "Healing Cancer World Summit"[7]

Kevin Gianni, a health educator and advocate, provided an online audio event "Healing Cancer World Summit" October 25-29, 2011, from interviews he conducted on www.renegadehealth.com. The following list of Alternative/Integrative Treatment Options are from that Summit and are not meant to be inclusive. They represent treatment options with a history of successfully treating some cancers and critical diseases, and have been operating for some time. In screening for treatment options, one should assess their track record for specific diseases as well as pros and cons of their protocols. Most approaches look to combine the best of Integrative, Western and Natural Healing.

Dr. Nicholas Gonzalez, M.D. PC is a physician who operates a clinic in New York City www.Dr-Gonzalez.com. He has been investigating nutritional approaches to cancer and other degenerative diseases since 1981 and has written two books. Dr.Gonzalez has identified three processes that must happen in order for the body to heal: 1. Adaptation of a diet that fits the individuals metabolic needs as established through testing; 2. Supplementation with essential nutrients including pancreatic enzymes; and 3. Detoxification with an emphasis on liver-gallbladder flushes.

Charlotte Gerson/The Gerson Therapy was developed by her father, Max Gerson, a German physician, in the 1920s. She was trained by her father and has carried his work forward. The Gerson Therapy Clinic is in Playas de Tijuana, Mexico www.gersonmedia.com. Charlotte has written several books that are comprehensive guides to the theory and practice of the Gerson Therapy. The Gerson Therapy is based on the belief that all diseases have the same underlying issues of toxicity and deficiency, and when corrected, the body has the ability to heal itself. The therapy activates the body's healing capacity through an organic-vegetarian diet, raw juices, coffee enemas and natural supplements.

Dr.Francisco Contreras, a Mexican oncologist and surgeon, oversees the operation of the Oasis of Hope Hospital in Tijuana, Mexico www.oasisofhope.com. 1-888-500-HOPE. The Oasis of Hope was founded by his father Dr. Ernesto Contreras, Sr. in 1963, and his son has followed in his father's footsteps. This Clinic provides a large variety of therapies. To name a few: Managed Nutrition, Mind-Body-Spirit Healing, Enzyme Therapy and the use of Laetrile. See www.oasisofhope.com/cancer_treatment.php.com for their list of treatment protocols under the collective name Integrative Regulatory Therapy (IRT). Noteworthy is the programs listing of statistics showing rates of success. www.oasisofhope.com/patient-survival-statistics.php.com.

Dr. Leigh Erin Connealy, M.D., M.P.H. is the medical director of the Center for New Medicine in Irvine, California. www.cfnmedicine.com. She is affiliated with the Oasis of Hope Hospital in Mexico. The Center for New Medicine provides therapies that support the body's innate defenses and healing mechanisms. The approaches and treatment entities are diverse and multiple. To name a few: Breathe to oxidize the body, remove chemicals from the water, alkalize the diet; increase absorption of nutrients, eliminate/ reduce sugar intake; add cleansing agents and beneficial supplements.

Dr. Thomas Lodi, M.D., Homeopathic Physician and Founder of the Oasis of Healing, Mesa, Arizona www.oasisofhealing.com 480-834-5414. Alternative cancer treatments and natural therapies to target cancer include:

- Insulin Potentiated Low Dose Chemotherapy

- High Dose Intravenous Vitamin C

- Oxidative Therapies such as Ozone and Hydrogen Peroxide Natural healing is promoted using cleansing, detoxification, stress reduction, exercise, nutrition with an emphasis on the bio-availability of the food, and supplementation. There is a spiritual component to the program.

Dr. David Getoff, Naturopath and Certified Clinical Nutritionist www.naturopath4you.com. He emphasizes the prevention of disease. In the interview with Kevin, Dr. Getoff said the following: "I think the most important way to help a body combat cancer is to reduce its toxic load. So we stop consuming foods that I believe lead toward the cancer and we replace them with foods which support the health of the body. We add in all the supplemental vitamins, minerals, enzymes, herbs, etc." He offers consultations.

Mike Adams is known for his consumer health advocacy. He calls himself a holistic health investigative journalist and he has authored several books. He is the editor of an on-line newsletter: www.NaturalNews.com. During the interview Mike was quick to highlight the negative impact conventional oncologists have on their patients by inducing fear and giving projected life expectancies. What a patient believes, he or she can make real- the "placebo effect." He then went on to talk about the outstanding and multiple benefits of vitamin D. Generally speaking he is positive about treatments that target the cancer cells and is extremely critical of the widespread use of chemotherapy and radiation. Mike puts emphasis on ridding the body of toxins and using natural supplementation.

Marcus Freudenmann is a German film producer who visited and conducted in-depth interviews at alternative clinics to understand their cancer treatment programs. He and his wife Sabrina, a naturopathic doctor, traveled around the world with their four children for three years to meet the experts. Marcus produced the documentary film called CANCER IS CURABLE NOW, which pulls together more than 30 international holistic professionals- doctors, scientists, researchers and writers. During his interview with Kevin, Marcus spoke about the negative impact that stress has on our bodies and minds. He was critical of programs that teach good nutrition but then serve unhealthy food. In any protocol Marcus emphasized the need to get a good history of the patient in the search for causes and problems and to implement life-style changes.

Burton Goldberg, a cancer survivor himself, has long been known as a strong voice for Alternative Medicine. He has authored 18 books and several videos on alternative treatment for cancer, heart disease and other degenerative diseases. Burton's Websites offer guidance for patients. www.BurtonGoldberg.com ,www.alternativecancerresources.com. During his interview with Kevin, he spoke highly of Suzanne Somers book KNOCKOUT because it emphasizes the emotional and physical components of healing cancer that need to be an integral part of any treatment regimen. Burton mentioned a laboratory in Germany with the capacity to scan blood for cancer cells and to test for which treatment option may be best. www.biofocus.de/de/onkonogie/ueberblick/ueberblick.com   English is spoken.

Two interviews featured cancer survivors. Both women said it is essential to have a team approach to gather information and to guide one through the treatment process. Karolyn Kloepping offers coaching. www.paradigmsofhealth.com.

Dr. Gregory Burzynski, M.D. is the son of Stanislaw Burzynski, M.D., PhD. who founded the Burzynski Research Institute based in Texas. Dr. Stanislaw Burzynski, a biochemist and physician, developed an innovative cancer treatment based on Antineoplastons. "Antineoplastons act as molecular switches to turn off cancer cells without destroying normal cells", see www.burzynskiclinic.com. Antineoplastons that are given intravenously are involved in a FDA clinical trial for specific brain tumors. The politics involved have been documented in the movie BURZYNSKI THE MOVIE www.burzynskimovie.com. The Burzynski Clinic offers Personalized Gene Targeted Therapy using molecular screening, activating one of the antineoplastons in the body, and then prescribing appropriate FDA-approved drugs. Currently they do not treat early- stage cancer, testicular cancer, and acute leukemia.

Summary Questions:

1. What is cancer?

2. How does holistic medicine complement allopathic medicine?

3. According to Dr. Tel-Oren, what is functional medicine?

4. What's a blockage and how does it cause disease?

5. How do you remove blockages?

6. If you had cancer, which treatment would you seek?

7. Why is energy medicine so effective?

8. Why are thoughts and emotions so important?

Chapter 9
Master Your Destiny

Overview

The goal of Hippocrates Approach to Optimum Health is to raise your level of Life Force Energy. This includes: visioning, cleansing and nourishing the body through proper eating, juicing, exercising, journaling, meditating, opening your heart and giving service. You have the innate ability to achieve optimum health and discover your true self.

The first place where health starts is in your head. Our beliefs and thoughts, which result in our habits, rule our current state of health. Mark Twain said, "It's not what we don't know that hurts us; it is what we know for sure that just ain't so". For example, TV commercials tell us "milk does the body good". Science shows us that "just ain't so".

Congratulate yourself on doing research to change your thoughts and beliefs.

What you will learn:

- How to integrate the "Hippocrates lifestyle" into your daily living.

- Importance of elimination of toxins.

- How to follow the timetables that govern your body.

- How to follow your food plan when with family, friends and eating out.

- How to love yourself.

- How to eat when travelling.

- How to encourage your children to eat a plant-based diet.

- How to gain weight on a plant-based diet.

- How to stay on a live food diet in the wintertime.

Master Your Destiny
by Betsy Bragg and Barry Harris

To master your destiny, you have to take responsibility for every aspect of what it means to be a human being. Let us take as a metaphor, the fruitfulness of a tree, which depends on the fulfillment of all the requirements necessary for its optimal growth. A tree is totally dependent on the blessings of nature, such as optimal rainfall, nutrients in the soil and sunshine. Whereas human beings have free choice and their fruitfulness is their responsibility.

Returning to the analogy of the tree, the seed contains the original potential of the individual. The roots depend on the soil in which the seed is planted; the soil is one's family and social-economic-political environment. Despite one's family and environment, unlike a tree, we are not limited to our growth depending on these external conditions. Humans need vision to grow. The extent of our vision determines our destiny, as Gandhi, in chapter one, states these ideas so beautifully. Now, that we've created a new reality of personal empowerment, there is nothing that can limit the extent of our vision.

The roots are our belief system. The Hippocrates belief system for personal empowerment incorporates the following:

1. Life Force Energy/Love

2. Laws of Nature – sunshine, oxygen and water

3. Nutrition based on a living food diet

4. Sleep and rest

5. Cleansing and limiting your exposure to toxins – exercise,

6. Mind-body connection and the wisdom within

7. Service

8. Consistent daily routine

9. Assessment of current health and its continual monitoring

The trunk of the tree incorporates all elements of a balanced health plan. The trunk is the source and foundation for the nutritional, physical, detoxification/regeneration, emotional and spiritual branches of health.

Nutritional Branch

The juice that flows through the nutritional branch must be alkaline to balance our overly acidic and polluted environment. For human beings, their alkalinity depends on a diet of sprouts and wheatgrass juice, both high in chlorophyll, with the addition of sea vegetables. It also depends upon an adequate intake of hormones, phytochemicals, enzymes and trace minerals. Humans, unlike the tree, learn to avoid excess protein, unhealthy fats, harmful sugars, all processed foods and cooking. For healthy fats, they can choose avocados, olives and coconuts. Healthy sugars come from sweet vegetables, such as carrots, beets, fruits and stevia. Water is essential for both trees and humans; humans need half their body weight in alkaline water. For humans, two pounds of leafy green vegetables are essential for optimal health, obtained from juice, salads and soups.

Physical Branch

One can have the best diet, but without exercise, results will be limited. Sitting behind a computer all day and lounging in front of TV will leave depleted life force. Stretching exercises for five to ten minutes on arising are recommended. Walk for at least a half an hour a day or do some other aerobic exercise. Strong people stay young. The body needs weight-training three times a week. Yoga and Pilates are forms of weight training.

Detoxification/Regeneration

No program of optimum health can be complete without addressing detoxification and regeneration. The Hippocrates program facilitates specific practices in this process. They are breath-work, skin brushing, exercise, juicing ("juice feasting"), enemas and implants.

Emotional and Spiritual Branch

Our lack of spirit is responsible for much stress and lack of ease (dis-ease) in our lives. A person who has a strong connection to the Divine has the advantage of a consistent state of peace and harmony. When we separate ourselves from spirit and the divine, it is like two cogs in a machine creating friction impeding its optimal functioning. When we set our will against God's, we are blocking the flow of the Divine through our being. This is not a metaphor, but this is the literal, physiological truth for we block God's breath with our ego control. This manifests as blocked emotions and a psychic state not at peace. No matter how excellent our diet and exercise program, the constant stress of working against God's energy wears us down and leads to bodily degeneration. The latest science has shown that peaceful vibrations can actually harmonize and transform the chaotic vibrations found in a diseased body. Intention and prayer has scientifically been proven to heal.

So, hang your heart on a star and go for it!

The Raw Food Choice
by Christine Lucas, HHC, AADP

Now that you've learned all of the wonderful benefits of raw cuisine and how to prepare this life giving, nourishing, energetic food, it's time to bring it all home and apply this eating style into your life. For many, the thought of this changeover can naturally bring up quite a bit of resistance and fear. There is the fear that you will fail or won't be able to sustain it; fear of going back to living in a society that doesn't understand it or support it. Soon, we begin to unconsciously come up with excuses why it won't work – I don't have time; I need to wait until I have all of the equipment; I need more protein; I can't eat raw in the winter; etc, etc… I've heard them all, and I've said them all. Even though so many before you have had incredible experiences living the raw foods lifestyle, there is still the fear that maybe it won't work for you, or that you can't give up your old favorite foods and attachments. As long as you allow yourself to continue to have these thoughts, you will continue to believe them to be true. The fact is… It's not the truth! Don't let it be YOUR truth!

In 2010, I was in the health food store, and I ran into an acquaintance of mine who is a 100 percent committed raw vegan. At the time I was about 70-90 percent, on a good day. I had never gone longer than two weeks at 100 percent raw. I, too, had some underlying resistance. I asked her how she was able to maintain 100 percent raw even during the winter. I'll never forget her answer, because it was a turning point for me. Her answer changed me forever. She simply said,

" It's a choice."

Plain and simple, it's just a choice. How profound!

Something shifted in me that day, as I pondered that simple statement. If she could make that choice, why couldn't I? From that moment on, I made the choice to go for it and live this beautiful, empowering, enlightening lifestyle all the way. Even though it was the dead of winter, I chose to take it on. I planned on going 100% raw for 38 days to celebrate my 38th birthday. Of course, I felt so amazing that I did not stop at 38 days. I continued on. Not only did I have abundant energy, look and feel great, and release 14 lingering pounds, my life started coming together in other ways that I had never imagined. Over the next few months, I got raw chef certified, had record income in my business, was cast to host my own online holistic lifestyle show and got paid to do so, and my boyfriend of six years finally proposed. I finally felt that genuine peace, grounding and happiness that had somehow managed to slip out of my life. As a side note, I also realized that the notion of 'eating raw in the winter will make you cold' is a total myth. I found the opposite to be true. When raw, I'm better able to maintain a comfortable body temperature. I attribute that to how beneficial living food is for your circulation.

When you're taking care of your body and giving to yourself, life just falls into place in a synergistic way. This is the life force energy we speak of, working it's magic. Now, as you go into your daily life dealing with naysayers, and are bombarded with questions from people who are far less educated than you on nutrition, remember why you are doing this – the health, beauty, glowing skin, youthfulness, energy, the list goes on – and stick to your guns. Remember…living the raw foods lifestyle is a choice. It's simply a choice. It's YOUR choice.

Eating with My Non-Vegan Family At Home

The best way to be with non-vegan family and friends is always remember not to impose your lifestyle on them. Do not lecture to them or you will alienate them. Let yourself be a role model for them. You can offer them a taste of what you are eating, but also continue to prepare, or better yet, have them prepare their own food. Have plenty of your food available for their snacks, such as dehydrated crackers, cookies, dips and fruit. Introduce them to transitional recipes such veggie burgers, eggless egg salad, linguini zucchini with marinara sauce and many others in the recipe section. Have healthy salad dressings always available and hide the carcinogenic store-bought ones. They should get the hint! They might even look at your live food literature and DVDs. So leave them around the house readily available.

Replace dangerous products that contain chemical additives from your refrigerator and pantry, with ones suggested in chapter 2 – The Living Foods Kitchen. Some reminders from Chapter 2 are to replace: ionized salt with Celtic or Himalayan Sea Salt; sugar with stevia, lucuma and yacon; vinegar with lemon juice (I juice one bag of lemons for the week and keep the jar in the refrigerator). Suggest removing the microwave or, like me, disconnect it and use it for storage. My oven is also used for storage.

When any family member feels bloated, nauseous or loaded with mucous, ask them what they've been eating. This has worked with my grandchildren when they have returned from a birthday party feeling "yucky" from ice cream.

By introducing delicious, nutritious and attractively presented dishes at all meals, almost all my students have slowly changed their families' eating habits. Remember "inch by inch, it's a cinch."

Eating Out

Call ahead or check menus on line when choosing an appropriate restaurant for dinner. The three magic words, when ordering your dinner are, "my doctor says". If the waitress or waiter doesn't understand you, it's advisable to have a little laminated card listing all the vegetables you can eat, which can be brought to the chef. On the card that I give to my students is written:

BY DOCTOR'S ORDERS

I eat exclusively Raw (uncooked), Plant-Base/Vegan Food

THIS EXCLUDES ALL MEAT, DAIRY, FISH, EGG AND BREAD PRODUCTS

I'd like a salad or vegetable plate with any of the following

ONLY FRESH, UNCOOKED ITEMS:

romaine, spinach, cauliflower, sprouts, kale, chard, arugula, bok choy, green beans, celery, zucchini, carrot, cucumber, broccoli, yellow squash, radish, cabbage, red bell pepper, mushroom, avocado, beets and snow peas

---

I keep one of these in my wallet. I have delicious meals from steak houses to Mexican restaurants. International cuisine that would best meet your vegan preferences are: Cambodian, Italian, Chinese, Middle Eastern, Greek and Mexican. Mexican is the best, since you can always order a salad and guacamole. I've always found most restaurants quite accommodating. I usually order a huge salad with lemons for dressing and all the cooked, lightly steamed vegetables available in the restaurant.

I recommend eating before going out, so you won't be as easily tempted to eat the rolls and nacho chips before dinner. I usually bring an avocado and crudité with me in my handbag.

As an extra precaution, I usually bring digestive enzymes to take before and after the meal.

Plant-based Live Food Travel Tips

Traveling can be a challenge, as most of you are aware. We all know that it can be difficult to find good plant-based live food on the road. I have put together a strategy, which works pretty well. I thought I'd share it with you. (I don't do all these things, all the time.) Feel free to chime in with any thoughts or ideas you have, because there is always room for improvement. Restaurants are very accommodating. Just say the three magic words "The Doctor says". Ask the waiter to give you all the raw vegetables they have available. I'm not 100% raw, so I will accept some cooked vegetables if they have them.

Before travel, research your destination:

- Contact your Hotel or B&B to find out if they can accommodate your dietary restrictions. Be specific. Ask if they have a blender and a juicer in the kitchen. Request a mini frig in your room.

- Find out which restaurants in the area are Vegan. Just google Vegan Restaurants to find the locations.

- Scope out the local health food stores, food co-ops, and farmer's markets. Note the addresses. You may even want to print out maps to help you, as the maps that you get from the car rental places can be lacking. It is convenient to do this before you leave home, because you will have access to a printer.

- If you are traveling outside the country, do research on local cuisines. Many cultures are not as meat and dairy-centric as we are, and you can find dishes based on lentils or beans. I've traveled in 52 countries and delighted in the delicious, beautiful fruits and vegetables in the local markets.

- When buying your plane ticket, request the vegan option.

- Always bring a backup of plant-based food to eat in the airport and on the plane. Let's face it, airport food leaves a lot to be desired, and delays are pretty commonplace. So it's always a good idea to be prepared. We usually bring along some combination of the following:

  - Two salads in Tupperware prepared in advance with a plastic knife, fork and cloth napkin. I hide a small bottle of salad dressing in the salad ever since I was held up for a half an hour when security thought it might be explosive. I put the Tupperware container in two double zip lock bags with rubber bands around them in case they leak.

  - A zip lock bag of sprouted mung, adzuki and lentils.

  - Fruit (if necessary, peeled and sliced).

  - Nuts and seeds.

  - Dehydrated crackers, kale and other veggie chips and dried fruit.

  - In cold weather, bring a small bottle of miso paste to add to hot water.

  - Herbal tea bags.

- Powdered core greens to add to your water.

- When travelling by plane, I've brought my hand cranked Healthy Juicer and my Tribest Personal Blender PB 100. When we went to an isolated beach house on a remote island in the Bahamas, we brought the Vitamix in the grandchildren's suitcase since they had few clothes to bring. We also brought almonds for almond milk and their favorite granola, seeds to sprout, crackers, raisins and figs.

- Pack your chef knife and cutting board in the check-in luggage. Last time I forgot and security kindly sent me back to check in to put my large chef knife in my check-in luggage. Security told me that ordinarily they would turn a person with a knife over to the police. I was very lucky!!

- When overseas, while in underdeveloped countries, try to buy hydrogen peroxide or vinegar, to wash your produce. Also, bring a special filtered, purifying water bottle to remove microbes from your drinking water. We did this in South Africa.

Strategies while you are on the road:

- Bring small ziplock bags of 1/3 cup mung, 1/3 cup adzuki and 1/3 cup lentils. You can put the beans in a nut milk bag, dip them in water morning and night and hang them in the shower. Or you can sprout them in any cup in your hotel room. You can usually eat them in three days.

- The coffee maker in your hotel room is your friend. You can boil water to reconstitute a number of different things. And you can use the pot to heat up soups – just be considerate of the next guests and don't put anything but coffee grounds in the basket – and clean out the pot well.

- Ask your hotel to empty out the mini bar so you can use the fridge for your food. We've had some success with this. Some hotels just won't do it. But they may be willing to provide you with a mini fridge if they have one on hand.

- Consider staying someplace with a kitchen for at least part of your trip. Being able to prepare your own food can be quite helpful.

- You can find food at any grocery store— salad ingredients, along with lemon juice that doesn't require refrigeration, are easily purchased.

Traveling by car opens up a wide range of options.

- I brought my Greenstar 5000 twin gear juicer and bought greens at all the local markets to juice.

- I also brought my Tribest Personal Blender 100.

- Bring a cooler with some large rectangular plastic containers for ice, which I bought at the Container Store. Bring plenty of Ziploc bags. You can get ice easily.

When staying with non-Vegan family/friends:

- Discuss in advance what you eat. When I returned to my French high school exchange family recently, I wrote them in advance and told them that I could no longer enjoy their wines, rich gravies and pastries. They were most understanding and they took me shopping the first day of my arrival. My daughter in San Francisco, who does not follow my food plan, also takes me shopping the first day of a visit.

- Offer to bring something to share. Or offer to prepare something, but make sure you can get your hands on the required ingredients.

- Regardless of how thoughtful your hosts are, always assume you will need to supplement your meal and bring vegetables. If it turns out, you don't need them, you can always bring them home again. But, it's far better to be prepared.

Ideas for Enjoying Winter Raw & Staying Healthy!

- Add warming foods to your diet such as garlic, ginger, onions, root veggies, cayenne and other spices.

- Warm items, such as raw soups, in your dehydrator, or with the double boiler method.

- Set items out from the fridge for a few hours before you eat them.

- Eat heavier raw food items when necessary such as nuts and seeds and more complex dehydrated items like pizza and breads.

- Increase your intake of dark green leafy vegetables like kale, chards, collards, spinach, dandelion, purslane, etc.

- Wheatgrass shots will warm you up and nourish you!

- Rest when needed – this is the time of year for it!

- Plan ahead, all meals and anything you may need to make your work week go smoothly.

- Twice a week, prepare a lot of food for yourself in advance.

- Have a few favorite recipes on hand to have as a treat or to bring to a function.

- Increase your immunity with supplements (if you take them) and/or immune boosting foods like garlic, onions, greens.

- Watch funny movies, or listen to a comedy CD, especially before going to a stressful event.

- Exercise, rest and treat yourself to your favorite bodywork of choice.

- Soak in a warm bath which has a cup of Epsom salts or Himalayan Crystal salts

- Take nothing personally and expect the best!

- Have fun!

Gaining Weight on a Raw Plant-Based Diet

For some, gaining weight is a real challenge, especially those on chemo. The following are a number of comments by people with the challenge of weight gain. These are personal, not medical, suggestions.

The following is from "How to Gain Weight on the Vegan or Raw Food Diet with Robert Cheeke – The Renegade Health Show Episode #335"

- A commonly asked question is "How do you get your protein?" Andrea replies on <u>December 31st, 2009</u> "Same place that bulls, horses, oxen, elephants, giraffes… get theirs! That makes people pause and think".

- To me building muscle is simply a matter of how much I want to workout (i.e. not directly related to protein intake). The body only needs 3% protein per day and most plant foods have around 5%." – Matt

- Sun Warrior Protein, Vega, greens, hemp seeds, chia seeds, blue-green algae, *spirulina*, chlorella, goji berries, various nuts & nut butters, various seeds, various sprouts, juiced wheatgrass, pea protein, sprouted barley protein powder, grains such as quinoa, brown rice, legumes, Manna bread, Ezekiel sprouted grain bread and pretty much everything else I eat that's raw vegan.

Randy Jacobs stabilizes his weight by adding manna bread and avocado to his diet and taking a protein shake during the day to which he adds hemp oil and lecithin (you can now get sunflower lecithin), Warrior Protein and stevia. Raw Hemp Seed Protein is awesome. Randy says, "There is something about it that fills me with energy all day long."

Bonnie Sinclair on August 9, 2010, says that even with chemo the next day, she is filled with enough energy to wash walls. See her Testimony in chapter 10 of the manual.

Lina Russo, a health consultant, recommends increasing your probiotics. She said, "take at least 100 billion colony forming units". Try many types of probiotics. Each will proliferate in your gut and clean you out.

Anne Marie Clement recommended the following for a senior who was 165 pounds and lost 45 pounds during seven months of chemo for esophagus cancer, which had spread to his liver. He could only take in food in liquid form through a straw. This is not medical advice.

- Nut almond milk with Sun Warrior in feeding tube

- 11 am juice made from sunflower, pea, cucumber and celery. The last two ingredients are added to make it palatable.

- 12:30 – 1:00: sunflower and pea sprouts blended and strained.

- 3 colonics and 2 enemas with 2 wheatgrass implants.

- Multivitamin 2x; iron, 2x; enzymes, 5x at meals.

- Sea Vegetables are highly recommended.

For those who can eat them, avocados help people gain weight, and they can be eaten in a variety of ways. However, they are too thick to go through a feeding tube.

Kids, Fruit & Veggies – An Awesome Combination

Vegetables. I know what you're thinking—"Great! I get to force-feed my kids two more times a day!" It's true—vegetables are usually the trickiest component to integrate into a kids' diet. But it's worth the effort, because veggies give them more nutritional bang for your buck than any other food group. What's best is, if both parents eat a plant-based diet and that's all that is available to the children since their birth. These children like vegetables. However, if the parents or just one parent has recently changed to a plant-based diet or when the children start to be exposed to processed and animal food, it's necessary to get creative. You can usually find a way to get your kids to eat vegetables without too much emotional scarring. Many dinner table disputes are about kids trying to assert their independence. You can get around this by letting your kids assist in the selection and preparation of the vegetables. If you take them to the farmers market and let them pick out the vegetables, learn about how they're grown, etc., you're more likely to get more acceptance back home when it's time to eat the vegetables. Encourage them to grow their own vegetables. You can also give them choices like celery sticks or baby carrots. But don't use dessert as a negotiating tool, as in the old standby, "no dessert until you eat all your vegetables." You just end up vilifying the vegetables and glamorizing empty calories—and those are values they'll take into adulthood.

Talk up the veggies and let them know all the health benefits they'll get from eating them. Karen Ranzi suggests "the use of puppetry with children, as it is an excellent way to introduce them to unprocessed fruit and vegetables, and to encourage discussion of healthful living topics in a non-threatening play situation."[49]

You can also serve veggies with hummus or guacamole. We made guacamole for my two grandchildren, Jane (6) and Ray (3) by mashing one avocado with a fork and adding one fourth teaspoon of onion powder and one eighth teaspoon sea salt.

Fruits. Fruits are a marginally easier sell than vegetables. They're sweeter and appeal more to kids' palates. Nevertheless, one thing to watch out for is fruit juice. A lot of people make the mistake of thinking a serving of fruit and a serving of juice are interchangeable. In fact, the American Academy of Pediatrics recommends limiting juice for kids to a couple of drinks a day, as juice is a contributing factor to dental cavities and gastrointestinal problems. Whole fruit, on the other hand, provides tons of fiber and other nutrients, and kids can partake of it quite freely, without any adverse effects. As with vegetables, if you have the patience and the knife skills, fruit can be carved into fun shapes or you can make fruit kabobs. You can also come up with low-fat healthy dips like guacamole and hummus that kids can dunk their fruit into. On hot summer days, try freezing some grapes or a banana as an alternative to a mid-afternoon Fudgesicle. With both fruits and vegetables, you might consider setting up a big "snack bowl" in the kitchen. Let the kids help choose which fruits and veggies go in the snack bowl, and then give them permission to grab what they want from the bowl, whenever they're hungry. This will help them feel like they're in control of what they're eating, but without giving them carte blanche to hit the sugar or the chips.

---

[49]Ranzi, Karen. "Creatively Fun Tips for a Healthy Family Lifestyle" www.vibrancemagazine.com accessed December 2010.

Presentation is everything. Cut apples into quarter inch slices and cut out shapes with miniature cookie cutters. Then spread them with almond butter and use raisins, cranberries, tiny slices of carrots or other veggies to create cat or other animal faces with whiskers. "Texture is very important if you don't want your children to fuss about eating their greens,"says Karen Regnante. She says, "a child may not like green leafy vegetables in a salad, but may love them in a green smoothie, green soup, green pudding, green dip, or green dressing." … "Name the food you make with lively or catchy titles. My kids created their own recipes, even from the time they were very little, and then gave names to the recipes."[50]

"Health Food Restaurant" is another idea that Karen has found successful with children – "Let your kids be the Chefs! If you set the example, your children will love setting up counters, and preparing smoothies, juices, fruit or veggie platters, guacamole, cole slaw and beautiful salads. My children often use a doorway as an ideal place to set up their restaurant. The ironing board, or a small table, was the counter. Even when we traveled, we bought food for them to prepare meals for us in our hotel room, and my husband and I would be the customers, paying them for our meals."[51]

"Equipment," Karen emphasizes, "is something that kids love – a saladacco for making veggie pasta; a snow cone maker for making ices from fresh fruit juice, for a special birthday party treat; a small juicer (such as The Healthy Juicer); a mini food processor, a juicer for making all sorts of recipes, especially banana ice cream; and a dehydrator, for making crackers, veggie burgers and chips, heated at low temperatures to preserve the enzymes, vitamins and minerals of the food."[52]

Smoothies. A lot of kids will refuse to eat any fruits or vegetables unless they've gone through a massive amount of processing. Here's where the blender or food processor can be your best friend. By keeping a few bags of frozen fruit on hand, you and your little kitchen helper can make your own smoothies. Just pick a combination of your favorite fruits, add some ice, some banana slices, and blend until smooth. It's a sweet, cold summer treat, and it gives your kids all the fiber and nutrients from fruit that a lot of fruit juices miss.

Healthy-packed cooler. It's summertime, which means it could be time for a family road trip. Hopefully, you'll have room in the car for a cooler packed with healthy snacks like the ones mentioned above.

Some of the favorite recipes of children are listed below and found in the recipe chapter.

- Green Juice
- Smoothies
- B.A.T.
- Guacamole dip for cut up veggies
- Ants on a Log
- Snowballs

- Black Snake Salad
- Veggie Burgers
- Banana Bread
- Apple Enzyme Pie
- Fruit Cream

---

[50] Ibid.

[51] Ibid.

[52] Ibid.

Khalsa Childcare - Starting Them Out Right
by Amar Fuller

Khalsa Childcare has a spiritual foundation. Like the nature of life and the children that we serve, our children's center is always evolving and growing. We are a blending of the experiences, influences and inspirations that I have been blessed to receive throughout my life. From the spiritual path we learn to maintain a healthy and clean body, mind and soul by taking care of ourselves through yoga, meditation, proper eating and positive thinking. From the Waldorf system of education, based on the teachings of Rudolf Steiner, we learn to flow with the breath of life, in-haling and exhaling with the coming and going of its many tides. From Hippocrates Health Institute, we learn that living foods promote optimum health and inspire us to nurture our planet.

I first met Drs. Brian Clement and Ann Wigmore in the 1970s at Hippocrates Health Institute in Boston. I was so deeply inspired by their teaching that I adopted the living foods lifestyle and brought it home to my family. Each day at Khalsa Childcare we produce a vast array of sprouts, fresh green drinks, sauerkraut and dehydrated foods. It takes organization and cooperation, and each person plays a role. My husband is the main grocery buyer. To supplement the produce form our own organic garden, we buy cases of organic produce from local organic farms and orchards.

My two assistants make wheatgrass juice, green drinks and a giant salad, and I make the dressings, snacks and lunches. The children love to help. They soak and sprout the seeds, and then plant them in the soil on sprouting trays. They pound the cabbage in the bucket for sauerkraut and even hull the buckwheat and sunflower greens for our salads. It's fun to work to lively, rhythmic music! One of the most precious moments of our day is when the children gather around the table, mouths wide open and heads lifted high to receive their gentle eyedropper squirt of wheatgrass juice.

Parents often ask for recipes for dishes we prepare. We are finishing two projects which celebrate our dining rituals a CD compilation of our favorite songs and blessings, and a recipe book – *Amar's Live Food Recipe,* featuring illustrations by the children and our "Very Berry Birthday Layer Cake." So yummy! At Khalsa's parent conferences we address the child's personal and social development, and discuss diet in relation to behavior and health. We have a lending library of books, audiocassette tapes and DVD's and we provide group and one-on-one food preparation instruction. Our newsletter features a regular recipe corner and health tips geared toward the living foods lifestyle.

In addition to responsible self-care, we also promote responsibility in caring for our group and our planet. Each day when a child comes through our door he or she becomes part of a larger family. Throughout the day we encourage an awareness of this family and an excellence in our interactions within it, from our speaking and eating, to our recreation. We strive to empower the children to take responsibility within the group in a graceful and confident way. They learn to speak, to listen and to work together. In all of our activities we talk about carefulness and appreciation for our earth through the materials we use and the ways in which we use them. As recycling keeps our rivers and streams unpolluted and the animal and plant life alive, eating living foods keeps our blood streams clean and continually oxygenated, helping us to feel and look our best.

At Khalsa Childcare, we are always open to insights, support and information to further our mission. The definition of success as Ralph Waldo Emerson expresses it, rings true in our hearts: "To leave the world a bit better, whether by a healthy child, a garden patch or a redeemed social condition: to know even one life has breathed easier because you have lived. This is to have succeeded." At Khalsa Childcare it is indeed our very joyous mission to succeed…one healthy child at a time.

Amar Kaur Fuller welcomes visitors. The address is 189 Long Plain Road, Leverett, MA 01054 Call Amar at 413-548-9841 or email her at amar.fuller@gmail.com.

Khalsa Childcare Update 2010
by Amar Fuller

The article for the Hippocrates Magazine "Healing Our World" was written in the year 2006. Now in the year 2010 we are putting into action the beginning steps of our future vision. The Khalsa Learning Center is a project to begin in Sept. 2011. It is not only an educational opportunity but a chance to live life as a community or village as a microcosm of how we hope to see the world in its full power. We have begun a leadership system at Khalsa Childcare. The children who are fortunate to stay with us which are six years and older become sprout helpers from the littlest sprout up. Starting with alfalfa all the way to sunflowers! Right now our youngest alfalfa sprout helper is helping juice the wheatgrass, green drinks, garnishing the open face kale wraps with sprouts, cutting fruit for smoothies and clearing the table after snacks and lunch, etc. Our 13 yr. old is already a sunflower sprout helper. She originally came with a health challenge to practice the basic Hippocrates program for her own healing and now all on her own can cut and prepare everything for juicing and even make luscious side dishes (walnut tacos, lasagna and onion bread are some of her favorites!) without any help!! She is artistic and will be illustrating our first published recipe book "Raw Power from the KHALSA KIDS KITCHEN!" The following is a little bit about our program for the older children after they graduate from daycare! You can email me at amar.fuller@gmail.com with any inquiries or for the PowerPoint presentation of the Khalsa Learning Center.

Khalsa Learning Center: An approach to education in the pioneer valley for children ages 5 through 13 that nurtures the spirit.

About Amar and Khalsa Childcare

- American Sikh
- Raw & Living Foods
- Certified Hippocrates Health Educator
- Licensed Daycare Provider for 25+ years
- Nurturing children from birth through adulthood for over 35 years
- Yoga, lessons, nature studies, circles, meditation, conscious toilet training

Inspirations and Vision for Khalsa Learning Center

- Siri Singh Sahib

- "Last Child in the Woods" by Richard Louv
- Native culture
- Non-Violent Communication - Marshall Rosenberg, Ph.D.

Mission Statement: Our mission for the Khalsa Learning Center (Khalsa means "pure one") is born out of the desire to create the healthy world in which we want to live. Our goal is to teach children 5 through 13 years old the values and skills to create a sustainable and peaceful present and future. Children will realize at a foundational age their own radiance and worth and the magic of learning and engaging.

All aspects of being - intellectual, physical, social, emotional and spiritual - will be nurtured and developed at the Khalsa Learning Center. "Lessons" come from natural learning opportunities woven into daily life, not isolated from their meaning or practicality.

A Day At Khalsa Learning Center:

8:30 a.m. morning circle

9:00 a.m. Seva/karma yoga

9:15 a.m. Snack

9:30 a.m. Lesson

10:15 a.m. Outdoor play

11:00 a.m. Gardening/Science & Food prep/Health Class

12:00 p.m. Lunch

12:30 p.m. Reading

1:00 p.m. Nature Class and Journaling

2:00 p.m. Music & Art

3:00 p.m. Talking Stick Circle/NVC/Drumming/Chanting

3:30 p.m. End of Day

Special Outings:

Horseback Riding (once per week)

Hiking (twice per week)

Fine Arts Center Performances (four times per year)

Summary Questions:

- Are you on a path to master your destiny? Explain.

- Do you experience life force energy?

- How are you integrating the "Hippocrates lifestyle" into your daily living?

- What are you doing to eliminate toxins?

- How do you follow your food plan when with family, friends and eating out?

- How do you eat when travelling?

- How do you encourage children to eat a plant-based diet?

- What are some ways to gain weight on a plant-based diet?

- What are some ways to stay on a live food diet in the wintertime?

DVD – "Practical Living"

How to really live the Hippocrates Lifestyle when you return home.

How to have what you need at home, work and in social situations.

47 minutes

1. What is the best source of nutrition in order to stay healthy?

2. What are the best nutrients to use in your green drink and the percentages of each?

3. Where do you get your amino acids from for living a healthy lifestyle?

4. What are the green drinks that best nourish the body for a healthy live food lifestyle?

5. If you are very anemic, what is the best thing you can do for your body that creates the best results for normalizing metabolism?

6. What is the best way to nourish the body and why?

7. What is the best investment you can make for your life with respect to your body, for living a healthy lifestyle?

8. What is the best type of juicer to purchase in order to obtain the best results from juicing?

9. Why is it better to use a masticating (grinder or auger) juicer, than a centrifugal juicer?

10. What is the temperature at which enzymes break down?

11. Why is it important to use a juicer that doesn't heat up?

12. What are two ways to grow sprouts?

13. Why is it better to use organic produce and support organic farmers, than non-organic produce?

14. Why is it better to drink the juices right away instead of making a whole lot ahead of time and drinking them later?

15. What is the importance and value of drinking juices, and what does it do to your organs and blood stream?

16. What is the best breakfast drink to drink on an empty stomach in this raw food lifestyle and why, and what drink would you follow up right after?

17. What are the heaviest detoxing hours in your body?

18. What is another drink that will help you cleanse after the green drink?

19. What does cayenne do for the body?

20. Why is it better to toast bread before you eat it?

21. What is the Hippocrates salad dressing?

22. Why is it better to dehydrate food, than to bake it?

23. List the four grains that Hippocrates recommends to use when dehydrating.

24. Why is it unhealthy to use whole wheat?

25. Describe a recipe for making veggie burgers in the dehydrator.

26. Describe a recipe for potato chips in the dehydrator.

27. List the five gluten-free grains that are recommended to use in this video.

28. Why is it important to purchase a dehydrator in which you can control the temperature?

29. Describe what irradiated spices are; are they healthy to consume?

DVD – "Bringing It All Home"

The various cycles of the healing process on the physical, emotional and spiritual levels. The importance of attitude and commitment to achieve your highest goals in life.Practical advice of integrating the Hippocrates Lifestyle.

47 minutes

1. How do I live in a sick world in a real and healthy way?

2. What is being committed to a "living food" lifestyle?

3. How do we convince ourselves to follow this lifestyle?

4. Do your family and friends discourage you from following a "living food" lifestyle, and if so, why?

5. How do you deal with family if they are uncomfortable with your "living food" lifestyle?

6. What is the name of the lifestyle you wish to achieve which is also the name of one of Ann Wigmore's books?

7. What are the three steps for reaching your goal in a "living food" lifestyle?

8. This is the first time you were told that gas is good for you. What do the initials G.A.S. mean?

9. Explain the process of regeneration in your body.

10. What is the foremost major challenge you'll have while creating a "living food" lifestyle?

11. What are the two basic areas in creating this lifestyle?

12. What are the challenges you'll face between the 7th and 14th year of this new lifestyle?

13. What are the challenges you'll face in dealing with the years between 14 and 21 years?

14. How are optimal health and wellness achieved by the Hippocrates "Living Foods" Lifestyle?

15. Compare how a vegan diet affects the environment versus animal-based diet. Answer is not in the DVD.

16. What's the difference between consuming salmon for your Omega 3's versus obtaining your Omega 3's in Blue-Green algae?

17. Explain the conclusions of T. Colin Campbell's "The China Study".

18. What do you think about the product "laetril" concerning cancer treatment?

19. What is the second evolution of the healing cycle called?

20. What is the third evolution of the healing cycle called?

21. What is similar to hemoglobin in the blood and chlorophyll?

22. What is the main method for killing microbes?

23. Why is the chlorophyll in wheatgrass important?

24. What are Phytochemicals? Not in the DVD

25. What happens to phytonutrients when heated over 115 degrees Fahrenheit?

26. Where are phytonutrients found?

27. What are the 3 types of sprouts that are anti-microbial, anti-carcinogenic and affective for cardiovascular disease?

28. What is the chemical "MTBE" and where is it used? Why is it dangerous to your health?

29. What are the two forms of filtration that create the best water and explain each type?

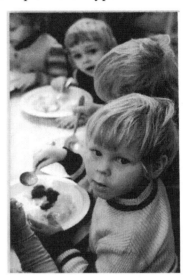

30. Does anything happen to vegetables if you freeze them and defrost them for consumption?

31. Describe a recipe with the gluten free grains Hippocrates recommends?

32. Describe the difference between white potatoes and sweet potatoes?

33. Describe the noodles that are recommended in this video, as well as why tomatoes are not a good sauce to use on pasta.

34. What is an excellent spaghetti sauce to use on pasta?

Chapter 10
Testimonials

My Journey to Health
by Betsy Bragg written in 2012

My journey in practicing the Living Foods Lifestyle began in 2006 when my son sent me to the three-week "Change Your Life" program at the Hippocrates Health Institute (HHI) in West Palm Beach, Florida. Through its holistic dietary, exercise, educational, therapeutic programs and loving atmosphere, I overcame lifelong persistent complaints of compulsive over-eating, Attention Deficit Hyperactivity Disorder (ADHD) accompanied by dyslexia, crippling arthritis and idiosomatic hypersomnia (falling asleep, even when driving a car).

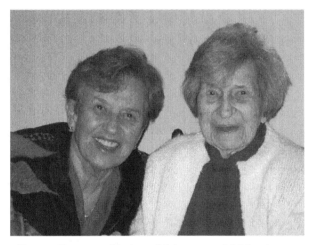

Betsy Bragg with her 104-year-old Mom

Like many Americans, my upbringing reinforced the myth that comfort food equals love. This myth led to my addiction to sugar, wheat, fat and, later, alcohol and pills. I turned to substances to fill my emptiness. I put down my last drink in 1980, and today, I take no drugs or medications of any kind. I attribute my success of overcoming my addictions to the 12-step AA program where I began my personal relationship with a Higher Power. My spiritual beliefs permcate and support every aspect of my life today. This is reinforced by the Hippocrates philosophy, which promotes a holistic comprehensive approach encompassing spiritual, emotional, mental, nutrition, elimination and exercise aspects of health.

During midlife, I developed severe arthritis due to various injuries and accidents as well as due to an acidic lifestyle. To change from being acidic to alkaline, water is an important component since the body is 70 percent water. In 2000, I installed an alkaline water ionizer. I also started drinking wheatgrass juice and adding more leafy green vegetables to my diet. Now I sleep through the night without pain and am filled with energy during the day. I still ski with my children and grandchildren, swim, bike, kayak and practice yoga. I maintain a busy schedule of teaching three simultaneous ten-week courses on "Life Force Energy – The Hippocrates Approach to Health," as well as public speaking engagements and individual health counseling.

In 1995 I was diagnosed by a neuro-psychologist as having ADHD. I believe this diagnosis was ultimately incorrect and that my behavior was due to my acidic diet. My ability to focus improved tremendously after practicing the living food lifestyle.

All these experiences led me to take the nine week Health Educator's Certification course at Hippocrates Institute. Upon its completion, I was selected to be the Executive Director of the nonprofit, Optimum Health Solution. Its mission is to eliminate obesity, chronic disease and malnutrition, especially in children, through education and advocacy of healthy living. To fulfill this mission, I first launched a thirty credit educational program for teachers at the Martin Luther King Jr. K-8 School in Dorchester, based on the Hippocrates Health Institute approach. This program included lesson plans for the students, as well as a gardening project. Support for this program came from the Life Force Energy Classes, Dinner Speaker Series and sales of health products. Now in 2012, we focus our energies directly on students in an after-school program, "Real Kids Real Food" (www.realkidsrealfood.org) in Somerville, MA.

At 78 years of age, I'm blessed to be doing my life's work healing myself and healing the planet through the Hippocrates Approach to Optimum Health.

In closing, let me quote the Director of Hippocrates Health Institute, Dr. Brian Clement: "Never forget that one step and one person at a time brings us closer to the world that we are meant to live in." My personal hope is that those lives I've touched, in turn, touch other lives, thus working in concert to make the world a better place.

The Turning Point toVitality,Inner Peace & Mindfulness: Overcoming Arthritis, Substance Cravings & ADHD

by Betsy Bragg, Waltham, Massachusetts

Published in *Healing Our World*, Hippocrates Health Institute, Volume 31, Issue 1, 2011

Growing up in my family, I was not allowed to show any feelings except happiness. Eating and drinking was my way to escape loneliness, emptiness and grief. My entire life I've struggled with compulsive overeating (at my highest weight I was 235 pounds!). Also, I began abusing alcohol at age 12 and later abused medications. Diagnosed with ADHD and dyslexia, I struggled through school. Even though I was expelled at the end of my freshman year of college due to poor performance, I returned and finished college with the help of many tutors. I married my eating and drinking partner and continued a downward spiral for 23 years. After that time when I became aware of my self-destructive path, I entered AA and OA, and the marriage ended. The only good to come from that union was my two wonderful children!

I put down my last drink in 1980, and today, I take no medications of any kind. I attribute my success of overcoming my addictions to AA, the 12-step program where I began my personal relationship with a Higher Power. In later years, I was struck with crippling arthritis and ideosomatic hypersomnia (the inability to stay awake, even while driving a car or teaching school). In 2006, my son, Tom Lindsley, offered to send me to the three-week "Change Your Life" program at the Hippocrates Health Institute (HHI) in West Palm Beach, Florida, and I jumped at the chance!

Each morning at HHI, I rose early to walk along winding paths of burbling brooks in tropical splendor, on my way to practice Qigong. This was followed by an invigorating shot of wheatgrass juice. Drinking only wheatgrass, green juices and water, eating sprouts and leafy greens and exercising eradicated my lifelong sugar/carbohydrate/alcohol/medication cravings, and filled me with vitality. Individual and group therapy released a lifetime of unexpressed tears and anger. At last I could sleep through the night without the severe arthritic pains which had resulted from years of an acidic diet.

Amazingly, I discovered that I was able to concentrate for hours, and my focus returned. I now believe that the neuro-psychologist's diagnosis of ADHD was incorrect, and that my behavior was due to my acidic, sugar-filled diet.

These miraculous life changes inspired me to take up the torch and implement Brian Clement's words "Heal Yourself and Heal the Planet." Therefore, I started the monthly Dinner Speaker series to help others learn about the living food lifestyle. These events offered gourmet raw vegan organic non-processed potlucks that also featured national and international speakers.

Education requires more than a monthly meeting. The word "education" is derived from the Latin word "educare," meaning "to draw out," while "e" means "from," and "duco" means "to lead, conduct, or guide." Everyone possesses the healing power of the life force within them, and my goal is to help people release that healing force and rebuild their immune system. A background of 55 years of teaching and counseling helped me accomplish this goal, and this background led me to take the nine-week Health Educator's Certification program at Hippocrates Institute in 2008. Combining the Hippocrates principles and methods with my intimate knowledge of the 12 steps, I wrote the syllabus and curriculum for the 10-week (30-hour) course "Life Force Energy – the Hippocrates Approach to Optimum Health."

I've been teaching the course four times a year ever since. Participants change their lives through yoga/meditation, hands-on food preparation, discussion of homework assignments in the manual and DVDs, weekly guest speakers and individual coaching between classes. (For program details see http://www.optimumhealthsolution.org).

Upon graduation from the HHI Health Educator Program, I applied, and was selected, to be the Executive Director of the nonprofit, Optimum Health Solution. Our mission is to eliminate obesity, chronic disease and malnutrition, especially in children, through education and advocacy of healthy living. To fulfill this mission, Optimum Health for Kids (a 30-credit teacher course based on the Hippocrates Health Institute philosophy) was launched at the Martin Luther King Jr. K-8 School in Dorchester, Massachusetts. With a donation of five dehydrators from the Excalibur Company, second graders created booklets on "How to Make Awesome Apple Crisps," and eighth graders took part in a blind taste test proving that dehydrated potato chips were "more yummy" than the cafeteria or store-bought ones. Students felt energized from chewing on wheatgrass and eating sprouts they grew in the classroom. (For details about the program, see http://www.optimumhealthsolution.org/kids.htm). This program is financed by the proceeds of the Life Force Energy classes, our Dinner Speaker Series, the sale of health products, auctions and donations.

I realized that the entire family needed to be educated if our goal was to effectively change the lifestyle of children. According to a recent study by the University of North Dakota School of Nursing, "obese parents have obese children, and warrant intervention." OHS is planning a study of parents who are struggling with obesity, and who have a three- or four-year-old obese child. OHS is offering a 10-week (30-hour) educational program for parents, and will then work to further support families by conducting a monthly "Healthy Eating Family Club" for the kids. Parents need to be educated about healthy nutrition and healthy living in order to properly guide their children. Part of the education they receive addresses real life challenges, such as how to keep the living food lifestyle going on a limited income. OHS plans to enlist:

1. A graduate student to do the statistical analysis and write up the study.

2. A medical facility to do pre and post blood tests, along with a six-month follow-up.

3. Funding for the study.

4. Community Supported Agriculture shares of food for families that can't afford them.

If you would like to help, please call 617-835-2913 or email bbski@stanfordalumni.org.

Thanks to the challenges I've overcome, and thanks to my recovery through the 12-Step AA and Hippocrates programs, with the help of a Higher Power, my life's work is to help others to heal themselves, and to heal the planet. I have been rewarded by seeing former students carry the torch. These students are now teaching this course in their areas. The goal is for these torchbearers to start a rippling effect, thus inspiring others to do the same. I am only one person in a long line of educators starting with Ann Wigmore's grandmother. Through the Health Educators program, we are helping each person fulfill their highest potential, and that is the sole objective behind my passion. My spiritual beliefs permeate every aspect of my life today. This is reinforced by the Hippocrates philosophy promoting a holistic approach to health and wellbeing, which is a comprehensive program encompassing the spiritual, emotional, mental health, nutrition, elimination and exercise facets of optimal health.

In closing, let me quote the Director of the Hippocrates Health Institute, Dr. Brian Clement, "Never forget that one step and one person at a time brings us closer to the world that we are meant to live in."

Curriculum Vita

All of my life experiences as an educator, counselor, chef and computer consultant have prepared me for my ideal position as a volunteer Director of *Optimum Health Solution (OHS)*. OHS is a non-profit organization dedicated to eliminating obesity, chronic disease and malnutrition, especially in children, through the education and advocacy of healthy living. Through OHS, I have:

1. Certified 171 health educators via the 10-week- course Life Force Energy / The Hippocrates Approach to Optimum Health, since 2008. These graduates have gone out and started their own way of healing the world.

2. Created the dinner speaker series, which brought to Massachusetts 65 national and international speakers since 2006.

3. Created a 30-credit/ one-year course, for teachers at the Martin Luther King School in Boston.

4. Created the *Real Kids Real Food* pilot program with 10 lessons given bimonthly to the children of the Elizabeth Peabody House in Somerville.

My work experience encompasses being a Director of Middlesex County Employment and Training Program for Refugees and Immigrants and numerous teaching positions from kindergarten through college. As a principal of Lindsley Associates with UN, USAID and CA contracts, I lived in the Philippines, West Indies and El Salvador. I have previously lived in Japan for one year.

My education includes a Bachelor's degree from Smith College in History & English, Master's in Counseling and Education from Stanford University and Harvard University, and Master's from Boston University in the Administration of Multi-Cultural Non Profit Organizations. I'm also certified as a Health Educator from the Hippocrates Health Institute.

Recovering from Lyme Disease
by Karen Regnante

Published in *Hippocrates Magazine,* Volume 28, Issue 1, pages 52-53, 2008

Reprinted with permission from the author and Hippocrates Health Institute

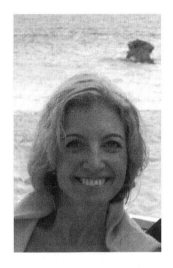

We hear about "miracles" every day, it seems, until we begin to doubt all the promises and cure the doctors and specialists offer us. This is my story of how I found my miracle at Hippocrates; of how it has brought me back to life. For the past seven years, I struggled with Lyme disease. For five of them, I haven't been able to work at all. Most of the time I was on the couch or in bed… in tremendous pain, utterly exhausted, anxious and mentally so confused I couldn't even balance my checkbook.

Prior to this, I led a very active life, working as a Business Development Executive in New York City, traveling extensively, skiing, windsurfing, hiking, biking and kayaking. My life was full spending time with family and friends and pursuing my spiritual path. I was at the top in my field.

Suddenly, in the fall of 2000, I developed incredible muscle pains, fevers, insomnia… the list goes on. My primary care physician said it was stress. Six months later, after seeing many doctors, I found a great Lyme doctor who properly diagnosed my condition and gave me a lot of oral antibiotics. It only helped to a point and my search continued. I then found another wonderful Lyme doctor who gave me antibiotics intravenously. I spent nine months with a pic line in my arm dosing twice a day. I also did a vitamin IV once a week. This and more oral antibiotics lasted for another two years. During this time, I worked with wonderful energy healers who gave their all to keep me going. Several of my friends were extraordinary in supporting me. I was so grateful for all the help and love I received but I was still barely surviving.

Finally, I had enough stamina to be up and around and financially needed to go back to work. I was lucky to get a job three days a week from one of my previous clients in NYC. I was so weak and the building was so large I couldn't walk to the bathroom in one stretch. I was living in Connecticut and had to take a car service to work and stay in a hotel one block away for these three nights just to be able to do the job. This lasted for a year and when I realized I didn't have the strength to work full-time in NYC, I took a job locally in Stamford. I was still very weak and had an ongoing lung problem that couldn't be diagnosed. Each day was a struggle to get out bed and go to work. Six months later, I was bitten again, and was totally back in bed and out of work! I went back on the antibiotics. With all the Candida that had developed, my digestive system was out of sorts. I ended up in the hospital having my appendix taken out. I was so sick of needles and hospital tests, I started taking anti-anxiety drugs just to get through the tests and treatments. Unfortunately, the drugs made me more anxious and my body couldn't stop shaking. At this point, my spirit and life totally fell apart.

This resulted in my moving back home with my parents to the home I grew up in. Quite an adjustment when you're 53 years old! I stopped taking some of the drugs the doctors had given me. I walked the beach every day, prayed a lot and did yoga. My Mom and Dad were great. In the spring, I went to a wonderful four-day course and became a raw food chef. I believed in the concept but I found that after three months of being raw, I couldn't stay on this version of a raw diet.

Shortly thereafter, I heard Brian speak and thought the Hippocrates lifestyle made great sense. For years I had wanted to go to Hippocrates, but many of the healers I had worked with told me a raw diet would be too much for my sensitive system. A few months later, I had a phone consult with Brian and it was one of the best consults I had ever had (and I have had many). Brian approached my challenge from all aspects – physically, mentally, emotionally and spiritually. He gave me a list of things to do including eating raw with no fruit, continuing to get off the medication and living life with more love and passion. It seemed impossible to do what he asked me but somehow I did it.

Seven months later, I decided to go to Hippocrates and stayed a month. Within a few days, I knew I had found my answer. I loved the food and could stay on the diet; the oxygen treatments made a huge difference; I got off more medication (yes, I was on a lot!) and over the month, I changed many of my perspectives and attitudes about life. I went through a tremendous detox and within two weeks my blood had changed dramatically. The people I met were so heartfelt and I knew several of them would become lifelong friends.

I left Hippocrates HEALTHY! I came home and started traveling and doing activities I hadn't been able to do in seven years! I am getting my life back. It's been several months and I'm now finding the diet is EASY. My body seems to crave this kind of food and when I eat something else, I notice a huge difference and go back immediately to what I know is best for me. For the first time in my life, I have the faith and courage to live my dreams. I'm much more comfortable stepping boldly into the unknown, letting the mystery of life unfold and handling whatever comes up along the way.This is a MIRACLE and I am ever so grateful to Brian, Anna Marie and all the staff and friends I made while I was there (as well as all my other friends and family I so dearly cherish). I highly recommend it to anyone and urge people with Lyme disease or an immune deficiency to come! There are no limits to what's possible for your life, especially once you've been to Hippocrates.

Update 2012:Karen has since been diagnosed with cancer and through the live food program has been fully restored to her optimal health.

Irritable Bowel Syndrome

Hippocrates Magazine, Volume 28, Issue 2, page 42, 2008

Reprinted with permission by Hippocrates Health Institute, Brian Clement

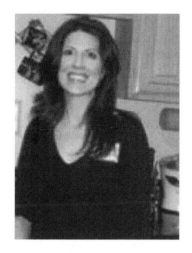

Well, just like many others before me, I can say that illness brought me to raw food. I spent over two years trying to work with numerous doctors to get a diagnosis for myself. All I knew was that whatever I put into my mouth caused me severe stomach pain and debilitating diarrhea. I spent years going from doctor to doctor, general practitioner, gastroenterologist, endocrinologist, etc. But no one could figure out what was happening to my body.

After numerous tests came out negative, I was told I probably had Irritable Bowel Syndrome (IBS) and was given medicine to help me live with it; however, the medicine's side effects cause not just drowsiness but actual sleep. This was not an answer for someone with two young children. I decided to find another way. I started to look into alternative medicine. I tried acupuncture, kinesiology, massage, reflexology, Chinese medicine, colonics, meditation and Qigong. I went to an osteopath, naturopath, chiropractor, and even a medical intuitive. I truly was desperate and was willing to try anything.

However, my weight kept on plummeting. I remember one day, I was getting out of the shower and I didn't even recognize myself in the mirror. I had lost thirty pounds and I looked like I was dying. People around me were scared and so was I. A doctor told me maybe I should start taking anti-depressants to calm my stomach, knowing that I wasn't even depressed! There were others who were convinced I was anorexic. At that time I was dabbling in raw food and was lucky enough to live by a raw food restaurant, and something just told me to stop. I'm so glad I did! Dr. Brian Clement, from the Hippocrates Health Institute was speaking.

Well, it was overwhelming, the knowledge he had about raw and living food. This man knew what he was talking about! I found out the institute had a three-week life-change program. I thought this would be great for my mother, who had pancreatitis. That night I called my mom and told her all about this interesting place called Hippocrates. The next day my mom called back and said my parents wanted to send ME to Hippocrates. I had a million excuses not to go. My mom said, "You just need to make the call." It took me months to make that call.

Then came my low point, one morning I got up feeling sick again. Feeling like I was again chained to the bathroom. I was home alone and I remember dropping to my knees screaming to God that I didn't want to live this way. I just wanted help. I kept screaming, "I cannot live this way, please help me." I cried so hard and for so long that I fell asleep on the floor.

That was the day things got better. When I woke up I had an amazing calmness. I immediately found the number to Hippocrates and called to make a reservation. The first date that was available was New Year's Eve. Looking back now I didn't realize how poignant that would be, a new start to a New Year and a new life.

The program was everything I needed to heal by body. I went down to Hippocrates thinking that my body wouldn't really detoxify that much because, I mean, I was a vegetarian. I didn't consume animal products, refined sugar, caffeine, or alcohol.

I was SO wrong! I couldn't even get through the first night orientation. I developed a migraine that was so severe. I had to be taken back to my room by golf cart! Boy, was I embarrassed. I had just as much to learn as everyone else.

The next day I was fine and over the next three weeks I learned to live the life that humans are supposed to live. I felt AMAZING! I can't imagine not having those three weeks. The first week was all about getting into the program, understanding how it all worked. The second week was more about how the physical manifestation of illness was being broken down. My body was HEALING. The third week was about strengthening my mind and awakening my spirit. I was no longer afraid of anything. I was not a diagnosis. I was not an illness. I was a human being, living and being supported by the earth and the people on it to become who I was supposed to be, a healthy individual. This is the right that we all are owed just by being born. I found a peace I had never known.

It has been a year since I left Hippocrates and my life has changed in such wonderful ways. I came home to teach my children and husband how to live a healthier life. I'm still working on transitioning them to a raw food lifestyle but I do it with love and compassion knowing that given the right options that their wants will change in time. They have come so far in one year. My kids now beg me for algae and my husband loves my collard green wraps! How wonderful is that? After hearing Gandhi's famous quote, "Be the change you wish to see in the world," I decided to start a monthly raw food potluck based on the teachings at Hippocrates. I am building the community that supports our family's lifestyle and it feels wonderful. I AM HEALED!

I want to thank Hippocrates, especially Brian and Anna Maria, for opening up my world to new possibilities and realizing that nothing is impossible. I also want to thank my parents, husband, and children as they continue to support me through this life-changing experience.

I continue to be well and healthy and wish the same for you and your families in this wonderful way of life.

Update 2012:Feeling Great!

Alkalizing & Embracing with Unconditional Love
Journey Through Cancer: Dorothy Torrey's Story
by Cheryl Kain, *Cape Healing Arts,* Autumn 2006

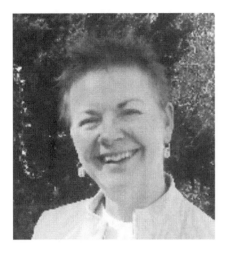

Dorothy Torrey's interest in health and prevention began over thirty years ago when she began talking with a neighbor about his healthy lifestyle; he added fresh vegetables and fruits to his diet and enjoyed just one 'special' cup of coffee a day. She wasn't interested in changing (she bought frozen vegetables and enjoyed coffee all day long) but continued talking with him, noticing his abundant energy, lean body and obvious joy.

Dorothy believed she was following the healthiest lifestyle possible – eating whole grain breads, organic yogurt, fresh fruits and vegetables, chicken, fish and dairy, taking vitamins and scheduling mammograms. She did what she was told to do by mainstream health practitioners.

Like most people, Dorothy was afraid of cancer. After hearing a woman's testimony about healing herself of cancer via adopting an alkaline lifestyle, Dorothy decided if she ever got "It" she would adopt a 100% alkaline lifestyle. Soon after, she purchased a recommended infrared comforter and felt she was doing the most possible to maintain her health. Little did she realize that she was barely touching the tip of the iceberg regarding balancing her body's alkalinity. After many years of a stressful, 'acidic' lifestyle, Dorothy speaks frankly. "This is a difficult thing to say, but today I know that I was 'doing cancer' for about 40 years. I had an extremely stressful first marriage to an active alcoholic; I gave myself very little sleep; overworked myself to prove myself worthy. I constantly sought approval, felt like I had no friends and spoke to no one about my pain. I hid, felt shame and blamed myself for everything." This kind of stress just creates an acidic environment in the body.

Dorothy was diagnosed with infiltrating ductal carcinoma of the breast in June 2003, confirmed by a Boston doctor. The immediate recommendation was lumpectomy, radiation and chemotherapy. Despite the doctor's recommendation, she decided to take three months to become more alkaline. On Dorothy's path she learned about Dr. Otto Warburg's – the only person to win the Nobel Prize twice in medicine – discovery that cancer does not grow in a highly alkaline/oxygenated environment; in fact, any cell deprived of 50% or more of its oxygen turns cancerous. Holistically, cancer is not local but systemic. Dorothy knew a person just doesn't cut out the cancer and think that it's gone. She knew she had to follow what was in her heart, a scary proposition since she had no idea where the money would come from to follow a holistic approach. Insurance would pay $150,000 to $300,000 for traditional standardized treatment covering lumpectomy, radiation and chemotherapy - not $10,000 to $20,000 for alternative or preventive treatment.

According to Dorothy, this was the first time she could remember standing on her own two feet to say no to something she did not believe in. Money or not, she would follow her truth, somehow finding the faith she needed to continue.

She found spiritual support at The Unity Church of the Light, where she was encouraged to 'come back home' to herself and be in integrity with what she deeply believed. At Unity, Dorothy learned it was not her job to figure out how she was going to do things. That was the job for God (the Creator, Source, Divine Father, Mother-God, whatever name you want to call this Energy).

At The Unity Church, she made a life-changing decision not to do God's job. She created a visualization of stepping out of her 'old box' and stepping into a 'new box' of personifying her truth and faith, and embracing her body's deep inner wisdom, no matter what it entailed. Pastor Steve Carty Cordry helped her process emotions and guided her spiritually throughout her journey with cancer. He continues to be a huge inspiration in her life.

"This is when the miracles started happening big time!" exclaims Dorothy.

Out of the blue, three weeks after Dorothy's diagnosis, she received a $10,000 check in the mail from her father. There was no note in the envelope, just the check. She had never received a check from her father in 45 years, and most interesting, her father did not know Dorothy had cancer. To Dorothy's and her siblings' surprise, he had sold some stocks and gave each of his children $10,000. What a serendipitous gift!

This was just what Dorothy needed to affirm that she was on the right path. Her mantra became, "Miracles are a natural, everyday occurrence when I follow my truth." She began to look for miracles each day. Somehow she knew that if she focused and committed to the truth, she would be all right.

Dorothy's two daughters were both entrenched in western medicine. They were very angry, believing their mother selfish for following her instincts. Dorothy's family wanted the lumpectomy, radiation and chemo. Understandably, they were scared that they would lose their mom. The ability to say no was difficult for a woman who never wanted to let anyone down.

"I did not have any identity from the day I was born, so I tried to please everyone in order that someone – anyone – would love me and not abandon me, or replace me. I needed to be perfect but was never good enough," she explains.

Resigning as a people pleaser was a daunting task. When Dorothy's daughter asked for help after a second caesarian, with a 2 year-old already at home, Dorothy said a gentle "no." She knew that with these words, she might never see her grandson, yet she opted once again to take good care of herself first.

Dorothy decided to live her life from a place of love, not fear. She would immediately replace fear with forgiveness of herself, knowing that fear and love could not exist at the same time. She continued to remove stress from her life as much as possible. Since her daughter didn't approve of Dorothy's treatments, she stayed away from her daughter's home, while still desperately wanting to help her.

The most powerful tool for Dorothy's healing was adding her name to prayer lists, along with consistent support from Pastor Steve. Falling asleep at night, it was profoundly nurturing to know friends, strangers, and health practitioners were praying for her when she was too tired to pray for herself.

She also attended a healing service at St. John's church in Sandwich. "When Father John McGinn puts his hands on my head and anoints it, I affirm that I am receiving the power of the Holy Spirit moving completely through my body. This healing experience is deeply moving," says Dorothy.

Dorothy became her own doctor; she couldn't find an oncologist who would track her progress. It was too threatening for most doctors to have a patient like her following non-traditional treatments and requesting tests out of their realm of experience.

At the suggestion of her naturopath, she found an oncologist in New Hampshire who said, "Yes, the treatment [we] oncologists recommend is barbaric, however this is the best we have today. From the studies that we have, the treatments show we get results. However, ten years from now doctors will not believe we put our patients through these treatments."

One Harvard doctor told Dorothy, "We have too much invested in keeping people sick. That is what our economy is based on." Yet another doctor said, "Cancer is a guaranteed salary." Dorothy's question remained, "What would happen if a cancer hospital says that there is a cure for cancer?"

Dorothy and her husband addressed previously unresolved issues, and he became her best friend and unending source of support. "I never thought it would happen! We're so different. Such unconditional love has come from him. We respect our differences and each other's boundaries now."

Women said to Dorothy, "I could never do what you did!" She replies, "This is not hard! Walking for 5 miles with a 50 lb. bag of cement on my back is hard work. Eating more green vegetables and drinking structured water is easy compared to that. My life is at stake. For me, going 'alkalarian' was much easier than surgery, chemo, radiation and drugs. Taking charge and responsibility for my health is a God-given gift."

Dorothy embraced a full commitment to changing her ways of eating, thinking and being. Her intention was to eliminate cancer and understand the root causes of sickness and disease. She drank six quarts of structured (pH drops added) water per day. She took many supplements – approximately 25 pills or drops. "Just the timing of the supplements and remembering were challenging!" laughs Dorothy. She ate organic and non-organic vegetables. For the first 21 days she ate only pureed foods, so her body's energy could be entirely focused on healing, not digestion.

Dorothy also completed a liquid cleanse to remove all yeast, fungi and mold from her system. She removed alcohol, coffee, sugar, grains, beans, and nuts from her diet, and took no drugs of any kind. She also ate lemons, limes, avocados and tomatoes.

She had a root canal extracted. Dorothy's holistic dentist, Dr. Tomasian, spoke about the connection between root canal and breast cancer. According to a study done by Dr. Rau in Switzerland, out of 150 women who had root canal surgery, 145 developed cancer. Sure enough, Dorothy's root canal was on the same meridian as her right breast. When the root canal was extracted, it was infected. There were no external signs or symptoms from this infection except the cancer.

Seven months after Dorothy's diagnosis, she had an Anti-Malignin Antibody Screen, a scientific cancer test developed by Dr. Samuel Bogoch, a Harvard-trained research neurochemist. The doctor said "Great news, you have no cancer cells. This test is 95% accurate." Dorothy's result was phenomenal. She felt overwhelming gratitude. "I was ecstatic!" she says.

Dorothy continues to alkalize and energize her body with her totally alkalarian diet. She enjoys Reiki, practices Tong Ren Healing (based on Carl Jung's theories), chiropractic, meditation, acupuncture, homeopathy and yoga. The 12-step program of Al-Anon has been extremely valuable to Dorothy (prompted by her first marriage to an alcoholic), assisting her in changing her patterns in relationships.

Perhaps most importantly, "I don't do any of this work alone. I call for help! I don't have any more faith, courage or inner wisdom than anyone else. We all have it," adds Dorothy.

For anyone with a cancer diagnosis, Dorothy recommends: "Go to the inner quietness deep within you and follow your truth. This is your path, no one else's! This journey can bring you unbelievable joy and peace." She adds, "I can finally be authentically who I really am. This is why cancer has been a blessed journey."

She battled with her cancer. She was not at war with her body; rather she concentrated on befriending her deepest self. She called cancer her "beautiful green healing crystals" and asked them what she needed to learn from them. "Sometimes we receive a gift, and we may not like how it was packaged or want what's inside. But does that mean that we deny or refuse the gift?"

The approach Dorothy chose contained no harmful drugs, treatments or tests. She had no side effects, and remarkably she also had no fear or doubt regarding the decisions she made.

Update 2012:

Canceling my Total Knee Replacement

For the past 10 years I have been bothered with arthritic knees. The orthopedic surgeons that I have seen over the years would say something like this to me: "Lady, look at your x-rays; you have bone-on-bone. From 1 to 10 you are a number 11, and you have bone spurs, too. You should have been in here for an operation a month ago. You must have great tolerance for pain". And, I would say to them, "No, I do not have great tolerance for pain; I just do not dwell on my knees being arthritic."

I would go home and clean up my diet more, eat more green leafy vegetables, alkaline smoothies, etc., and do those things that focus on prevention and well-being. However, during this past year, I allowed the stress in life to affect me, and so in January, I scheduled a total knee replacement. In moving forward on the operation, I attended the pre-operative education class for total joint replacement, visited the rehab center, spoke to physical therapists, and arranged support for good, fresh food and the right water to be brought in for me. In no way did I want to eat hospital or rehab food, processed and having GMOs, or to drink regular water.

Then all of a sudden, one evening, it was like a light bulb that went on within me, and I received this message, "This is not for you to do." I did not question this "clear knowing" that I received because it resonated within me as the Truth. I just clearly knew! So, the next morning, I told my husband I was canceling the operation. I told myself, "If I reversed breast cancer and other diagnoses, I can reverse this too. I am going to build cartilage!" Do I know exactly how I am going to do this? NO! However, I do know that God is in the unknown, and that I will gladly go into the unknown with God. I started to do a couple of different things:

1) Meditating and visualizing Healing Angels building cartilage in my knees. I said to myself, "Why not believe in this instead of believing that there is no cartilage being built?"(I was not about to hang onto any limiting beliefs.) I also began to do mind-body techniques in which I would visualize myself already healed and doing the things that I love to do, like biking and walking the beach, and hiking in Nepal in the near future. And I began to love my knees and say "Thank you for serving me so well today. "I would bend over and give them a kiss.

Well, all I can say is, "Wow, what energy returned!" To my surprise, one day I pedaled down to the beach and even walked the whole beach that is over 1- 1/4 miles!. Was I ecstatic! I decided to visit another orthopedic doctor see if there are any studies being done in the Boston area with mind/body techniques for building cartilage. The surgeon said, "No, there aren't." However, this visit was most interesting. After the doctor examined me, followed by looking at my x-rays, he said: "There is no question that you have arthritic knees — however, the person, you, sitting in front of me, does not match her x-rays."

He also said: "Do not underestimate the power of the mind. Your body wants to heal. Give it those thoughts and that support that attracts healing. Do not have any knee operation until the pain is so great that you cannot get out of bed to walk to the bathroom. You are not there yet, and you may never be there. I do not operate because of what x-rays tell me, I look at the whole person. You are vibrant. Keep doing the thing that you are doing. Your knee wants to build cartilage. Believe that it can and it will!"

Today, I am as happy and as joyful as I can be, knowing that I am building cartilage and this is the right thing for me to do. I know that I am a "Miracle Worker" when I allow myself to come home to the magnificence of who I am (spiritual being). Today, I choose to step into that magnificence because it demonstrates the workings of the Divine Intelligence who has created each and everyone of us. We came to the Universe to be healers and not tobe separate from the Divine. This is the most joyful path that I can be on. And I invite you to join me. Thank you!

Dorothy Torrey

Alkaline Health Coach, Certified Wellness Cuisine,

508-888-6677

dorothy@PathToVibrantHealth.com

Alternative Treatment for Cancer
byKaren Calise Woeller

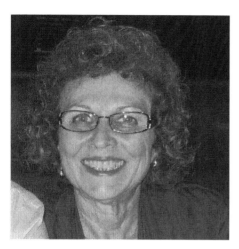

I was diagnosed in January of 2007 with DCIS Breast Cancer. But my journey to health began, as I discovered, sometime earlier.

In February of 2005 my mother had decided that she was going to enter into a hospice program. She had bravely lived with many illnesses and now that there was nothing that could be done she wanted to be home and live the rest of her life on her terms. And she did just that!

I moved in with her and stayed with her until she passed in July of that year. What I'd like to share with you is the gift she gave me about a week before she died. She was in a coma and I sat with her and talked to her about many things, then I just held her hand in silence and she said three things to me.

1. Love unconditionally, yourself and others.

2. Karen, trust your gut feelings your inner knowing and trust in God.

3. Have Courage and face life with your head held high.

I am very grateful for that powerful exchange, but at the time didn't realize how much that gift would impact my life and my journey.

Getting my life back together in the following year brought a weight gain of about 20 pounds and a knee injury. That brings me to the next milestone.

A torn ACL required surgery in December 2006. That's when a friend loaned me a book, "Prepare for surgery, Heal Faster," by Peggy Huddleston.I followed all the recommendations, speaking to doctors, meditating, and visualizing. I intuitively knew **"trust your gut feelings"** that everything was going to be fine and it was, but the best part was that the doctor was amazed at how well and how quickly I healed.

Now comes January 2007 and a diagnosis of breast cancer in both breasts. There were three sites in the left breast with one area that was considered invasive and one larger site in the right breast. After the initial shock, I knew in my inner knowing that this was just a bump in the road of life and that all would be fine. Again I had to" **trust my inner knowing and in God. "**My biggest question at that time was "What was the message that I was supposed to get from this experience?" "What information is in this for me?"

A month or so of testing and decision making followed and in March I had a bilateral mastectomy. Of course I once again followed Peggy's book with a great outcome.

I'd like to share this little story with you. As I was preparing for surgery and doing meditation and visualization, I visualized the invasive cancer as soap bubbles. Every time I did the visualization exercise I would systematically take a pin a break each bubble until there were no bubbles left and the area was squeaky clean.

On my follow up visit post-surgery, the doctor had a little story of her own. As she was affirming to me that everything had turned out well and all reports were good, she said an unusual thing had happened. She said that she was initially concerned when the pathology report had only shown that there were two sites in the left breast. The one site that they considered invasive was not there; the pathologist couldn't find a trace of it.

She had the lab going crazy checking everything. Yes, the surgery was perfect, all tissue was removed, it was my tissue, but that area was not there. What she believes happened was when I had the biopsy done they must have removed it all.

I know what really happened! My only thought at that time was, "why didn't I do that with all the sites? Duh!"

No chemotherapy, radiation or hormone therapy was recommended at that time. The surgery was a success with good margins and the chance of recurrence with only 2 to 3 percent of breast tissue remaining, was very low.

So I cleared that "bump in the road" that took up most of 2007 and now I could get back to living my life. And that I did.

The next chapter began three years later in April of 2010. I was taking a class in yoga and nutrition, an advanced polarity therapy class, when I began to think, "I have been living and eating exactly the same way I did before the cancer." What's the definition of insanity? Doing the same thing over and over and expecting different results. Duh! A light went on in my brain!

As each student presented research on different diet programs and or specific foods such as meat and dairy products and how they affect us, I began to think that now is the time to make some changes. There was a wealth of information in this class but the thing I kept hearing was make those changes and avoid any further "bumps in the road."

The one presentation that fascinated me the most was on Living on Live Food. It made so much sense. We are always trying to enhance our life force energy, why not do it with food that contains life force energy? The presenter actually made recipes from Alissa Cohen's book, "Living on Live Food." And so began my journey and my lifestyle changes.

I bought Alissa's book and read it. In it she recommended a 30-day commitment to eating raw in order to make an informed and intelligent decision about how you feel while eating an all-raw diet. So that's what I did. With great enthusiasm on my part, I might add, but not so much on my husband's part. He thinks I'm a bit crazy and likes to give me a hard time sometimes, especially when I have unconventional ideas. But being the wonderful and supportive guy he is, he agreed to try some of the recipes as long as he could still have his steak.

At about the two-week mark I became very ill. I felt nauseous, tired, and foggy, just all around miserable. In her book, Cohen mentioned these symptoms and that they could be the effects of the body detoxing and that it should pass in a few days. Well, it lasted for a week and I thought I couldn't make it one more day if I kept feeling that bad. But I had made a commitment to 30 days and kept going. On approximately the twentieth day, I felt fabulous. I remember waking up and feeling like something was very different then I realized I was breathing without wheezing. I had mild asthma but always had a slight wheeze in my breathing. It was gone! At that moment, I gave up dairy forever. The fog had lifted and I felt human again. Only now I felt even better. I made it 100 percent raw for eight weeks and have continued to eat mostly raw (approximately 80 percent) and totally gave up eating dairy and other animal products as well as processed foods.

My concern at that point was how do I know whether I'm getting all the nutrition I need? How do I find that information? And I don't know a single person who eats this way.

In August 2010, a small tumor appears under the skin on the right breast. In September, pathology report says it's cancerous. Doctors get into high gear about treatment, surgery, radiation, hormone therapy and try to convince me that we need to get started and as soon as possible.

I, on the other hand, listening to the words of my mother, am **listening to my inner knowing**. Diet and nutrition is what I think I should do. Where do I find the information I need?

A friend had loaned me the DVD "Healing Cancer from Inside Out" and I had watched the day before I got the news from the doctors that the cancer had returned. (Interesting timing) On that DVD I remembered Brenda Cobb who cured herself of cervical and ovarian cancer. "That was where I could get the information I needed!"

I received a flyer about the Health Expo in Sturbridge, Massachusetts (about 25 minutes from my home). Brenda Cobb just happened to be one of the speakers talking about her experience and her Institute in Atlanta, Georgia. I was not able to make it. A friend did go and was so impressed with Brenda that she bought her book and called to tell me about her. (Not knowing about the cancer returning – again, interesting timing.) She gave me the book, which eventually led me to a 12 day retreat at The Living Foods Institute in Atlanta.

My time spent at The Living Foods Institute was very well worth it. Besides learning more about the living foods lifestyle and how to prepare any number of recipes from breakfast to dessert, I came away learning a few important things about myself.

1. In the emotional healing classes that we had one of the topics was "forgiveness." I realized that I was able to forgive everyone but myself. That night I gave myself permission to not be perfect. Then I woke up in the middle of the night and cried for what seemed like hours.

My mother's words **"Love unconditionally, YOURSELF and others."**

2. The second one came in an energy session. When I was in high school I spoke to my Dad about going to college. He very lovingly said that the family could not afford to send both my brother and me to college. And since Vinny was the boy and would be the bread-winner in his family, it would be more important for him to go to college.

At the time I just accepted this and went on with my life. What I realized in the session was that what I "heard" is, you are not as important, not as worthy as your brother to receive an education.

Now I want to be clear that I know intellectually and in my heart that my father didn't feel that way. But what I learned is that we are affected in profound ways not by the words that are spoken but rather by the way we hear them.

At that moment I was freed of the feeling that "I'm not worthy."

Both those realizations have changed me tremendously.

Other benefits of being immersed in the living food lifestyle for 12 days were:

- Loss of 10 pounds

- Increase in energy

- Elimination of medication for hypertension

- Knowledge and confidence on how to live this lifestyle

- A happier and more positive outlook on life which has given me the "courage" to face all the challenges that have come my way **"with confidence and my head held high."**

Returning from Atlanta and on my own again.

Not long after returning home I realized that I needed to connect with other like-minded people and to continue to learn and integrate this into my life.

Up popped Betsy Bragg. I received her newsletter from "Optimum Health Solutions" giving the dates of her upcoming class from "Hippocrates Institute" on raw foods. Coincidence? I don't think so! Blessing? Absolutely!

I signed up the next day and took Betsy's class twice and could do it again. Thank you, Betsy.

In the last two and a half years that I have followed this lifestyle, my bloodwork has improved and my health will continue to improve every day.

How I maintain this lifestyle.

1. Take one day at a time

2. Love myself unconditionally.

3. Forgive myself when I'm not perfect

4. Stay connected to others that believe in this lifestyle

5. Remember it's a process

6. Try to keep a routine

7. Cleanse – enemas and colonics. I have committed to do at least 2 cleanses and 10 colonics a year for 2 years.

8. Drink and use alkaline water

9. Read and reread all the information that I have processed in the past 2 ½ years and continue to learn and grow

10. Expand my horizon

11. Enjoy life

12. Be grateful for all that there is

13. Share what I have learned

14. Don't expect – especially that my husband follow my path, let him find his own

15. Trust my "gut" feelings and trust in God, for He only gives us what we can handle and from that we learn and grow.

16. Have "Courage" and face life with my head held high.

So back to one of my first questions, "What was the message I was suppose to get from this experience?" I believe it was to "Open my heart;" I needed to learn to love myself unconditionally. "Connect with God;" I had questions about my spirituality that were answered, and "Share my blessings with others" by being a good role model.

So in closing I'd like to say my journey has been a combination of physical healing, emotional, energetic, and spiritual healing.

A Testimonial About The Living Food Lifestyle
by Bonnie Sinclair

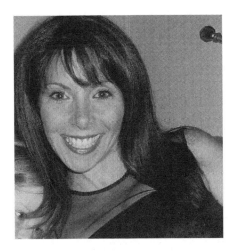

Bonnie Sinclair is a super testimonial about practicing the "living food" lifestyle. Bonnie attended the 2009 spring class, "Life Force Energy: The Hippocrates Approach to Optimum Health," then attended the Life Change class at Hippocrates Health Institute. She's a single mom with 6-year old twins – an absolutely super mom. Bonnie has become an excellent raw food chef and gardener. She wrote the following to me:

July 31, 2009, was a very important day for me. It was the one-year anniversary of the diagnosis I received in 2008. I believe this made me a one-year survivor of fallopian cancer.

In this past year, I have learned a lot about nurturing and alkalizing my body and eating live raw food, wheat grass and mixed green vegetable juice. I have met a whole new group of people because of this transition. I have released nearly 20 lbs and am happier with the way my body feels and looks than I have been in many years. My cholesterol has dropped enormously. I think I just might be healthier than I have ever been.

I have a much deeper appreciation for most things – even the most mundane. I feel an inner strength and acceptance I didn't have before. I pray every day now. I don't take much for granted. I recognize more keenly how fragile most of life is.

I feel love more deeply and feel upset less often or deeply. My daughters, my parents and my friends supported me in numerous and profound ways, which encouraged me to keep going and move forward with health into the future. For that, I thank you so much, and I want to tell you that I appreciate you dearly.

I just wanted to share the good news with you on this very important day for me. By the way, I still plan on having a 95th birthday party – December 2051.

Postscript: Bonnie's oncologist congratulated her for conquering cancer and congratulated her for conquering chemo. Bonnie called me from the 2-day Food and Wine Trade Show in Atlantic City, where she is working. She maintains her Hippocrates raw food lifestyle in New York City as Executive meetings, Atlantic City and on a small Maine island. If you are willing to live the straight and narrow, it's not easy but you can reap the greatest benefits possible.

Toxemia, Hypoglycemia, and Vocal Cord Weakness
By Barry Harris

It was easy for me to become a vegetarian because my mother was such a horrendous cook. All week, we had Chef Boyardee Meatballs and Spaghetti, Swanson Big Beef TV Dinners, and, of course, the once a week big treat, Kentucky Fried Chicken. Once a week, she cooked, and she made Chef Boyardee look good, and what was served up by the Kentucky Colonel as the height of haute cuisine.

I come from a Jewish background, so it would be embarrassing for my mother if she didn't cook Friday night's Shabbas dinner. She cooked tough and stringy beef, her specialty, and vegetables that had been so boiled, there was no nutrition left in them. She had so little practice during the week to improve her cooking skills, it was easy to understand why I was too embarrassed to invite friends over for Friday night's dinner. Then, Saturday at lunchtime, she would cut the leftover beef into big chunks, stuff it between two slices of Wonder Bread, and put congealed fat and Heinz Ketchup on top.

It should come as no surprise that at the age of 24 I got very sick. I started losing weight, spitting up blood, and I had bad chest pains. I went to the library to investigate what these symptoms could possibly mean, and the option that I was hoping for was "tuberculosis," because this was usually less lethal than the other two possibilities of leukemia and lung cancer. It also made some sense, since my father had been a doctor at a tuberculosis sanitarium, and I spent one summer there washing test tubes, etc.

My macrobiotic brother introduced me, at that time, to the awesome powers of the body to heal through natural methods and a superior diet. This was the first time I experienced what could be called a healing miracle. He convinced me that I should try a macrobiotic ten-day brown rice fast before I check it out with the doctor. Within three or four days, eating nothing but brown rice, the bleeding had stopped, and the chest pains began to subside. Armed with the knowledge I had gained from experience, I felt empowered when I visited the doctor. His diagnosis was that my symptoms and miraculous recovery were indicative of such extreme toxemia, my tonsils had become engorged and were leaking blood. In addition, the toxins had inflamed my chest and were causing the pain, and my toxic gut wasn't assimilating my food. This explained the weight loss.

Let us jump forward seven years to the early 1980s. I had improved my diet, and had become a semi-vegetarian, but considering the self-destructive dietary habits I had formed in childhood, my improvement wasn't enough to even be in the ballpark of what was necessary for optimal health. At that time of my life, I had been training to become an opera singer. Through overuse, emotional blocks and poor technique, I had been insidiously and unconsciously weakening my vocal cords. And then one day, while practicing, I felt something snap, and afterwards, I couldn't even talk above a whisper without jaw pain. Doctors said I would never regain the strength of my previous speaking voice, let alone sing again.

A good friend, knowing my condition, suggested I read Arnold Ehret's book on the "Mucusless Diet Healing System." This was my first introduction to living food (ie.,a raw, plant-based diet). He claimed that anything could be cured with living food. One sentence particularly caught my eye. Right there on the page, he had written. "I have helped singers restore the lost voice." At that point I had no faith, and I was a beggar as to what miracles I would let into my life, so, I didn't take the claim seriously. However, I did consider his regimen might help me get back my speaking voice. I went on his month-long program of alternating three days raw food, with four days, green juice fast, and then doing a 10-day juice fast. He recommended breaking the fast with a week of fruit. Mucus came up in buckets. And then, I discovered my speaking voice was clear and strong, and the full miracle became evident when I started singing, and I sounded better than I had in quite some time.

Several years later, in 1985, '86. I'm working at the Hippocrates Health Institute in Boston, editing health booklets for Dr. Ann Wigmore. This was such a fertile environment to grow miracles, they started to become commonplace. There were not only miracles of physical healing, but also miracles of transformed consciousness, and miracles of personal empowerment. I had previously been diagnosed with the pre-diabetic condition of hypoglycemia, and thus much of the time, I had been too tired to be very productive during the day. In less than two weeks on the living food diet and lifestyle, this fatigue had become a thing of the past, never to return. Ehret had claimed that after detoxification and regeneration of one's body, there would be new experiential insight about the true source of happiness. We are all looking for the key to happiness. Little had I realized, until then, that the source of much happiness comes from being optimally healthy. Western medicine surely hasn't understood that equation – being healthy equals being happy.

Now that I had clean blood, and thus no toxicity affecting the brain, I had a mental clarity and peace that I had never before experienced. I would still get appropriately angry or sad in certain circumstances, but the peace behind these so-called negative emotions were a form of happiness. In short, I was happy, because for the first time I felt fully alive and not numbed to life. I found my sentiments reinforced by the many guests who had recovered from serious, often life-threatening illness, using the Hippocrates program. They would often say that the terminal diagnosis which led them to Hippocrates was the greatest gift of their life.

There is one final influence from the past that woke me up to the power of a live food diet and lifestyle, and indelibly imprinted on my consciousness the importance of always being responsible for one's own health. The year is 1988, and my mother has just experienced a stroke. After several months of taking toxic drugs and totally allopathic care, the condition has now magnified to include congestive heart failure. I feel so deeply grateful to the Hippocrates Institute, and blessed by my stay there, because I know that I have the knowledge and experience that can save my mother's life. On several occasions, I had seen guests diagnosed with congestive heart failure hobble into the Institute with assistance, gasping for breath, and leaving three weeks later, without assistance, breathing normally.

I felt honored to give this gift to my mother, and I told her that I would be happy to come to St. Louis and prepare the diet for her, and give her all the spiritual exercises, so she could experience the miracles I had observed in others with congestive heart failure. She got angry, and she asked me where I had gone to medical school. She said I was insulting the memory of my dead father, the doctor. I told her that I might not have all the medical knowledge, but I had the experience of what works. She refused my offer, and continued to get worse, and when her breathing was so painful, there was no quality to her life, she committed suicide. All these experiences make it understandable why I have dedicated my life to empowering those who feel victimized by illness. It is tragic that most people in our culture feel so powerless, both in making the choices that prevent illness, and in recovering once they experience a life-threatening or serious condition.

Dangers of Our Toxic Environment

(Chemical Sensitivities)

as experienced by the author (2010-2011)

Is it real to talk about the dangers of a toxic environment, or are these merely scare tactics by environmental Jeremiahs, foretelling an environmental apocalypse? The new burgeoning specialty known as environmental medicine should give us the answer. However, many symptoms — such as, in my case, headaches, nasal decongestion, stomach discomfort and difficulty in breathing are misdiagnosed as diseases without any environmental component, and I was advised to take pharmaceuticals or have surgery.

After seeing a number of doctors, I was finally diagnosed with a mold allergy by an Ear, Nose, Throat (ENT) doctor at New England Medical Center. At that time (2000), I was teaching at Framingham's Fuller Middle School, and this created for me a health disaster, for it was built on a filled-in swamp. I lost my voice and had severe flu symptoms. I had to resign that job. Although many teachers and students got sick, the union and school department would not admit that mold was in the heating/air conditioning system.

My problem resurfaced in 2011, following heavy March rains. In July, when I turned on the central air conditioner, I started experiencing sinus congestion and a constant headache. First I tried natural methods and visited a highly recommended herbalist who suggested the following very comprehensive regimen:

- Use Essential Oils in an "ionizer aromatherapy diffuser" with a combination of eucalyptus, frankincense and lavender.

- For sleeping, put three drops of these oils on a tissue and place over the face breathing in for six minutes before sleeping.

- Have an energetic chiropractor adjust the hiatal valve in order to correct an unbalanced stomach meridian and an overly acid condition.
- Have laser treatment by the energetic chiropractor.
- Use a Nettypot and fill it with ½ teaspoon of sea salt and ½ capsule of goldenseal to 8 ounces of warm water twice a day on rising and on retiring.
- Gargle three times a day with goldenseal/saline solution.
- Take 2 capsules of astragalus three times a day at each meal for a month.
- Deep massage to remove the blockages in L5 related to 2nd and 3rd chakras, which affect digestion and throat.
- Allow images to come up in meditation and see what parts of the body to which they are related.

Although following these suggestions improved my condition somewhat, my symptoms still bothered me, so I decided to see an ENT physician. Unable to find the excellent ENT specialist I had in 2000, I went to another specialist, who declared it was a mechanical, not environmental, problem and recommended some pharmaceuticals, surgery or continuing to use the Nettypot, as I had been doing.

Even though this doctor denied that my sickness had an environmental source, I wanted to investigate further. Therefore, my next step was to have my blood tested. Not surprisingly, the tests showed a strong allergy to mold.

To remedy the situation, I interviewed seven mold/basement contractors and hired a contractor who installed French drains, a sump pump and a new bulkhead to replace the one that had leaked and had flooded my basement. A central air and heating contractor installed a new HEPA filter, ultraviolet lighting and a pure air filtration system in the central air-conditioning/heating system.

My next step was to hire Jeff May, an indoor air investigator, who had written "My House Is Killing Me," and a number of other books on the same subject. This should have been my first step, as it would have saved a lot of time, money and aggravation.

Jeff took microscopic samples, which showed that mold spores were rampant.

The following were Jeff's instructions:

- Remove the furniture, rugs, wooden bookcases, bureaus, boxes of teaching materials and 15 boxes of other books.

- Replace the wooden bookcases with metal wire shelving on wheels to hold the plastic totes for the remaining books, children's games, crafts, contents of bureaus etc.

- Clean and insulate the dirt crawl space under my office, which used to be a porch, and leave the crawl open to the cellar.

- Cover the open insulation in the basement ceiling with sheetrock, plaster, and then paint it.

- Paint the fieldstone walls and floors.

- Urethane bare wooden shelving.

- Remove fabric treads on stairs and replace them with vinyl treads. Paint stairs.

- Buy a HEPA vacuum (I traded in my Miele), and vacuum and wash the baseboard heating fins in the apartment and basement.

On February 10, 2011, while the "Tom Sawyer" crew was beginning work on the crawl space, I had a severe allergic attack. The dusty mold had seeped through the floorboards. My sinus infection, drippy nose, and headache worsened immediately. That day, while my guest speaker shared her knowledge with my class, I had to lie on the sofa covered with a comforter, for I was chilled and unable to stay awake. After the class left, I moved into my neighbor's home, and, almost immediately, my breathing improved. I believe this was due to the healthy air oxygenated by the many leafy plants filling her rooms.

I slept Thursday through Saturday night, only rising to go to the bathroom and to drink water. Greatly improved, I was told by my friends that the spark had returned to my eyes. My sinuses were no longer congested; my nose stopped running; and my headache almost disappeared. I remained weak, however, and was wobbly, achy and nauseous, with a croaky voice and a deep, hacking cough. I wasn't at all hungry, but maybe I was just weak from drinking only water for five days. I had a follow-up visit with the ENT doctor who said that I had miraculously recovered and he, finally, agreed that my allergy was indeed due to mold.

When the Tom Sawyer construction crew completed Jeff's list, I turned on the air purification system and I immediately got sick again. This was not my overly sensitive system, for many participants in my class also became ill. I called Jeff May again. He asked me when the ducts were last cleaned. I called and asked the air conditioning contractor who, to my astonishment and fury, stated that it wasn't their job to clean the ducts and they do not send annual notices to remind people to have them cleaned. The dust and mold of the last 12 years covered the apartment. I sneezed, blew my nose continually, my eyes stung and at night I couldn't breathe. Once again I was forced to move. Meanwhile, I had to hold my classes elsewhere.

I went back to following Jeff's recommendations: Clean the five ducts and the baseboard heating; seal off each room; put a blow-out fan in the window; and thoroughly HEPA vacuum everything in each room. I also followed Dr. Tel-Oren's recommendation of using a Bioactive Plant Fraction Therapy ultrasonic diffuser. This inhibits microbial growth. I have felt better ever since.

Experiencing such a health crisis can be a blessing or curse depending on whether you take responsibility for getting well. There are many who have seen it as a blessing, because they now feel more empowered in regard to their health. They will tell you, they've become "weller than well."

Overcoming Crohn's Disease & Ulcerative Colitis and Discovering a Life of Service
By Paul Nison

At age 20, Paul Nison was diagnosed with inflammatory bowel disease (also know as Crohn's disease and ulcerative colitis) – a potentially deadly diagnosis.

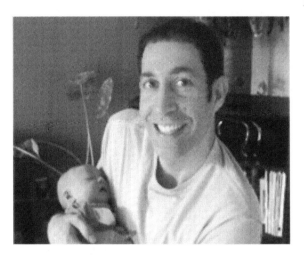

His search for a cure began with medical doctors, but they didn't have the answers he needed. After trying almost every so-called cure to overcome his pain and suffering, Paul finally discovered the benefits of eating more simply. He started by getting rid of foods that were no good for him. Simplifying his diet was the first step in his cure.

"I was eating so much unhealthy food, but didn't care because I felt great. When I got sick, I finally realized health doesn't start with what we add to our diet, but with what we leave out."

Paul started to leave out all unhealthful foods, and the healthful foods he was left with were raw, ripe, fresh, organic fruits, vegetables, nuts and seeds.

After turning to a more simple diet called "the raw food diet" consisting of just that, raw foods, Paul was amazed at how quickly his health returned. He was even more amazed because doctors told him raw foods would not help his condition. In fact, they warned him by saying a diet of raw fruits and vegetables would be harmful to anyone with inflammatory bowel disease.

This led Paul to simplify all areas of his life. With his new understanding of "less is more," Paul left his office job in the financial industry on Wall Street in New York City, wrote some books about health, and started traveling, giving lectures about health and living simply.

Paul didn't know it at the time, but his return to health and a simpler life were just the beginning of a path that would bring him to see the connection between today's fast-paced urban lifestyle and the sadly diseased state in which so many people find themselves. "The more I started to realize what was really going on, I would see most people moving around like robots, barely surviving while I was thriving."

This led Paul to continue to search for an answer. He realized that people are being controlled by the world. Most of the people in control do not have the best interests of the people they are controlling at heart.

As Paul continued to study, he was led to read the Bible. When he saw that it clearly said, we should not be controlled by the people of the world, but by the Master Creator, Father YHWH (יהוה). Everything made perfect sense.

As a definitive confirmation that Our Creator had all the answers and not the world, Paul found Genesis 1:29: *"See, I have given you every plant that yields seed which is on the face of all the earth, in which there is life, every green plant is for food."*

"Discovering healthful eating was a big step for me, but finding and building a personal relationship with Our Creator was the biggest. My life has definitely changed and is better than it ever was."

Paul's life is now dedicated to studying and living according to the Scriptures and to developing his relationship with The Most High. It is Paul's prayer to help as many people as possible to see the amazing health message of the Scriptures, and to help them get to know and understand their Creator. According to Paul, the Scriptures comprise the greatest book on health ever written.

To convey his message, Paul will travel wherever he must. He spends most of his time on the road. Paul explains that the hectic life on the road, working many hours, is only possible with the help of Our Creator (יהוה).

"There is so much to get done, but each second I spend working on this is a joy because I know it's not for me, it is for Our Creator (יהוה) and it is helping people."

Paul will speak anywhere and is accepted everywhere. He usually speaks at health food stores, retreats, churches, Messianic assemblies, yoga studios, parks, and corporate offices. Paul says there is no place he wouldn't speak, as long as people are interested in helping themselves get better.

Paul is on a mission to bring the message of health and healing to the world. His experiences and background in raw food nutrition, along with his study of the Scriptures, have helped him develop a unique teaching style that is fun, simple and to the point. Paul has helped people in several countries achieve their goals while pleasing their Maker.

He's known among his peers as one of the most humble, enjoyable people to be around, while, at the same time, he speaks boldly and to the point. He has a unique style combining humor and boldness to get his message across to everyone. From children to seniors, men and woman, everyone stands to benefit from Paul's message.

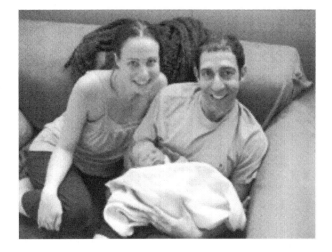

Paul grew up in Brooklyn, New York. He is married to Andrea and they have a daughter Noa Raquel. The Nison family all shares the same passion for health and the Scriptures.

http://www.paulnison.com/index.html

www.PaulNison.com -Official website of Author Paul Nison

www.RawLife.com -Health E-store for all your health needs

www.RawLifehealthShow.com - Videos added daily

www.twitter.com/Paulnison

www.facebook.com/paul.nison

www.myspace.com/therawlife

Reversing Diabetes

By Diana Bronner

I have been a Type 2 diabetic for 28 years. I am not and never have been overweight, so that was not my problem as it is for most diabetics. Until recently I was taking three different kinds of medication, each of which served a different function in the control of my blood sugar. Over the many years various doctors have suggested that I go on insulin, but that was never an option for me – I always said I would try harder to control the numbers with my diet. I was on minimal dosages, but at times I would get low blood sugar from either over-medicating or not eating enough carbs. I was on a real rollercoaster and it was not a good ride at all. The longer one has diabetes, the harder it is to control, and I was getting terribly frustrated and down from the continual fight.

Recently, my son brought to my attention the name of this place in Florida called Hippocrates Health Institute. He wanted me to go there to investigate how a raw foods diet could help control my diabetes. I signed up, then chickened out! But I continued to pursue the idea of raw foods on my own and did a lot of Google research, and jumped in feet first, little knowing what I was doing.

Somehow, in my Google research, the name "Waltham Raw New England Community" jumped onto my screen and before I knew it, I was calling Betsy Bragg, raw food coach, and suddenly my new life began. Betsy has encouraged me, teaching me sprouting at her home and coaching me regularly by phone and email. She also urged me to go to Hippocrates to learn more about raw foods.

It is now about three or four weeks later; I am doing 100 percent raw and I haven't looked backwards. Incredible as it sounds, I am off most of my of my diabetes meds (I sometimes have to take a minimal dosage of one med first thing in the morning) and low blood sugars are a horror of the past. I continue to research online, read my recipe books, talk to Betsy – and yes, I am going to Hippocrates to further my education. This raw stuff really works!

July 14, 2008

I recently wrote of my experiences as a Type 2 diabetic and the raw food diet; it is time to update my report. In the past, one of my biggest problems with my blood sugar numbers was that in the very early morning hours I would get what the doctors called the "dawn phenomenon" – my blood sugar would rise 20-30 mg for no apparent reason, certainly not from anything I ate as I hadn't eaten breakfast yet. I was on an evening dose of 1500mg of metformin to try to control that rise. Those high numbers at the start of the day always put me behind the eight ball because I had to work hard to get them down. After three weeks at Hippocrates Health Institute, my follow-up blood tests showed a blood sugar reading of 140, even after being on the raw foods for weeks. By this time I was off all diabetes medication including metformin. My numbers, except for that dawn phenomenon, were great.

Now, I am happy to report that I no longer get that early-morning rise. I can take my blood sugar reading at 3 a.m., go back to bed and when I get up five hours later, the reading is the same! This is progress and I could not have achieved it without being on the raw food diet.

Recovery from Ulcers
By Dr. John Duffy

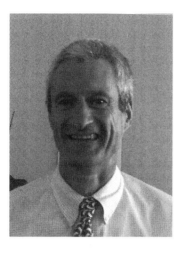

I was given a recipe for my ulcers while taking Betsy Bragg's class, "Life Force Energy." My ulcers have been chronic and severe for many years. I had been carrying a very heavy schedule as a chiropractor, father, employer, landlord and student, and with this combined with eating meat five to seven days a week, my ulcers had become very severe. At that point I started throwing up no matter what I ate. This motivated me to take the Life Force Energy class, which provided a living plant based diet. During this class, we had the opportunity to work with a volunteer Life Force graduate. I experienced an ulcer attack and was about to go to the hospital when I consulted with my Life Force coach concerning my crisis. He sent me the following recipe:

- ½ cabbage
- 2 apples
- JUICE AND DRINK twice a day

He recommended that I do this for a whole month; I compromised and did it for three weeks as needed. It was phenomenal! Since going 80 percent raw and continuing cabbage juice and apples as needed, my ulcers have become a distant memory. I had been taking Tagamet as needed and antacids prescribed by my primary care physician. In order to sleep, I had to exhaust my body. I would typically run 5 miles a night just to ease the pain caused by my ulcers. If I didn't run, my ulcers would keep me awake all night.

My coach learned this from Dr. Garnett Cheney, of Stanford's School of Medicine, who had considerable success treating ulcers with cabbage juice. The key component was believed to be the amino acid glutamine, which cabbage juice is rich in.

Other Sources:

www.truestarhealth.com/members/cm_archives14ML3P1A22.html accessed November 15, 2012

Traditionally, raw cabbage juice has been used for stomach ulcers and raw potato juice for duodenal ulcers. In the 1950s, Dr. Cheney studied 181 patients and found one liter of raw cabbage juice daily to be highly beneficial. Green cabbages are best, but red cabbages can also be used, and they can be mixed 50:50 with carrot and/or celery juice for flavor.

www.doctoryourself.com/colitis.html accessed November 15, 20121

To give you an idea of the therapeutic potential of vegetable juices, we should look further at the work of Dr. Cheney. He had 100 peptic ulcer patients drink a quart of raw cabbage juice daily.The patients reported dramatically less pain, and X-ray examination confirmed faster healing time.There was no other change in their diet, and they did not have drug therapy. Eighty-one percent of the patients were symptom-free within one week and two-thirds were better in just four days, whereas the average healing time for patients given standard hospital treatment was more than a month. (Cheney, G: "Vitamin U Therapy of Peptic Ulcer,"*California Medicine*, vol. 77, number 4, October 1952)

Dr. Cheney used cabbage juice to also treat gastric ulcers and duodenal ulcers. He clearly was onto something, which he called "Vitamin U" (for ulcer) for lack of a better name. Today, the cabbage family (cruciform) of vegetables, including Brussels sprouts, cauliflower and broccoli, are finally being recommended to help prevent diseases, including cancer. Dr. Cheney was getting therapeutic results in four days with cabbage juice OVER FORTY YEARS AGO! Do we really have to wait for orthodox medical approval of vegetables?

I know of people who have used cabbage juice along with vegetarian diet and fasting to heal all forms of gastrointestinal diseases without drugs and without surgery. One person even cured her untreatable rectal bleeding with cabbage juice. The attending physician confirmed her excellent but unexplained progress, asking her what she was doing. She told the doctor of her diet and about cabbage juice. His response was, "No, that couldn't be it."

I highly recommend the book *Cabbage Cures to Cuisine* by Judith Hiatt, Naturegraph Publishers Inc., Happy Camp, CA, 1989

Chapter 11
Recipes

In the Living Food Cuisine

Tastes for Every Meal/Support Your Organs

SALT	SOUR	SWEET	PUNGENT	BITTER
Kidney,	Liver, Gallbladder	Spleen, Pancreas, Stomach	Lung, large intestine	Heart, small intestine
Miso	Lemon	Apple juice	Garlic	Broad leafy greens i.e. Kale
Sea salt	Lime	Dried fruits: dates, raisins, cherries, coconut, apricots etc.	Ginger	Dandelion greens
Miso	Orange juice		Horseradish	Cilantro
Umebosha plum	Grapefruit	Beet	Mustard	Parsley
Sundried olives or brine	Cranberry	Bell Pepper	Leek	
	Umebosha plum	Cherry Tomatoes	Onion	
	Sauerkraut	Coconut water	Watercress	
		Stevia	Daikon	

Tastes of an International Cuisine

*Most Used

Italian & Sicilian	Thai & Balinese	Mexican & Spanish	Moroccan & African
Herbs & Spices	Herbs & Spices	Herbs & Spices	Herbs & Spices
Garlic*	Basil*	Cilantro*	Cilantro*
Basil*	Lemongrass*	Cumin*	Ginger*
Olive oil*	Tamarind*	Garlic*	Cinnamon*
Oregano	Curry*	Olive oil*	Cumin*
Rosemary	Ginger	Coriander	Coriander
Thyme	Lime leaves	Onions	Mint
Pepper	Cilantro	Parsley	Saffron
Onions	Mint	Paprika	Chives
Parsley	Turmeric	Chiles	Fenugreek
Sage	Coriander	Cinnamon	Rose
Marjoram	Cumin		
	Sesame		
	Chiles		

Japanese & Chinese	Middle-Eastern & Greek	Indian	American
Herbs & Spices	Herbs & Spices	Herbs & Spices	Herbs & Spices
Cilantro*	Garlic*	Garlic*	Garlic*
Garlic*	Mint*	Ginger*	Onions*
Sesame*	Oregano*	Cardamom*	Basil*
Miso*	Dill*	Curry*	Oregano*
Basil	Cinnamon*	Cumin*	Dill*
Miso Tamari*	Parsley*	Garam	Cinnamon*
Basil	Anise	Masala*	Marjoram
Cardamom	Chiles	Cinnamon	Bay leaf
Coriander	Cilantro	Clove	Allspice
Scallions	Saffron	Chiles	Chiles
Star anise	Sesame	Fenugreek	Poppy
Lemon Juice	Thyme	Fennel seed	Caraway
Wasabi	Marjoram	Mint	Thyme
	Clove	Mustard	Vanilla
	Poppy Seed	B. pepper	Nutmeg
	Fenugreek	Tamarind	
	Onion	Sesame	
	Rosemary	Turmeric	
		Onions	
		Saffron	
		Rose	

Recipes

The following are food demonstrations presented in the Life Force Energy course:

Week One – Eggless Egg Salad rollup

Week Two – Learn to prepare healthy, delicious breakfasts: Chia porridge with almond milk and smoothies

Week Three – Juice: wheatgrass, Hippocrates Green Drink and smoothie

Week Four – Nori Rolls/Vegetarian Sushi and taste treat appetizer of Red Pepper and Sunflower Pate

Week Five– Spinach Avocado Soup or Sweet Potato Corn Chowder

Week Six– Kale Avocado Salad

Week Seven– Marinara Sauce and preparation of many different types of pastas using many gadgets and gizmos

Week Eight – Dehydrates: flax crackers, kale chips and green beans
Fermentation: Sauerkraut and other fermented vegetables to get your probiotics

Week Nine – Fermenting Veggies

Week Ten – Lemon Cheesecake

Beverages

Note: Hippocrates only endorses the HHI drink. The others are added as transitional drinks for those transitioning from a Standard American Diet to a Hippocrates Diet.

Abbreviations:

c = cup   T = tablespoon   t = teaspoon   g = gram

Hippocrates Green Drink

Green Drinks are a major component of the Hippocrates Health Institute (HHI) Program, so much so that HHI provides three opportunities for guests to drink them daily.

The formula for a 12-ounce green drink is 6 ounces of sprout juice and 6 ounces of vegetable juice.

To generate 6 ounces of sprout juice, start with one-half tray of sunflower greens and one-third tray of pea-greens. Be sure to cut as close to the soil as possible. It is not necessary to remove the black hulls before juicing. You might want to rinse the sprouts before juicing them. For the 6 ounces of vegetable juice, use 1 large cucumber and 2 stalks of celery. Several cloves of garlic, a piece of ginger, etc. can be added, as desired, for flavor and health. Run the vegetables through the juicer first; follow with the sunflower greens and lastly add the pea-greens. Use the plunger during the entire juicing process.

Coffee Substitutes

It's best to buy an organic, no-coffee substitute that is grain-based (e.g., barley) or plant-based faux coffee made from chicory, dandelion, or something else. Below are some possibilities with brand information.

1.Dandy Blend Instant Herbal Coffee Substitute—Dandy Blend, a healthy herbal coffee substitute, is similar to Postum and is gluten-free. www.dandyblend.com/

2.Teeccino Caffeine-Free Herbal Coffee—Teeccino Herbal Coffee is naturally caffeine-free, non-acidic and tastes just like coffee! www.teeccino.com/

3.Cafix All Natural Caffeine Free Beverage —All Natural Caffeine Free Instant Beverage.www.cafix.com/

Almond Milk

Makes 2 cups, 4 servings

Advanced Prep:

Soak 1 c almonds for 8 hours, or overnight.

Equipment:
- Blender
- Spatula
- Fine-mesh strainer or nutmilk bag
- Medium-size bowl
- Measuring cups and spoons

Ingredients:
- 2 1/2 c water
- 1 1/2 c soaked almonds (1 cup before soaking
- 1/2 t vanilla extract
- 3 chopped pitted Medjool dates (optional)

Directions:
1. Place 1 ½ c water, soaked almonds, and vanilla extract in a blender.
2. Blend on high speed until smooth.
3. Add the remaining 1 c water and blend until smooth.
4. Pour the almond mixture through a fine-mesh strainer set over a medium-sized bowl. Using a spatula, stir and press the pulp that is caught in the strainer, to extract as much milk as possible into the bowl.
5. Discard the pulp left in the strainer, and store the milk in a sealed container in the refrigerator.
6. Almond milk keeps for five days. It naturally separates, so shake well before using.

Eggless Egg Nog
by Tom Lindsley

Blend all these ingredients:

- 8-16 oz. water
- 1 T hemp
- 1 T sesame
- ½ T chia
- 10 almonds (soaked)

- 3 pitted dates or 3 stevia drops
- ¼ - ½ t turmeric
- ¼ t nutmeg
- ¼ t cinnamon

Green Smoothies
by Victoria Boutenko, www.rawfamily.com

What do I mean by a green smoothie? Here is one of my favorite recipes: 4 ripe pears, 1 bunch of parsley and 2 cups of water. Blend well. This smoothie looks very green, but it tastes like fruit. I enjoy green smoothies so much that I bought an extra blender and placed it in my office, so that I could make green smoothies throughout the day. Green smoothies are very nutritious. The ratio that is optimal for human consumption is about 60 percent ripe organic fruit mixed with about 40 percent organic greens.

The Hippocrates Institute does not recommend smoothies. If you have health challenges, you should eliminate fruit. However, smoothies are a good drink to transition from a Western diet to a raw one. I reverse the ratio and have 60 percent greens and 40 percent fruit.

Victoria Boutenko recommends smoothies for the following reasons:

1. Green smoothies are easy to digest. When blended well, most of the cells in the greens and fruits are ruptured, making the valuable nutrients easy for the body to assimilate. Green smoothies literally start to get absorbed in your mouth.

2. Green smoothies are a complete food because they still have fiber. Consuming fiber is important for our elimination system.

3. Green smoothies belong to the most palatable dishes for all humans of all ages. With a ratio of fruits to veggies as 60:40 the fruit taste dominates the flavor, yet at the same time the greens balance out the sweetness of the fruit, adding a nice zest to it. People who eat a standard American diet enjoy the taste of green smoothies. They are usually quite surprised that something so green could taste so nice.

4. A molecule of chlorophyll closely resembles a molecule of human blood. According to the teachings of Dr. Ann Wigmore, consuming chlorophyll is like receiving a healthy blood transfusion. Many people do not consume enough greens, even those who stay on a raw food diet. By drinking two or three cups of green smoothies daily you will consume enough greens for the day to nourish your body, and all of the beneficial nutrients will be well assimilated.

5. Green smoothies are easy to make, and quick to clean up after. To prepare a pitcher of green smoothie takes less than five minutes, including cleaning.

6. Green smoothies have proven to be loved by children of all ages, including babies of six or more months old. Of course you have to be careful and slowly increase the amount of smoothies to avoid food allergies.

7. When consuming your greens in the form of green smoothies, you are greatly reducing the consumption of oils and salt in your diet.

8. Regular consumption of green smoothies forms a good habit of eating greens. After a few weeks of drinking green smoothies, most people start to crave and enjoy eating more greens. Eating enough greens is often a problem with many people, especially children.

9. While fresh is always best, green smoothies at cool temperatures will keep for up to three days, which is convenient for work or when traveling.

Start playing with green smoothies, and discover the many joys and benefits of this wonderful, delicious, and nutritious addition to your menu. You may find many more amazing facts about green smoothies in Victoria Boutenko's book, *Green for Life,* available at www.rawfamily.com.

Below are five of Victoria's green smoothie recipes. They are merely basic ideas for your green creations. Feel free substitute these ingredients with your own choice of greens and fruits. Enjoy!

Apple-kale-lemon

- *4 apples*
- *½ T lemon juice*
- *5 leaves of kale*
- *2 c water*

Pear-kale-mint

- *5 leaves of kale*
- *4 ripe pears*
- *½ a bunch of mint*
- *2 c water*

Peach-spinach

- *6 peaches*
- *2 handfuls of spinach leaves*
- *2 c water*

Mango-weeds

- *2 mangos*
- *1 handful of edible weeds,such as lambsquarters, stinging nettlespurs-lane, etc.*
- *2 c water*

Breakfast

Hippocrates only recommends any of the breakfasts in this section for those underweight or with certain medical conditions. For the rest, HHI recommends wheatgrass juice and the HHI green drink.

Chia Berry Porridge Servings: 2 -3
by Joseph Lucier www.livefoodcuisine.com

Ingredients:
- 1 c chia seeds ground into a fine powder.
- 1 c blueberries, raspberries or straw-berries
- 1 c water, filtered, fig juice or coco-nut water

Toppings:
- ½ c coconut flakes or2 T Yacon syrup, better with 6 drops stevia, or 1 T lemon or orange zest (optional)

Directions:
1. Put the ingredients into a bowl.
2. If you want warm water, mix 1 part heated water to 1 part room-temperature water, to get about 118 degrees
3. Add the water to the chia and mix well
4. for a few minutes until porridge is thick.
5. Mix in the berries.
6. Add toppings and serve.

Chia Berry Porridge

Alternate Versions:
- Include 1 c mashed avocados, do not add water and add additional ingredients and blend until smooth.
- Top with nut milk.

The Basic Gel

To make a basic chia gel, simply add 1/3 cup of seeds (2oz) to 2 cups of water. Stir the mixture well, to avoid clumping, then leave it in your fridge, in a sealed jar. This will yield around 17oz of chia gel. You can begin to eat the gel almost immediately if you like. Just 10 minutes is enough time for the gel to be formed. More of the nutrients will be easily accessible after a few hours, however, so many people like to make up a batch like this and leave it in the fridge. It will stay good for about three weeks. Then you can just reach into the fridge and take out some of the ready-made gel whenever you need it. You might add it to smoothies, mix it with salad dressings, puddings or granola, or simply take it by the spoonful.

As mentioned above, chia will absorb anything, it doesn't have to soak in water. We like soaking it in things like apple juice for example. That way, the intense sweetness of the apple juice is also offset by the chia and it tastes yummy. We also often blend fruits; for example bananas and persimmons, then stir the chia into that mixture. Again, the longer the seeds are left to soak, the more their nutrients will be readily available to you, yet you could easily eat a meal like this 10 minutes or less after preparing it.

You can also sprinkle the dry seeds onto salads or add them to granola mixes. You may also want to experiment with grinding them first in a coffee grinder, to make a 'chia flour' you can then add to smoothies, soups and so on.

Basic Chia Gel

Ingredients:
- Chia
- Water

Directions:
1. Mix 1/3-cup chia seeds to 2 cups water. Stir. This is the 'basic gel' recipe that can be stored in your fridge and used as required.

Fruity Chia

Ingredients:
- 3 small or 2 big apples
- 8 dates, pits removed or 4 drops of stevia
- 4-5 T chia seeds
- 1/4 c dried mulberries

Directions:
1. Blend the apples and six dates.
2. Transfer that mixture into a bowl and stir in the chia seeds and mulberries.
3. Chop down the remaining 2 dates into pieces and stir those in too.
4. Soak for at least 10 minutes before consuming.

Banana-Nut Bread

Ingredients:
- 2 c vegetable juice pulp (preferably at least half carrot)
- 8 T ground chia
- 3/4 c chopped walnuts
- 3/4 c raisins
- 5 bananas

Cream cheese:
Blend 3 avocados, 9 dates or 6 drops of stevia and juice of 2 lemons.

Directions:
1. Mix the veggie juice pulp and bananas in a food processor.
2. Add in the ground chia and let the food processor run until the seeds are completely mixed in.
3. Transfer the mixture to a bowl with the walnuts and raisins and mix them in thoroughly by hand.
4. Shape into a loaf.
5. For major yumminess, top with 'Cream Cheese'

Appetizers

Crudites with Guacamole and Raw Hummus

VEGGIES – Carrot sticks, celery sticks, julienne red bell pepper, broccoli, cauliflower, cucumber, radishes, black olives only in oil etc.

GUACAMOLE – My grandkids like the first simple recipe. I just use mash avocado and salt. For company, I use the second more elaborate recipe.

Guacamole I

Ingredients:
- 1 avocado
- ¼ t onion powder
- 1/8 t. sea salt

Directions:
1. Mash together with a whisk or fork

Guacamole II

Prep Time: 20 min

Ingredients:
- 3 avocados, halved, seeded and peeled
- 1 lime, juiced
- 1/2 t kosher salt
- 1/2 t ground cumin
- 1/2 t cayenne
- 1/2 medium onion, diced
- 2 Roma tomatoes, seeded and diced
- 1 T chopped cilantro
- 1 clove garlic, minced

Directions:
1. In a large bowl place the scooped avocado pulp and limejuice, toss to coat.
2. Drain, and reserve the limejuice, after all of the avocados have been coated.
3. Using a potato masher add the salt, cumin, and cayenne and mash.
4. Fold in the onions, tomatoes, cilantro, and garlic.
5. Add 1 T of the reserved lime juice
6. Let sit at room temperature for 1 hour and then serve.

Hummus - I yields 5 ½ cups
by Jenny Robbins

Ingredients:
- 4 c sprouted chickpeas
- 1 ½ c olive oil
- 3 cloves garlic
- 4 oz. lemon juice
- 1 T Miso Tamari
- 1 T kelp powder

Directions:
1. In a blender, combine all ingredients.
2. While blending , stir vigorously with the stirring rod.
3. Season to taste

Hummus - II
by Jenny Robbins

Ingredients:
- 5 c zucchini, peeled and cut into chunks
- ½ c tahini
- 4 cloves garlic
- ½ c lemon juice
- ¼ c olive oil
- ½ t paprika
- 1/8 t cayenne
- 1 ½ t sea salt

Directions:
1. Blend all together in food processor until smooth. If too thick can add a bit of water. If too thin, you can thicken it with 1-2 T ground flax seed.

Raw Sunflower Seed Paté
by Becky Tucker

Ingredients:
- 1 ½ c sunflower seeds soaked 8-12 hrs
- ⅓ or ½ c fresh squeezed lemon juice
- 3 T tahini
- 1 T "Miso Tamari"
- ⅓ c water
- pinch sea salt to taste
- pinch cayenne pepper to taste
- 1 t extra virgin olive oil

Directions:
1. Soak sunflower seeds, drain and rinse them.
2. Add all ingredients together in a food processor or blender and blend into a smooth paste.
3. Will keep in refrigerator for one week.

Stuffed Portobello Mushroom

Ingredients
- Portobello large mushrooms

Marinade:
- 1 cup sesame oil
- ¼ cup tamari
- ¼ cup lemon juice, freshly squeezed
- ½ tsp coarse black pepper

Directions:
1. Clean 2 or 3 portobello mushrooms with wet towel and remove stems. Set steams aside for future use.
2. Place marinade ingredients into a plastic resealable bag along with portobellos. Shake bag several times to completely coat mushrooms.
3. Place mushroom with marinade in refrigerator for 6-8 hours or overnight. Once mushrooms have marinated, remove from bag and put in a pyrex dish with the marinade and place in the dehydrator at 115 degrees for 4 to 6 hours, basting when dry.
4. Stuff with guacamole, garnished with a sprig of cilantro.

Veggie Pate
by Karen Woeller

Ingredients:
- 2 c sunflower seeds (soaked over night)
- 1 c almonds (soaked over night)
- 1/4 c lemon juice
- 1 T Miso Tamari
- 1/4 c fresh parsley or 1 T. dried
- 1 c red pepper
- 1 c zucchini or yellow squash
- 1/2 c sun dried tomatoes (soaked 4 hours or overnight)

Directions:
1. Mix all ingredients in food processor (put nuts in last).
2. Taste and add additional seasonings if necessary.
3. Serve with veggies such as: cucumbers, zucchini, bell pepper, squash, carrots, celery.

Nori Rolls

From *Healthful Cuisine,* pp 35-36
by Anna Maria Clement & Chef Kelly Serbonich

Ingredients:

- 1 sheet nori

- ⅓ c nut/seed pate or guacamole

- Any 3 or 4 of the following vegetable ingredients: marinated chopped salad, leafy sprouts, shredded carrot, squash, rutabaga, radish, asparagus spear, scallion, any julienne strips - red bell pepper or zucchini, sun flower sprouts, alfalfa or broccoli sprouts, horse-radish

- Instead of rice, chip cauliflower, celeriac or jicama in the food processor.

- Serve nori rolls with your favorite dip or dressing- wasabi sauce (wasabi powder mixed with water) and/a dipping sauce (blend 4 oz. Miso Tamari, 1 t sesame oil, 1 clove of garlic, 1 T of slivered ginger).

Directions:

1. A bamboo sushi mat is very handy for this task, although not absolutely necessary. (Whole Foods sells them; they're located on the shelf below the nori and other sea-weeds.) Lay the sushi mat on a flat surface. Line the edge of 1 sheet of nori up with the edge of the mat that is closest to you. You will be rolling away from yourself.

2. All ingredients will be placed on the nori in horizontal lines, so that if you were to cut into the completed roll at any two points, you would see the same interior. Start with the moist ingredient first (pate, avocado or marinated salad) and place a plump line of it across the nori parallel to the edge of the mat nearest you.

3. Next place the other ingredients you wish to include, making a line of each across the sheet of nori.

4. Prepare to roll!! Use your fingers to wet the edge farthest from you with pure water. This will seal the roll upon completion of the rolling process. The initial roll over and tuck is the most critical part of the rolling process. Lift the mat along with the nori and other roll contents up and over the piled ingredients and tuck tightly to complete the first rollover.

5. At this point, release the mat, pulling forward and rolling the remainder of the nori. When you lift up the mat, be sure the nori sheet is tucked completely under so that you can finish the rolling process. Voila!!

6. Allow the completed roll to sit for 5 to 10 minutes before cutting. This will soften the nori a bit and make it easier to cut cleanly.

7. Slice and serve!

Note: Whole Foods carries 2 packages of Organic Pacific Nori by Emerald Cove.The green package is raw/untoasted; the orange one is pre-toasted.

Soups

Avocado, Spinach and Sprout Soup
by Tom Lindsley

Ingredients:
- 1 c water
- 2 to 3 handfuls of baby spinach
- ½ chopped cucumber
- ½ or 1 avocado
- ¼ red pepper (optional)
- 1 T Miso Tamari (optional)

Directions:
1. Blend all ingredients.
2. Put a handful of mung, adzuki, lentil or other sprouts in a bowl.
3. Pour the above blended mixture over the sprouts.
4. Top with dehydrated sprouted dehydrated buckwheat, oats or other sprouts and dulse and or other seaweed

Vegetable Barley Soup

Learned working in kitchen at Hippocrates. Served at HHI to guests on a special diet.

Ingredients:
- Make stock with carrot, celery, red onion the day before
- Mushrooms - sauté in stock (no oil). Use medicinal mushrooms such as shiitake or portabella
- Barley
- Kombu
- Red onion, carrot, celery chopped fine

Hippocrates tips
1. Fresh herbs – parsley, dill, basil
2. Keep raw soups simple
3. Carrots, onion, celery
4. Avocado to make creamy
5. Kelp, cayenne
6. Garlic, cilantro if people like it
7. Put water equal to contents, add as blending to right consistency\
8. Lemon, lime

Corn and Sweet Potato Chowder —Serves 4. Preparation time: 30 minutes
by Joe Lucier Inspired from a different recipe at www.SpaFinder.com

Ingredients:
- 2 c sweet potato, peeled
- 1 whole avocado
- 1 T Miso Tamari
- 1 small knob ginger (finely chopped), about 2 inches square, start off with half
- 1/2 c leek or 1/4 cscallions
- 1 dash Celtic sea salt to taste
- 1 dash cayenne or black pepper
- 1 c water
- 2 c fresh corn

Directions:
1. Peel, wash, and chop the sweet potato and onions.
2. Place all the ingredients except the corn in a blender and blend until the texture is smooth.
3. Taste and adjust the seasoning if necessary. I like a good ginger flavor.
4. Remove from blender and put in a bowl with the corn

Chia Gazpacho Soup   serves 4
by Susan Allison created for the OHS/RNEC Dinner Speaker July 2009 Event

Ingredients:
- 3-4 medium tomatoes, blended (2 cups)
- 1/2 cucumber, peeled
- 2 stalks celery
- 1/2 red bell pepper
- 1/2 c fresh basil
- 1/2 c fresh cilantro leaves
- 2 T dried dulse seaweed
- 3 cloves garlic, peeled
- 1/3 c fresh lemon juice
- 1/4 c extra virgin olive oil
- 1 T chili powder
- 1 t ground cumin
- 1 t Himalayan sea salt
- 2 T chia seed

Directions:
1. In a high speed blender, combine all ingredients and blend until smooth.

Optional garnishes: sprouts, cilantro, chopped red peppers

Chunky Miso
by Joseph Lucier inspired by Jonathon Batchelder at Tree of Life

Ingredients:
- 1/2 c barley miso
- 2 c sea palm fronds
- 1/2 c hijiki seaweed
- 1 c broccoli
- 1 1/2 c carrots
- 1/2 c cabbage, purple
- 1/2 c sweet potato cubed, optional
- 1/4 c scallions (green parts)
- 4 c water
- 1/2 c shitake or mitake mushrooms (optional)

Directions:
1. Soak sea veggies 1 hour before using.
2. Mix 1/2 boiling water and tap water for warm soup.
3. Add all ingredients together.
4. Mix well.

Borscht Soup
From *Healthful Cuisine*, Hippocrates Health Institute Yields 5 cups

Ingredients:
- 1 c shredded green cabbage
- 1/2 t fresh chopped thyme
- 1/2 c finely diced red onion
- 2 c water
- 2 3/4 c chopped red beet
- 1/2 avocado
- 1 1/2 T fresh lemon juice, optional
- 1 1/2 t Miso Tamari
- 1/2 c chopped red onion
- 1 stalk celery, roughly chopped

Directions:
1. In a mixing bowl, combine cabbage and diced onion. Set aside.
2. In a blender, combine the remaining ingredients. Blend well and season to taste.
3. Pour over the cabbage and onion mixture and mix well.

Squash soup
by Linda Schafer

Ingredients:

- 1/2 buttercup squash
- 1 c butternut squash
- 2 carrots
- 1 c zucchini
- 3 basil leaves
- 1 T flax oil
- 1 T almond butter
- 1 T parsley
- 1 T Miso Tamari
- 3 c water
- Pinch of cayenne

Directions:

1. Blend all ingredients in mixer or food processor until creamy.
2. Garnish with more parsley or sprouted adzuki beans.

Salads and Salad Dressings

Betsy's Salad with Hippocrates House Dressing

Salad Ingredients:

- Sunflower, mung, adzuki and lentil Sprouts
- Mixed Greens
- Carrots shredded in food processor
- Red Cabbage shredded in food processor
- Avocado chunks

Hippocrates House Dressing
(Yield 1.5 cups)

Ingredients:

- 1 c Extra Virgin Cold Pressed Olive Oil
- 2 T lemon juice
- 2 T Miso Tamari
- 2 t ground mustard seed

Directions:

1. In a blender, combine all ingredients. Blend well, add 2 to 4 T water as you blend.

Kale Avocado Salad - serves 4
by Betsy Bragg

This is a great way to prepare kale, being difficult to eat raw for most people "transitioning" to the raw foods diet, when Celtic Salt is used and the kale is massaged, the kale "wilts" making it easier on digestion and definitely more palatable. This salad has grown to be a staple dish for many.

Ingredients:
- 1 Head of kale, any variety is great, shredded
- 2-3 carrots shredded
- 2-3 avocado chopped
- 1 ½ T lemon juice
- 1 t Celtic salt

Directions:
1. In mixing bowl toss all ingredients together, squeezing as you mix to "wilt" the kale and creaming the avocado.
2. Serve immediately.
3. As variation, add chopped fresh herbs

Asian Coleslaw
by Diane Willmont

Ingredients:
- ½ red cabbage shredded
- 2 large carrots shredded
- 2T olive oil
- 2T lemon juice
- 2T Miso Tamari
- 2T dark sesame oil
- 2T sesame seeds
- Pepper to taste

Directions:
1. Put cabbage and carrots in a bowl.
2. Blend olive oil, lemon juice and Miso Tamari for sauce.
3. Mix sauce, sesame seeds and pepper into cabbage and carrots.
4. Serve.

Rainbow Salad serves 8
by Elaina Love www.PureJoyLivingFoods.com

Ingredients:
- 1/2 red cabbage, shredded
- 2 large carrots, shredded
- 3 broccoli stalks, and 1 ½ heads, shredded
- 4 scallions, thinly sliced
- 1 c raisins
- ¼ c almonds
- 1 ½ c almond mayonnaise (see next page)
- ½ t mustard powder
- ½ t ginger
- ½ t garlic powder
- 1 -2 t Celtic sea salt or 4-6 T Miso Tamari

Almond Mayonnaise

by Elaina Love

Ingredients:

- 1 c soaked almonds (½ cup before soaking)
- ¾ c water
- 1 clove garlic
- ½ t Celtic sea salt or 1 T tamari
- 3 T lemon juice
- ½ t Italian seasoning
- 3 large dates or 2 drops of stevia
- Dash of cayenne pepper
- 1 ½ - 2 c flax or olive oil

Directions:

1. Peel almonds for a whiter mayonnaise.
2. Place all ingredients except the oil in the blender and blend until creamy.
3. Put your blender on a low speed, and drizzle the oil through the hole in the blender lid.
4. Add oil until the mixture becomes thick.

Tips: Use extra mayonnaise for avocado sandwiches using lettuce leaves in place of bread. The mayonnaise will last in a glass jar up to 2 weeks.

Sunburst Salad and Dressing

by Jonathan Fang

Ingredients:

- ½ red cabbage
- ½ green cabbage
- 2 carrots
- 2 apples peeled and sliced like match-sticks
- 2 kiwi peeled
- 2 bananas
- 2 slices of ginger
- 2 peeled oranges
- 1/3 c olive oil
- Pinch of salt

Directions:

- Thinly slice all ingredients.
- Marinate sliced cabbages and carrots (not in water) with 1 T sea salt and massage for 5 minutes. Let stand for 1 to 2 hours.
- Put apple slices in salt water for 1 – 2 minutes to prevent oxidization (turning brown) and then combine with drained cabbage/carrots.
- Blend at high speed the remaining ingredients to make the dressing.
- Mix the dressing into the cabbage, carrots and apple and serve yummy dish.

Mock Potato Salad
by Aimee Perrin

Ingredients:
- 1 head cauliflower
- 2 stalks celery
- 3 green onions or 1/2 leek
- 2 dill pickles (Real Pickles brand in the refrigerated section of your Health Food store)

Mayo:
- 1 c cashews, soaked
- 2 T. lemon juice
- 1/4 to 1/3 c of filtered or spring water
- 1 1/2 t Celtic or Himalayan salt
- 1 t dry mustard
- 1 t turmeric

Directions:
1. Process cauliflower with S blade in food processor.
2. Chop celery, green onion, and pickles.
3. Cream mayo in blender until creamy.
4. Adjust water.
5. Stir mayo into vegetables.
6. Wrap in romaine leaves.
7. Sprinkle with paprika.

Sea Vegetable Salad with Sesame/Ginger Sauce -yield 1 quart of sauce
by Rawbert Reid www.organicgardencafe.com

Rawbert Reid, Chef and owner of Rawbert's Organic Garden, which was awarded Best of Boston 2009, gave a sensational food demo of a Sea Vegetable Salad at the OHS/RNEC Dinner Speaker series.

Ingredients:

- 1/2to 1 c (2.1 oz Pkg) of Arame
- 1/2 to 1 c (2.1 oz Pkg) of Hijiki
- 2 T to 1/4 cup of dry dulse flakes
- 1 c olive oil
- 1 c water
- 1/2 c lemon juice
- 1/4 c Miso Tamari
- 1 t sesame oil
- 1 c hulled sesame seed
- 1/3 c ginger

Directions:

1. Soak (re-hydrate) equal amounts of Arame & Hijiki sea veggies for 20 minutes in purified water.
2. Drain, rinse and drain for 10 to 20 minutes in strainer/colander
3. Add dulse flakes and use or store in refrigerator where it will keep for a couple of weeks. Give seaweed a fresh rinse before use after a week passes.
4. Blend other ingredients to make sauce.
5. Top or mix with sesame/ginger sauce before serving. The sauce also makes a delicious salad dressing or dip for other veggies.
6. Garnish with sesame sprinkles, or diced red pepper.

Stuffed Avocado
Prepared while assisting in the Hippocrates Kitchen 7-16-07

Ingredients:
- 1 avocado, halved
- ¼ c chopped alfalfa sprouts
- 2 T shredded zucchini
- 2 T shredded carrots
- 2 T minced dill or parsley
- 1 T extra virgin oil
- 1 clove garlic pressed
- Miso Tamari, Dulse
- Kelp granules

Directions:
1. In a bowl, combine all ingredients except the avocado. Mix well and season to taste.
2. Stuff each avocado half with the mixture and serve on collard leaf.

Easy Caesar Salad Dressing
by Elaina Love

Ingredients:
- ½ c extra virgin olive oil
- 2 T lemon juice
- ¼ -1/2 c water
- 1 T light miso
- 2 pitted dates chopped or 2 drops of stevia
- 3 medium crushed cloves of garlic
- ¾ t mustard powder or1 ½ t prepared Dijon mustard
- 2 t dulse flakes
- ¼ t Celtic sea salt

Directions: Blend all ingredients.

Hearty Dishes

Note: Hippocrates recommends these as small side dishes to your main dish of sprouts.

Veggie Mix
by Jasmine Hsu inspired by www.about.com.

Ingredients:
- 2 zucchini, sliced into strips with a vegetable peeler
- 2 large handfuls of bean sprouts, approximately 2 c
- ¾ c chopped nuts (use almonds, walnuts or cashews)
- 1 red or yellow bell pepper, sliced into strips
- 1/2 c fresh chopped cilantro
- Juice from one lime
- 1 T olive oil
- ¼ t sea salt

Directions:
1. Toss all ingredients together in a bowl until well coated.
2. Add a dash of salt. Enjoy!

Veggie Burgers–yield 36
by Ken Bleu, Head Chef at Hippocrates who taught Betsy Bragg

Ingredients:
- 2 c of walnuts, soaked overnight
- 2 c of pumpkin seeds, soaked overnight
- 2 shredded large carrots
- 2 chopped scallions or an onion (optional)
- 2 stalks of celery
- 2 T flax flour

Directions:
1. Use Twin Gear Juicer with pate attachment for nuts. If nuts are dehydrated, add water.
2. Using food processor with S blade, chop up onions or scallions, celery and carrots.
3. Combine pate and vegetables in a bowl and mix in the flax flour.
4. Make patties, by making a little ball and flattening out, so they are the size of your palm.
5. Put on teflex sheets in the dehydrator over night.
6. The burgers may be frozen and then heated up without teflex sheet for 5 hours when taken out of freezer

Ketchup
Inspired by Ani's Raw Food Kitchen http://therawtarian.com/raw-ketchup-recipe/

Ingredients:
- 1 1/2 c diced Roma tomatoes
- 3 T Medjool dates (do not soak) or 4 drops of stevia
- 1/4 c olive oil
- 1 t sea salt
- 1 T lemon juice
- 1/2 cup sun dried tomatoes (do not soak)

Directions:
1. Blend everything except the sun dried tomatoes.
2. Add the sun dried tomatoes in last and blend until desired consistency.

Living Raw Pizza
by Betsy Bragg inspired by *www.RawGuru.com*

Crust Ingredients:
- 3/4 c golden flax seeds (ground fine)
- 2 c almonds (ground fine)
- 2 c sunflower seeds (ground fine)
- 2 T olive oil
- 2 t dried basil
- 2 cloves fresh garlic (chopped)
- 1 1/2 t salt
- 3-4 T honey or 8 drops of stevia
- 1/2 c water or as needed

Tomato Sauce:
- 8 Roma tomatoes (chopped)
- 1 c sun dried tomatoes (soaked for 2 hrs., save soaked water)
- 3 t dried basil
- 1 t dried oregano
- 1/2 t thyme
- 2 cloves garlic (chopped)
- 2 T olive oil
- 3 dates (pitted) or 6 drops of stevia
- 1 T lemon juice
- Salt-to-taste

Ricotta Cheese:
- 8 Roma tomatoes (chopped)
- 1 c sun dried tomatoes (soaked for 2 hrs., save soaked water)
- 3 t dried basil
- 1 t dried oregano
- 1/2 t thyme
- 2 cloves garlic (chopped)
- 2 T olive oil
- 3 dates (pitted) or 6 drops of stevia
- 1 T lemon juice
- Salt to taste

Crust Directions:
1. Put the water, honey or stevia, salt, basil and olive oil in a food processor.
2. Pulse everything till smooth. Set aside.
3. In a large mixing bowl combine the flax, almonds, and sunflower seed powders.
4. Pour the water mixture on top, using your hands, form into a big mound.
5. Add more water if necessary.
6. Knead the dough to form a smooth round.
7. Give it a taste to test for seasonings. If it needs more salt add some.
8. Divide the mound into four equal sections.
9. Form mounds into balls. Put the balls onto a dehydrator tray without the teflex sheet. Shape them into thin rounds, about ¼ inch thick. Make the "lip" (crust) around the pizzas a little thicker. Use a rolling pin for a thinner pizza without the lip.
10. Place each tray of pizza into a dehydrator set to 105 F. for 10 hours or up to two days.

Sauce Directions:
1. Put everything in a blender, add the tomato soak water and blend till thick. Set aside.

Ricotta Cheese Directions:
1. Blend everything till smooth and thick.
2. Add more salt if needed.
3. Put mixture in a glass bowl and cover with a clean cloth.
4. Let stand for 6 hrs. at room temperature.

Toppings:
Chopped sun dried olives, fresh herbs, zucchini slices, chopped tomatoes, slices of avocados, pesto, chopped pineapple, slivered red onions, edible flowers, etc.

Assemble:
1. If possible serve the pizzas in pizza boxes. Take one pizza, put it into the box.
2. Spread the tomato sauce on the pizza crust.
3. Add dollops of cheese all around and then throw some toppings on top.
4. Garnish with edible flowers and close the lid of the box.
5. Decorate the box if you like! Enjoy warm with a light salad.

Raw Pad Thai

by Sparkle Richardson
Note: This dish is particularly open to modification. Substitute ingredients to suit your tastes or based on availability. As long as the general formula is followed, you will end up with a sumptuous dish.

Ingredients:
- 2 carrots
- 4 summer squashes
- 2 bell peppers
- 1 red onion
- ¼ c red cabbage
- ½ c pineapple
- ½ c garbanzo sprouts
- 1 avocado
- 1 minced sprig of fresh basil
- 2 tomatoes

Directions:
1. Blend all sauce ingredients until smooth.
2. With a potato peeler, make carrot and squash "noodles."
3. Thinly slice remaining vegetables.
4. Combine everything.
5. Use the tomatoes to garnish.

Sauce ingredients:
- ¼ c Miso Tamari
- ¼ c oil oil
- ¼ c walnuts
- ¼ c ground flaxseed
- ½ c raw almond butter
- ½ c water
- 1 hot pepper
- 1 squeezed lemon
- 2 cloves garlic
- 2 T of minced ginger

Croquettes with Ravy Gravy
by Aimee Perrin

Ingredients:
- 3 cloves garlic
- 3 T fresh sage
- 3 T rosemary
- 1 T thyme
- 1/2 bunch parsley
- 2 c soaked walnuts
- 2 c soaked almonds
- 2 c soaked sunflower seeds
- 1/4 c Miso Tamari
- 1 white onion, chopped fine
- 5 stalks celery, chopped fine
- 1/2 c water
- 1/3 c olive oil
- Himalayan salt to taste

Directions:
1. Place seasoning in food processor and process well.
2. Add walnuts, almonds sunflower seeds and Miso Tamari and process again.
3. Add olive oil and enough water to blend so that the mixture will stick together.
4. Turn out into large bowl.
5. Add onion and celery and salt.
6. Shape into croquettes and place on Teflex sheet.
7. Place in dehydrator at 110 degrees, for 3-4 hours.
8. Carefully turn over while removing teflex sheet and dehydrate for another 6 hours, or until dry on the outside.
9. Serve with Ravy Gravy.

Ravy Gravy
by Aimee Perrin

Ingredients:
- 1 c soaked cashews or pecans
- 1/2 c water
- 3 T hemp oil
- 1 T onion powder
- 2-3 T Nama Shoyu
- 1 T rosemary
- 2 T hemp seed butter
- Himalayan salt
- Chipotle

Directions:
1. Blend all ingredients in blender until creamy.
2. Taste and adjust ingredients.
3. Add Himalayan salt or cayenne, if desired.
4. Warm in dehydrator.
5. Serve over Mashed Taters.

Chow Mein Memory
by Beth Scoular

Ingredients:

- 4 c butternut squash, cut into thin strips
- 6 or more fresh shitake mushrooms, thinly sliced, or 1 package enoki mushrooms
- 1 T ginger juice (grate ginger and squeeze juice out)
- 1 large clove garlic, pressed
- 1 T Miso Tamari or additional salt to taste
- 1 t Celtic sea salt
- 3 T olive oil
- 4 green onions, finely chopped
- 1/2 cup cilantro leaves
- 3 T pine nuts, for garnish
- Sesame seeds for garnish (optional)

Directions:

1. Toss the squash spirals with the mushrooms, ginger juice, garlic and Miso Tamari
2. Add the sea salt and olive oil to taste.
3. Top with green onions and cilantro leaves.
4. Garnish with pine nuts and sesame seeds.

Portobello Mushrooms with Guacamole

Ingredients:

- 3 Portobello mushrooms or box of Baby Portobellos
- 1 c sesame oil
- ¼ c Miso Tamari
- ¼ c lemon juice
- 1 t oregano
- 1 t rosemary

Directions:

1. Clean mushrooms with wet towel and remove stems. Set steams aside.
2. Place marinade ingredients into a resealable bag along with portobellos and stems.
3. Shake bag several times to completely coat mushrooms.
4. Place mushroom with marinade in refrigerator for 6-8 hours.
5. Place mushrooms, stems and marinade in Pyrex baking dish on dehydrator tray without teflex
6. Set the dehydrator temperature at 115 F. Check on them occasionally, to mix and add more marinade if needed. In about 2-4 hours your mushrooms will be done. Serve with guacamole garnished with dulse and sprig of parsley or cilantro.

Fermented Foods

Veggiekraut yield 2 quarts

by Sharon Kane taught to me by Sharon A. Kane in her excellent highly recommended Fermenting class www.Sanctuary-Healing.com, 508-881-5678

Ingredients: (1 or more of the following vegetables)
- cabbage, green, red or savoy (curly)
- carrots
- daikon
- any other vegetable

For leaf layer:
- 3-4 whole cabbage leaves peeled from the outside of the cabbage

For the brine:
- 2 quarts filtered or spring water
- 3 T pure salt, kosher, pickling or coarse sea salt, with no additives

Equipment:
1. Large pot for boiling water
2. 2 wide mouth quart canning jars
3. 2 canning lids and rings
4. 2-4 rocks that easily fit through the mouth of the canning jar.
5. Small pot for sterilizing the canning lids, rings and rocks
6. Wooden pressing tool
7. Wide mouth funnel (optional) for filling the jar
8. Ladle

Directions:

Making the Brine:
1. Bring the filtered water to a boil for 4 minutes.
2. After it's cooled a bit add 3 tablespoons of salt and stir to dissolve.
3. Allow brine to cool to near room temperature (2-4 hours or
4. overnight)

Sterilizing:
1. In small pot sterilize lids, rings and rocks by boiling for 4 minutes.
2. Let them cool about 10 minutes and pour out the water to let them cool further.

Leaf Layer:
- Peel off, wash carefully and set aside a few outer leaves of the cabbage for the top leaf layer (you can also use horseradish leaves, raspberry leaves or grape leaves instead of cabbage).

Filling the Jars:
1. When the brine is almost cool, chop or grate vegetables to desired size.
2. If using herbs or spices put them at the bottom of the quart jars.
3. Start layering the cut cabbage into the jar an inch or two high at a time, gently pressing it down with wooden pressing tool.
4. Keep adding 1-to 2 inch layers of vegetables, pressing down each layer until about 2 to 3 inches of space is left at the top.
5. Press it down again.

Leaf Layer:
1. Fold a cabbage leaf, or other leaf to fit over the top layer of cabbage and press it in.

Brine into Jars:
1. Ladle brine into the jar leaving about 1 inch of space from the top. Let sit uncovered for 10 minutes to allow air bubbles to escape. If the brine level drops below 1 inch from the top add some more brine.
2. Wipe any brine off top of jar, put lid on jar, and screw on band.

Rocks:
1. Place a rock or rocks on top of the leaf.

Fermentation
1. Allow to ferment on kitchen counter or shelf for 3 days at room temperature, approximately 72 degrees.
2. Gently move to the refrigerator for 3 weeks. Taste after 3-4 weeks.
3. Store in refrigerator. Taste gets better with time.
4. Lasts 3-6 months in refrigerator.

Dehydrated Living Foods
The Joy of Dehydrating

by Betsy Bragg

Sun drying is the oldest known way of preserving food and predates smoking, salting, pickling, or fermenting. Since prehistory people have extended the "shelf life" of fresh foods by drying food to preserve it.

Early travelers would live off dried food when exploring inhospitable terrain. Farmers and primitive gardeners would protect their crops from spoilage by drying them at harvest.

Drying had a setback with the industrialization of agriculture and new technologies for preserving food replaced the labor-intensive hand drying of food. Freezing, canning, and vacuum packing have largely replaced the drying of many foods.

By the 1960's drying was nearly a lost art and journals like the Whole Earth Catalog featured do-it-yourself dryers made out of screen windows, etc.

However, now with the growing interest in raw foods and whole-food cooking developing a health-conscious niche in the consuming market, drying or dehydrating food is making a comeback. A dehydrator is the raw foodist' oven.

Sun drying, especially in hot dry climates, is still a viable option. But the wonders of modern technology have provided us with a new generation of dehydrators complete with fans, thermostats and timers. Also, some of the newer ovens have "bread-warmer" settings that may be good for dehydration.

What is the best temperature?

The application of heat to food (cooking) breaks down cell membranes and eases digestibility. However, valuable nutrients and enzymes are damaged or destroyed by heat. Not all sources agree on the correct temperature for dehydrating your raw food. The range of temperature discussed in raw food literature and recipe books is from 105 degrees to 120 degrees.

Anything under 105 degrees will not damage your food. Anything over 120 degrees will almost certainly destroy the food and nutritional value. The lower the temperature the longer the dry time but the less heat damage to the food. Many folks use a mid-point between 105-120 as their temperature setting.

What type of dehydrator to get?

The cheapest dehydrators lack a thermometer and often provide uneven drying temperatures. Consider getting a dehydrator with a thermometer and fan for convenience and more uniform drying.

The round models, with stackable trays, are simple and rather elegant looking. The square box models are less attractive but allow the use of sheets that the round dehydrators do not. This is important if you plan to "bake" raw crackers or make raw pizza, etc. Furthermore, sheets can be removed in order to heat casseroles.

The Excalibur brand, with three models, is the most commonly endorsed dehydrator by raw food chefs. It provides uniform temperatures and has removable sheets.

Why dehydrate at all?

A food dehydrator can expand your raw food menu options considerably. It is also a way to enjoy warmed food, important in the winter for many folks. Dehydration is really the ultimate in slow cooking and converts raw food into cooked food taste-a-likes without really cooking. Flavors are enhanced by dehydration and textures can be achieved that your cutting board and food processor cannot provide.

In order to consume nuts in the healthiest way, raw food experts advise soaking the nuts to remove the enzyme inhibitors. Nuts must then be dehydrated overnight to be ready for storage without the risk of spoilage by molds. They must be kept in tight glass containers. After a few days I put them in ziplock bags and store them in the freezer so they won't turn rancid.

A dehydrator is actually an essential kitchen gadget for raw food enthusiasts, not just a novelty or luxury item. However, luxury foods can be prepared. If you have never enjoyed munching on a slab of dried honey-dew melon (which you won't find in your local grocery store) you have one of life's little joys waiting for you.

How long does it take to dehydrate?

Dehydrated food is not fast food. Most items can take up to 24 hours of dry time so it is important to plan ahead. Most items may take an additional day. A wise raw foodist keeps his or her dehydrator in use, preparing food for the next day or preparing surplus items for future use.

If you have too many tomatoes from the garden to eat at once, dry them. By shopping in discount bins, etc. you can stock up on yummy food at good prices and then preserve the morsels with your dehydrator. Dried food can also be rehydrated with soaking.

Apples take about 12 hours depending on thickness and temperature. Bananas take longer, about 18 hours. Edible flowers only take a few hours and should be kept to 98 degrees to preserve color. Mangos and melons take about 24 hours. Onions take about18 hours. Peaches take about 18 hours while pineapples take about 24 hours. Tomatoes take about a day. Experiment, less time is needed if you are soon to eat the dehydrated goodies.

Dehydration Does and Don'ts

+ Remember, seasonings will be twice as strong after drying.

+ Dried food that is too thick will be hard to chew.

+ Food not completely dried will soon mold in storage, get the moisture out.

+ Heat rises, the upper layer of your dehydrator will be warmest.

+ Clean your dehydrator periodically, even if in continuous use.

+ Start simple and build your dehydration experience before tackling complex recipes.

+ Experiment, you will be surprised at the diversity of foods you can dehydrate.

+ Your oven, when not in use, is a good place to store your dehydrator.

Recipes For Dehydrator

Kale Chips

Ingredients:
- 2 bunches of kale (Dino or Curly)
- ¼ c olive oil or coconut oil
- Celtic sea salt
- 1/2 a lemon
- 2 drops of stevia

Directions:
- Wash and dry your kale.
- De-stem the kale and break or cut into 2 inch square pieces.
- Put into a large mixing bowl.
- Pour oil, salt and lemon over the kale and massage it for about 3 minutes.
- Add stevia.
- Place it on dehydrator trays at 115 degrees F. Two bunches of kale will probably take up 2 dehydrator trays. It will take about 8 hours to become crispy.

Cheesy Kale Chips
by Carla Finn

Ingredients:
- 1 large bunch of curly, green kale, washed, large stems removed, torn into bite size pieces
- 1 ¼ c cashews (you can substitute another creamy nut like pine nuts or macadamias)
- 1 red pepper, seeded and chopped
- 1 c water
- Juice of 1 lemon (ca. 2 T)
- 1 T nutritional yeast
- 2 pinches of garlic powder
- 2 pinches of cayenne pepper
- 3 pinches of sea salt

Directions:
1. Soak cashews for 2 hours.
2. Blend together all ingredients except for the kale
3. Massage blended ingredients into the kale getting it inside of the curls
4. Put on teflex sheets (don't worry about flattening them, they'r better bunched up)
5. Dehydrate kale at 110 degrees overnight or until the coating in dry.
6. Slide onto mesh screens and dehydrate 12 hours, or until very crispy.

Onion Bread
Makes 9 servings

Ingredients:
- 3 large yellow onions,
- ¼ c Miso Tamari
- 1/3 c olive oil,
- ¾ c ground flaxseed,
- ¾ c ground sunflower seeds.

Directions:
1. Soak ground sun-flower seeds for 2 hours
2. Shred onions and in a bowl mix other ingredients into the onions
3. Mix well and spread on Teflex sheets to ¼ inch thickness,
4. Dehydrate at 100 degrees for 12 hours then flip over and dehydrate for another 12 hours.
5. Cut to desired shape or size.

Red Bell Pepper-Beet Flax Crackers
by Amar Fuller

Ingredients:
- ½ red bell pepper
- 2 ribs celery
- ⅛ medium onion
- 3 cloves garlic (optional)
- 1 peeled lemon
- 1 large beet peeled
- ¼ c Miso Tamari
- ½ t cayenne
- 1 t Italian seasoning
- ½ cups water or more if needed
- 2 c golden flax seeds

Directions:
1. Soak 2 c of flax seeds for a minute or 15 minutes in enough water to cover seeds.
2. Blend all other ingredients .
3. Mix dressing with flax seeds after they have absorbed all the water and spread onto teflex dehydrator sheets
4. Dehydrate 12 – 16 hours at 105 degrees until almost all the way dry. Turnover and re-move teflex and score into squares. Continue drying until crisp. Break into squares and voila!

Flax - Chia - Sesame Crackers

Ingredients

- 1 c sesame
- 2 c golden flax
- 1 c chia
- Juice carrots, pea or sunflower sprouts, celery and cucumber and use just the pulp
- Choose spices from *Tastes of an International Cuisine* (pages 279-280)
- "Miso tamari" to taste

Directions:

1. Soak seeds in 8 c of water at least 15 min. or overnight
2. Mix pulp and miso tamari into the seed mixture thoroughly
3. Spread out on teflex trays
4. Heat at 118 degrees in dehydrator overnight
5. Turnover and remove teflex and score into squares. Continue drying until crisp. Break into squares and voila!

EZ Dehydrated Soup

by Sergei Boutenko – very funny and educational

http://www.youtube.com/watch?v=weoWS0NMZ9Y

Green String Beans or any other Vegetable

Ingredients:

- Zucchinis
- Yams
- Any other veggies – choose a variety of colors such as beets

Directions:

1. Chop ends off the string beans.
2. Massage with coconut oil.
3. Sprinkle with sea salt.
4. Dehydrate at 115 degrees F for several hours if desired to be eaten hot or longer to store as dried.

Desserts

Lemon Cheesecake
by Café Gratitude

Ingredients:

The Crust

- 2 c almond
- 1/4 t vanilla
- 1/8 t salt
- 1/4 c chopped dates

The Filling:

- 3 c soaked cashews
- 1.5 c almond milk
- 1 c lemon Juice
- ¾ cup of Yacon syrup or coconut nectar or 20 drops of stevia
- 1 t vanilla
- 2 pinches salt
- 3 T lecithin
- ¾ c raw unscented coconut butter

Garnish: Top with lemon slice or fruit of your choice.

To make the crust:

1. In the bowl of a food processor fitted with the S blade, process almonds, vanilla, and salt until finely crumbled.
2. Continue processing while adding small amounts of the dates until crust sticks together.
3. Press crust onto bottom of greased (with raw unscented coconut butter) 9-inch spring form pan.

To make the filling:

1. Make Almond milk first according to recipe in **Beverage** section- Blend all ingredients except lecithin and coconut butter until smooth.
2. Add lecithin and coconut butter and blend until well incorporated.
3. Pour into the pan with prepared crust and set in fridge/freezer (about an hour) until firm.

Banana Coconut Cream Pie
by Katia Zarrillo

Crust Ingredients:
- 2 c of soaked walnuts (can sub. almond, pecan, etc.)
- 2 c of raisins (can sub. dates)
- 1 c cups dried coconut
- cinnamon and salt to taste

Directions:
1. Process until well mixed but may not be totally smooth.
2. Cover the bottom of a pie pan with dried shredded coconut.
3. Press crust into pan and up sides. (Optional: put in dehydrator at 105 for 30 minutes)
4. Place crust in refrigerator.

Filling Ingredients:
- Flesh of 3 young coconuts
- 3 - 4 bananas
- 1/2 cup coconut oil (approximately)
- Juice from 1 lemon
- Zest from 2 lemons and 1 lime
- pinch of salt

Directions:
1. Process or blend until smooth.
2. Pour into crust and place in refrigerator and let set overnight.

Top with:
Juice from 1 lime and 1/2 bunch of peppermint blended with 1/2 banana and 3 - 4 tablespoons of coconut water; or sliced kiwi, raspberries and banana.

Carob Mousse with Fruit
by Betsy Bragg

Ingredients:
- 5 6 dates, soaked for a few hours
- 2 avocados
- 1 t coconut oil
- 2 T heaping of carob powder
- 1/4 c date soaking water

Directions:
1. Blend avocados, dates, coconut oil and carob powder in a food processor or blender.
2. Thin mixture with soaking water from dates to desired consistency.
3. Serve with fresh, ripe fruit or berries of your choice
4. Enjoy right away or refrigerate.

Banana Pecan Cookies yield: 12 large or 24 small cookies
by Joe Lucier, adapted from The Creative Health Institute, www.chiDiet.com.

Ingredients:
- 8 medium bananas
- 1 1/2 c pecans, ground or chopped fine
- 3 T raw carob powder
- 1 dash Yacon (origin CHI recipe calls for Honey)

Directions:
1. Mash the bananas into a cream. Use a potato masher so some small chunks are left. This will make the cookie thicker.
2. Add other ingredients and mix well.
3. Spoon small amounts onto dehydrator sheets and mash down.
4. Dehydrate for about 24 hours.

Snowballs
by Amar Fuller

Ingredients:
- 1 c dried fruit soaked min. 5 hrs.
- ¾ c fresh cranberries or a mix of
- cranberries and other berries
- shredded coconut
- 1 t vanilla

Directions:
1. Strain away soak water from dried fruit. (You can use soak water for something else)
2. Put all fruit in food processor with vanilla.
3. Add coconut to processor until mixture is thick enough to form balls.
4. Roll in coconut for a dusting of "snow".

Chapter 12
Resources

Overview

We are truly blessed in this age of the Internet. Anyone who seriously wants to pursue a comprehensive living-food lifestyle will find almost all questions answered. In addition, every facet of this new way of living is addressed on-line. It's your choice and your responsibility to be informed. You are your own best doctor. Take the time to investigate. The following are just a few suggestions.

You will learn:

- Local educators and practitioners
- Local suppliers of sprouts and green drinks
- Relevant websites
- Restaurants
- Lending DVD/CD Libraries

Equipment & Living Food Sources

In our Optimum Health/ Raw New England Community

Betsy Bragg - Tribest Equipment – especially for juicers- 10% discount on all equipment if purchased through Optimum Health Solution

781-899-6664 OR cell 617-835-2913

E-mail betsy.bragg6@gmail.com **(www.optimumhealthsolution.org)**

Joseph Lucier - Live Food Cuisine (all equipment & much more)
Founder and Director of Raw New England Community
33Nightingale Ave, Quincy, MA 02169
PHONE Cell 617-276-5603

E-mail: joe@LiveFoodCuisine.com or joe@tongrenhealer.com

or joe@rawnewenglandcommunity.com

www.LiveFoodCuisine.com, www.TongRenHealer.com, www.RawNewEnglandCommunity.com

For any member of Raw New England Community and Optimum Health, Joseph will match any price. For members and graduates of Life Force Energy class, Joe will give a further discount and volume pricing.

Randy Jacobs – Life Force Growers (wheat grass, sprouts, seeds & equipment)
781-492-7624
lifeforce1@rcn.com

Larch Hanson – Maine Seaweed
P.O. Box 57, Steuben, ME 04680
(207) 546-2875
hanson.larch@gmail.com
www.maineseaweedcompany.com

LifeAlive Café – Cambridge
Heidi Feinstein, owner
765 Massachusettes Ave.
Cambridge, MA 02139
617-354-LIFE
www.lifealive.com

LifeAlive Café - Lowell
194 Middle St.
Lowell, MA 01852
978-453-1311

LifeAlive Café – Salem
281 Essex Street
Salem, MA01970
(978) 594-4644

Organic Garden Café
Rawbert Reid –
294 Cabot St., Beverly, MA 01915
978-922-0004
rawbert@organicgardencafe.com   www.organicgardencafe.com

Green Force Juices
Brian Axelrod, Life Force Health Educator
551-265-9482
babaxelrod@gmail.com
*www.facebook.com/**GreenForceJuice***

Organic Living Superfoods.
Bruce Namenson, previous owner of Prana Cafe **& Craig Singer**
617-510-1203
http://www.organiclivingsuperfoods.com

Recipe and Sources for Food Links

http://www.living-foods.com/recipes   - The creators of this website attempt to offer support to raw-foodists in every way, from linking them to others who have a similar interests to generous amounts of easy recipes and lots of articles that may be helpful in understanding the raw and living foods lifestyle. While we have not read all of them, we can say that several have informed us well or connected us to other websites that have interesting information. And their list of links is certainly worth checking out.

http://www.bakingforhealth.com/veganrecipes.html - healthy snacks and treats purchased on line

http://www.chetday.com/bethrecipes.html - look at soups, salads and dressing (breads are baked); 80% raw and 20% cooked

http://www.fromsadtoraw.com/RawRecipes.htm - another database of raw food chefs

http://www.goneraw.com - sweeten up life with these 3 to 4 step recipes that will have you asking yourself, "I can't believe it's raw"

http://www.healthfree.com/raw_food_recipes.html - Ron Radstrom, the founder of Health Freedom Resources and Southern Botanicals offers recipes.

http://www.nevermorefarm.com/ ,530-574-3597, Email: nevermorefarm@gmail.com- raw almonds

http://www.nutsinbulk.com - almonds are pasteurized, but others are not; located in Cambridge but must ship. Excellent prices for raw nuts. Call 1-800-988-7136 http://therawchefblog.com/category/raw-recipes - presentation is everything - fantastic recipes to impress your friends but take time

http://www.rawfoodlife.com - select tab BARFAQ for raw recipes for dogs

http://www.rawganique.com/recipes.htm - recipes and healthy comfortable lifewear

http://www.rawguru.com- several nuts and nut butters are sold via this link. While they may be good, we encourage checking several to obtain the best prices.

http://www.rawsacramento.net/recipes.htm - Doug Graham's 555 raw food kitchen rule = 5 ingredients, 5 minutes to make and doesn't cost more than $5

http://www.rawtimes.com/recipes.html - database of leading raw food chefs

http://www.shazzie.com/raw/recipes - Shazzie will talk you through delicious recipes shown on her TV show

http://starwestbotanicals.com - Herbs and natural body care

Other Links

http://action.foodandwaterwatch.org

http://www.allrawdirectory.com/rawfoods.asp?topic=rawfoodrecipes

http://www.angrymoms.org

http://www.cancerproject.org

http://www.chiphealth.org

http://www.foodstudies.org

http://www.goldminenaturalfoods.com/ for kelp noodles

http://www.healthyjuicer.com - least expensive hand juicer

http://www.hippocratesinst.org- great for books, DVDs, supplements

http://kgi.org/world-kitchen-garden-day

http://www.mountainroseherbs.com/

http://www.renegadehealth.com/bloodtests/ Readyourblood.com – How to read your own blood testing lab in Salem, NH.

http://www.mercola.com/ - Dr. Mercola is the most read natural health website. He provides up-to-date information on health and longevity.

http://www.naturalnews.com - Mike Adams (Health Ranger) an online news source covering all areas of personal and planetary wellness from nutrition to renewable energy. Here, he's written thousands of articles and built a following of over 800,000 people across the globe.

http:/www.renegadeHealth.com (Video Blogs & Store) Kevin and AnnMarie Gianni

naturalzing.com

http://www.optimumhealthsolution.org - check it out; it's me – Betsy Bragg

http:/www.paulnison.com   – Raw food - Messianic.

http://www.realfoodreallife.tv/realhealth -Donna Gates – "The Body Ecology Diet" – has helped to heal children from autism. Her information on eating not just fermented foods, but fermented foods with beneficial bacteria strains in them are very important.

http://www.seaweed.net-Mendocino Mendocino SeaVegetable Company. Great herb resource.

http://www.southrivermiso.com (local)

http://www.sprouthouse.com - good source for seeds

Sunorganicfarms.com – For excellent olives Greek International located in West Roxbury, MA

Vitacost.com – Reasonably priced supplements

Vitamin Code (brand name vitamins) - Raw vitamins recommended by Brian Clement

http://www.youtube.com/watch?v=V_hvLvS2dgY&feature=related - Daniel Vitalis tests water

http://www.youtube.com/watch?v=XbBKcysyMTk&feature=related-h20magic(listen to allparts)

www.mayindoorair.com I highly recommend Jeff May as an Indoor Air Quality Consultant and his book, *Healthy Home Tips – A Workbook for Detecting, Diagnosing & Eliminating Pesky Pests, Stinky Stenches, Musty Mold and Other Aggravating Home Problems*. I bought this book as used for $1 on Amazon. I would have saved a lot of money if I had called him as soon as my basement was flooded instead of half way through the work.

http://www.yoursafeandsoundhome.com/ Important to eliminate toxins in your home. Call Phyllis Traver, Owner, Safe & Sound Home LLC, 204 Surplus St., Duxbury, MA 02332, 781-934-5659.

http://www.youtube.com/watch?v=35k2SKUQfHA - Dr. Brian Clement lecture (listen to all parts)

'Lick the Sugar Habit' by Nancy Appleton

An in depth, scientific approach to convince the reader to 'lick' the sugar habit.

Nature's First Law by Arlin, Dini and Wolfe

The raw food diet is the **only** diet that will restore health and well-being.

www.therawdivas.com

learn about colon health and other subjects relating to health

www.alkalizingforlife.com

http://glutenfreesourdough.com If you want to learn how to ferment veggies, take a class with Sharon Kane in Ashland, MA 508-881-5678

Healthy vegan living, politics and environment. **Free podcast downloads from his Progressive radio show. For $5 you can download a full movie on health.**

www.rawveganradio.com

Podcast free, great shows with Steve Prussack.

www.immunolabs.com

http://theveganpact.com Lisa Kelly is a Life Force graduate who prepares delicious cooked and raw dishes in the Boston area at a reasonable price.

Parent Resources - Raising Children on Raw Food and/or Vegan
by Lisa Edinberg

Websites and articles

www.superhealthychildren.com

www.kidsgoneraw.com

http://www.therawfoodfamily.com/

http://www.vegfamily.com/

http://www.peta.org/living/vegetarian-living/raising-vegetarian-kids.aspx

http://www.veganhealth.org/#kids

http://www.npr.org/templates/story/story.php?storyId=129137062

http://thefeelgoodvegan.com/

http://www.shazzie.com/life/articles/raw_vegan_children.shtml

http://www.squidoo.com/EasyRawFoodRecipesforKids

http://www.terawarner.com/monkey-mike (used to be called rawmom.com)

http://livingfoodvillage.com/raw-food-and-kids/69-helping-your-kids-to-enjoy-raw-foods

Ebooks:

Smoothies Gone Raw – Elizabeth Fraser and Maggie Knowles

Books

Ranzi, Karen – **Creating Healthy Children**

Boutenko, Victoria – **Raw Family Signature Dishes: A Step-by-Step Guide to Essential Life-Food Recipes**

Boutenko, Sergei and Valya - **Eating without Heating** (written by teenagers)

Stephens, Tino Jo - **Real Life Raw: Kids in the kitchen: Make wonderful memories by getting your kids in the kitchen, creating healthy versions of the delicious foods they love most**

Lynn, Michaela - **Baby Greens: A Live-Food Approach for Children of All Ages**

Stoycoff, Cheryl L. and Sananda, Solomae – **Raw Kids: Transitioning Children to a Raw Food Diet**

Newell, Joanne – **Monkey Mike's Faw Food Kitchen, an Un-Cookbook for Kids**

Shazzie – **Evie's Kitchen**

Fuhrman, Joel – **Disease Proof Your Child – Feeding Kids Right**

Villamagna, Andrew and Dana – **The Complete Idiot's Guide to Vegan Eating for Kids**

McCann, Jennifer – **Vegan Lunch Box**

Olson, Cathie – **Simply Natural Baby Food – Easy Recipes for Delicious Meals Your Infant and Toddler Will Love**

Naturopaths/Doctors

Dr. Brian Clement

Hippocrates Health Institute

1465 Skees Road

West Palm Beach, Florida 33411

561-471-8876

hdirector@hippocratesinst.org

Dr. Brian Clement, Ph.D., N.M.D., C.N., has spearheaded the international progressive health movement for more than three decades. By conducting daily clinical research as the director of the renowned Hippocrates Health Institute, the world's foremost complementary residential health Mecca, he and his team have developed a state of the art program for health maintenance and recovery. His Florida center has pioneered a program and established training in active aging and disease prevention. With hundreds of thousands of people participating in this program over the last half century, volumes of data have been accrued giving Clement a privileged insight into the lifestyle required to maintain youth, vitality and stamina For his superb, in-depth phone consults, send your blood tests and medical history.

. **Dr. James Belanger, Naturopath**

442 Marrett Road (Rte 2A) Suite 8,

Lexington, MA 02421,

Phone: 781-274-6190

http://www.lexingtonnaturalhealth.com/pages/Personal.html

Licensed Naturopathic doctor, Bastyr University 1998. Bachelors in Medical Technology UMASS-Lowell 1994. He currently teaches nutrition at the New England School of Acupuncture and is a guest lecturer in oncology at the University of Bridgeport College of Naturopathic Medicine. In 1990, he was diagnosed with cancer and is now cancer free because of the combined use of conventional and alternative medicine.

Dixie J. Mills, MD, FACS

djmsurg@aol.com

http://www.drdixiemills.com/

is a Harvard-trained general surgeon who has been specializing in breast care since 1989. She has worked with Dr. Susan Love at her breast clinic and with the Mind-Body Clinic in Boston. She believes in working with women to understand, clarify and trust their choices relating to breast care, whether it is performing self examination, treating breast pain, getting a mammogram, or obtaining breast cancer options. Viewing breast diseases as messages to women's nurturing strengths, Dixie urges women to find their own guidance and power through political, spiritual, physical and/or psychological means. Using her surgical and medical tools, Dr. Mills sees herself as an ally with each woman's unique healing process. Before attending medical school at the University of Massachusetts, Dixie worked at a nationally known education / prevention program as a teacher trainer. While practicing in Boston, she was co-founder of the Breast Cancer High-Risk Clinic at the Dana Farber Cancer Institute.

Dr. N. Thomas La Cava, MD – specializes in Lyme disease

360 W. Boylston St., Rm 107

W. Boyalston, MA

508-854-1380

referred by Ellen Simoneau

Mark Mincolla, Phd is a nutritional and natural health therapist.

Santi Holistic Healing: http://www.santiholistichealing.com

12 Parking Way

Cohasset, MA 02025

Telephone: +1.781.383.3393

Fax: +1.781.383.1047

E-mail: wuway1@gmail.com

Sales: sales@markmincolla.com

http://www.markmincolla.com/site/

Colonic Therapist

Stephanie Dumas

Healthy Spirit

16 Clarke St

Lexington, MA

781-860-5116

www.i-act.org

Stephanie, a Certified Colon Hydrotherapist by the International Association for Colon Hydro-therapy.

Meghan Sylvester

ISIS

One Harvard Street

Brookline Village

617-734-4708

www.isisboston.com.

Meghan Sylvester is a Licensed Practical Nurse, Holistic Health Nursing, Colonic Hydrotherapy, Lymphatic Drainage, Prenatal Specialist, Cleanse Coaching.

Dentist

Dr. Ekkasak Sornkul,
Prosthodontist and General Dentistry
209 Harvard Street
Suite 406
Brookline, MA
617-975-0337
General dentistry with an emphasis on all restoration such as fillings, crowns, implants, partials and fixed bridges. Replaces amalgam fillings with composite. Appointments Saturdays and Sundays

Chiropractors

Dr. John Duffy
Waltham Chiropractic
136 Bacon Street
Waltham, MA 02451
781-894-4270
jduffy@walthamchiropractic.com
www.walthamchiropractic.com/

Dr. Nina Englander
244 Bedford Street
Lexington, MA 02420
781-274-6462
doctornina@msn.com,
www.englanderchiro.com
Graduated from Tufts University in 1987, BS Biology and Psychology. Chiropractic degree 1992 from Western States Chiropractic College in Portland, Oregon. Post-graduate education focused on children and pregnant women. Dr. Nina combines several adjusting techniques such as KST, Applied Kinesiology and Activator. Nina also works with nutrition and detoxification to help facilitate the healing process.

Dr. Andrew Kulick
Doctor of Chiropractic
140 South Street
Jamaica Plain, MA 02130
617-477-8617
foresthillschiro@doctor4u.com
Cleveland Chiropractic College-1980
Kent State University-BBA
Nutritional Response Testing (NRT) Certification 2010
Active Isolated Stretching - AIS

Dr. Yasaman Vafai, D.C., M.S.
66 Leonard Street, Suite 3
Belmont, MA 02478
617-855-5161
lightchiro@gmail.com
www.ltchiropractic.com
Bachelors Arts Brandeis University, University of Bridgeport College of Chiropractic. Ten years extensive post graduate education in network spinal analysis, certified in basic and advanced care. Takes some insurance, reasonable out of pocket rates. Gentle, non force approach to clearing tension and reorganizing the human frame.

Careers of some of Life Force Energy Graduates
All are recommended practitioners who will be glad to help you.

Axelrod Brian, Health Educator, Juice Distributor
Life Force Juice
117-Amory St
Cambridge 02139
551-265-9482
babaxelrod@gmail.com
http://lifeforcejuice.com

Marlene Campbell, Health Educator
Ripple Effects Workshop
176 North Street
Shrewsbury, MA 01545
marlenec@townisp.com
www.rippleeffectworkshops.com

Dr. John Duffy, Health Educator, Chiropractor
Waltham Chiropractic
136 Bacon Street
Waltham, MA 02451
781-894-4270
jduffy@walthamchiropractic.com
www.walthamchiropractic.com/

Mark Karmel Gorman, Health Educator, Trager practitioner Medical Clown, nutritional teacher/coach, chef both catering and preparing for individual needs
68 Bob-o-link Lane
West Yarmouth, MA 02673
617-771-2381
Markkarmel@gmail.com

Barry Harris, Health Educator
"Beggars at God's Banquet: Miracles are our Birthright"
40 hour course taught in 2 full weekends or 16 evenings, once a week
857-600-5247
barrymh2002@yahoo.com

Randy Jacobs, Health Educator, Grower
Life Force Growers
781-492-7624
lifeforce1@rcn.com

Lisa Kelly & Jim McIver, Health Educators and Chefs
67 South Main Street, apt 1a
Natick MA 01760
781 228 9200
LisaKelly1085@gmail.com
www.theveganpact.com

Kate Kilmurray, Health Educator, Consultant on Lifestyle Changes, Yoga Teacher
214 Crosby St
Arllington, MA 02474
781-643-0117
katekilmurray@yahoo.com
www.katekilmurray.com

Dr. Andrew Kulick, Health Educator, Chiropractor
Forest Hills Chiropractic
140 B South St.
Jamaica Plain, MA 02130
617-477-8617
hu4love@gmail.com
www.yournextsteptohealth.com

Chris Lucas, Health Educator, teacher of 10 week course Life Force Energy
8 Nashua Avenue
Marblehead, MA 01945
christine@completemindandbody.com
www.CompleteMindandBody.com

Meizler, Lauri, Health Educator, JOOS Distributor
Newton, MA
617-571-5101`
lauri@drinkjoos.com
www.drinkjoos.com

Alev Orgad, Health Educator, Massage Therapist and Breathworker
Zanjabee
300 Trade Center
#4750
Woburn, MA 01801
781-933-7000
www.zanjabee.com

Marcia Ouellet, Health Educator, Chef and Zumba Tcacher
36 Barnard Ave
Watertown, MA 02472
617-678-1963
 marciaouellet@gmail.com
www.busymomschef.com

Cindy Soby, Health Educator
103 Snake Pond Road
Forestdale, MA 02644
508-477-1622
cindy1724@comcast.net

Jacyntha Kamor Taylor, Health Educator, Energy Healer, Nutritional Coach, Personal Chef

88 Quincy St, Unit 1
Medford, MA 02155
206-877-3353
jacynthakamor@gmail.com
http://www.jacynthakamortaylor.com

Becky Tucker, Health Educator, Massage Therapist, and Bodyworker
Main Street Massage and Wellness
11 Main Street
Watertown, MA 02472
617-744-6021
www.mstreetmassage.com

Karen Calise Woeller, LMT, CPP Level III Life Force Graduate teaches Life Force Course,
The Wellness Center for Holistic Therapies - Polarity and Massage Practitioner
19 South Street
Northborough, MA 01532
Office: 508-320-8711
kwoeller1@verizon.net

For Chefs according to Hippocrates see www.optimumhealthsolution.org

Optimum Health Solution

TRIBEST PRICES

www.tribestlife.com

OPTIMUM HEALTH SOLUTION

10% DISCOUNT for items over $100 subject to change

All proceeds benefit RealKidsRealFood

Product Description	TRIBEST Sale Price	OHS 10% Discount	MA SH&H	Total
Green Star Elite 5000	$549.00	$494.10	$36.00	$530.10
Green Star 1000	$485.00	$436.50	$36.00	$472.50
Z-Star Manual Juicer	$98.10	$88.29	$15.00	$103.29
Citristar Juicer	$44.99	$40.49	$14.00	$54.49
Personal Blender & Grinder PB 250	$69.95**		$14.00	$83.95
Personal Blender PB 100	$49.99**		$14.00	$63.99
Freshlife Sprouter	$108.00**		$16.00	$124.00
Choisons 6" Original Ceramic Knife	$62.95		$12.00	$74.95

**No discount on smaller items

NOTE: If you order several items, shipping is: $20-30 = $11; over $30 = $10 & 5% of total. If ordering more than one knife, add only $1 for each additional knife.

To order: call Betsy Bragg, 781-899-6664 or cell 617-835-2913 or email betsy.bragg6@gmail.com.

Optimum Health Solution Products

Sale Prices subject to change

1/8/13

		Sale Price
Clement's		
	Longevity	$15.00
	Life Force	$20.00
	Healthful Cuisine	$22.00
	Killer clothes	$14.00
	7 Keys to Lifelong Sexual Vitality: The Hippocrates Institute Guide to Sex, Health, and Happiness	$11.40
	Killer Fish: How Eating Aquatic Life Endangers Your Health	$10.65
	Food Is Medicine: The Scientific Evidence -Volume One	$26.50
Eating DVD		$15.00
Healing Cancer From Within		$10.00
Nut Milk Bags - Hemp		$12.00
Nut Milk Bags - Nylon		$8.00
Supplements 15% off retail		
	Lifegive Systemic Enzymes 120	$40.00
	Lifegive Biotic Guard 180	$64.00
	Lifegive HHI Zyme 90	$18.00
	Ocean Energy B12 90	$20.00
	Phyto-Tumeric 90	$35.00
	Women's Formula	$60.00
	Sun D 180	$60.00
	CardioKick 90	$25.00
	Chlorella 1500	$60.00
Enema Bags		$5.00
Skin Brush		$10.00
Permacharts		
	Food Combining	$8.00
	Lifestyle	$8.00
	Wheatgrass Juice, Green Drinks, & Sprouts	$8.00
	Detoxfication	$8.00
	Juicing	$8.00
	SuperFoods	$8..00
	How to Store Goods	$8.00
	The Raw Kitchen	$8.00
	Dehydration	$8.00

"Eat to Thrive" DVD Assignments

Procedure:

Class members make a $30 refundable deposit that allow them to borrow up to three DVDs per week. DVDs may be renewed for up to two weeks. If DVDs are overdue there is a fine of one dollar per DVD per week that will be taken from the deposit. DVDs may be returned by mail to Optimum Health Solution, 337 Newton St. #4, Waltham, MA 02453.

Non-class members may rent DVDs by making a refundable $30 deposit and paying $2 per copy. Originals may be rented for $10 a week. If DVDs are overdue there is a fine of one dollar per DVD per week that will be taken from the deposit. DVDs may be returned by mail to Optimum Health Solution, 337 Newton St. #4, Waltham, MA 02453.

Week	DVD Titles
1	Principles of Health
1	Eating
2	Water- Boone #25
2	Food Combing
2	Meatrix
3	Delicate Balance
3	Sprouting
4	Fasting
4	Internal Awareness
5	Detox
5	Making A Killing
6	Living Matrix
6	Self Help
7	Supplements -Lecture 3
7	Supplement 2009 Lecture
8	Healing Cancer
8	Simply Raw
9	Practical Living
9	Bringing It All Home
10	Food Matters
10	Beyond Raw 1

Additional Options

Processed People
Beyond Raw 2
Breakthrough
Overcoming The Food Imprint
Food Inc.

Derrick Brockie Library

The Derrick Brockie Memorial Library of DVDs and CDs has the following guidelines for borrowing: a deposit of $35 when the DVD is returned in good condition within one week. If a DVD is not returned within the week, there is a fine of $1 per week.If the DVD is damaged, the $35 deposit will be used to replace the DVD and pay for shipping and handling. You are welcome to read books here at Optimum Health, 337 Newton Street #4, Waltham, MA (Betsy's home), but they are not lent out.

Hippocrates Health DVD Series – Viewable on www.hippocratesinst.org
SKU: 878801001249
PRICE:299.95

Hippocrates Health DVD Series Description:

Lecture 1:

Principles of Health

A brief history of how Hippocrates came into being. A comprehensive explanation of the food groups in the Living Foods diet.

Lecture 2:

Internal Awareness

The basics of the digestive/eliminative system and how to detoxify.Instruction in the proper way to use enemas and implants.

Lecture 3:

Supplements, Algae, Herbs and Homeopathy

A guide to supplements and their benefits.Also alternative options to complete the needed consumption that our human body requires.

Lecture 4:

Ancient and current self-help techniques

Many helpful at home healing techniques. For cuts, burns, impaired vision, infection, pre-mature gray hair; and many others.

Lecture 5:

Fasting on Liquid Nourishment

The benefits of fasting on green juice rather than water.A review of the physical, emotional, mental, and spiritual benefits of fasting.

Lecture 6:

Questions and answers 1

Questions on the science, psychology, and food of the Living Foods Lifestyle. The responses provide clear and thoughtful information.

Lecture 7:

Detox & Elimination

The workings of the elimination systems (Lymph, Liver, Lung, Kidneys and Skin) and your bodies' reactions to a detoxifying program)

Lecture 8:

Practical Living

How to really live the Hippocrates Lifestyle when you return home. How to have what you need at home, work, and in social situations.

Lecture 9:

Questions and Answers II

Questions of the participants are posed. The responses provide clear and thoughtful information.

Lecture 10:

Bringing it all home

The physical, emotional and spiritual healing process.How to achieve your highest goals in life. Applying the Hippocrates lifestyle at home.

Lecture 11:

Food combining

Proper combining of foods for good digestion.Foods that should never be eaten together.Key information for optimal health.

Lecture 12:

Questions and answers III

Questions of the participants are posed. The responses provide clear and thoughtful information.

A Delicate Balance-the Truth

A Delicate Balance picks up where Al Gore left off…Backed by scientific data, and eminent world authorities, this crucial message is very convincing. The camera work is brilliant. It is wonderful to see so many people determined to save the planet. (84 minutes)

A New Approach for Diabetes

This DVD provides a guide for moving beyond simply managing diabetes. It will help you turn the disease around. It delivers medical results: weight loss, blood glucose control, and reduced heart disease risk, and may even reduce or prevent the need for some medications. This empowering program offers new hope and scientifically supported guidance from a caring team committed to your success. (3 hours 10 minutes)

Beyond Raw: A Philosophy with Dorit

You will feel honored to be part of this wide ranging discussion about Raw Foods, Life, Vibrational Energy, Health, Illness and more, in a way that you have never experienced before.

Burzynski-Cancer is Serious Business

(1 hour 48 minutes)

Burzynski is the story of a medical doctor and Ph.D biochemist named Dr. Stanislaw Burzynski who won the largest, and possibly the most convoluted and intriguing legal battle against the Food & Drug Administration in American history. His victorious battle with the U.S. government were centered around Dr. Burzynski's belief and commitment to his gene-targeted cancer medicines he discovered in the 1970's called Antineoplastons

Change your water change your life

Pat Boone and his special guest Bob Gridull for an inside look at the Anagic SD 501 and the 7 special types of water it makes.

Crazy Sexy Cancer

A story about looking for a cure, and finding a life

Diagnosed with a rare, incurable cancer, 31 year-old actress/photographer Kris Carr exits her career and dives head-first into an epic journey, becoming a "full-time healing junkie." What follows is a four year adventure of mind, body and heart as Kris explores a colorful variety of treatments, both east and west. Along the way she meets four other survivors, her posse of soul sisters, who refuse to be defined by the big "C".

Hip and humorous, intimate and empowering, this cutting-edge documentary shatters old stigmas with a force of spirit, redefining what it means to truly live—not just for those struggling with cancer, but for anyone who needs a personal revolution. (90 minutes)

Creating Healthy Children

Karen Ranzi will guide you on the path to creating happy and healthy children, confident of their disease-free future. Rather than medicate your child's asthma, ear infections, chronic allergies and other illnesses, Karen's holistic approach simply eliminates the causes of health problems through the healthful raw food lifestyle. (45 minutes)

Eating 3rd Edition

SKU: 9780972659024

PRICE: 14.00

It's the biggest cause of disease, disabilities and death in the U.S. today. Discover why we eat like robots and die like robots. Learn how to unplug your eating habits and reverse the damage that's already been done to your health.

Food for Life

Unlocking the power of plant-based nutrition

The leading killers in the Western world—heart disease, cancer and stroke—can be prevented and even treated with dietary and lifestyle measures. Explore nutrition's role in combating specific health problems, from arthritis to diabetes to high blood pressure. (63 minutes)

Food, Inc.

Food, Inc. lifts the veil on our nation's food industry, exposing how our nation's food supply is now controlled by a handful of corporations that often put profit ahead of consumer health, the livelihood of the American farmer, the safety of workers and our own environment. Food, Inc. reveals surprising – and often shocking truths- about what we eat, how it's produced and who we have become as a nation.

Forks Over Knives

(96 minutes)

Forks over knives examines the profound claim that most, if not all, of the degenerative diseases that afflict us can be controlled, or even reversed, by rejecting animal-based and processed foods. The major storyline traces the personal journeys of Dr. T. Colin Campbell, a nutritional biochemist from Cornell University, and Dr. Caldwell Esselstyn, a former top surgeon at the world-renowned Cleveland Clinic.

The Future of Food

There is a revolution happening in the farm fields and on the dinner tables of America, a revolution that is transforming the very nature of the food we eat. The Future of Food offers and in-depth investigation into the disturbing truth behind the unlabeled, patented, genetically engineered foods that have quietly filled grocery store shelves for the past decade. The Future of Food examines the complex web of market and political forces that are changing what we eat as huge multinational corporations seek to control the world's food system.

Going Raw with Ronnie and Minh

Totally Awaken Your Mind, Body and Spirit with Raw and Living Foods. Easy delicious step by step raw and vegan recipes.

God's Way to Ultimate Health Seminar

In this dynamic 2 ½ hour seminar, Rev. George Malkmus tells how he healed his own colon cancer and other diseases more that 20 years ago by simply switching to the diet God gave mankind in Genesis.

Greens Can Save Your Life

An Inspiring and Informative Lecture with Victoria Boutenko

In this inspirational lecture, Victoria addresses some of the most intriguing questions regarding health such as: is anything missing from in the raw food diet, what is green smoothie and what are its benefits and why is healthy soil more valuable than gold? (3 hours)

Grow Your Own Greens-Loreta's Living Foods

(118 minutes)

Using simple techniques, Loreta shows you how to awaken seeds, optimize nutrients and understand the fundamentals of living food preparation.

Growing Wheatgrass, Sunflower, Pea, & Buckwheat Sprouts DVD

by Michael Bergonzi
SKU: 978801005732
PRICE: 26.95

Michael has been a master grower / sprouter for over 18 years and has spent most of that time growing wheatgrass. So if anyone knows how to grow good grass, he does! Michael is also featured in the book, "Wheatgrass, Nature's Finest Medicine" by Steve Meyerowitz.

www.hippocratesgreenhouse.com for more!

The focus of this DVD is for home growing of wheatgrass, sunflower greens, pea greens, and buckwheat lettuce. These four seeds are grown in trays, in soil, which is also explained in detail. Learn everything you need to grow all your greens at home just like the pros! Total run time is 2 hours, 6 minutes.

Another product you may be interested in is "Sprouting the Easy Way" DVD by Michael Bergonzi which covers how to grow sprouted seeds and green sprouts. This product is currently only available through the Hippocrates Store and Mail Order. For more information or to order, please call Hippocrates Mail Order Dept. 561-471-8876.

Healing Cancer From Within:

Most valuable DVD you will ever watch, The cancer industry is insidious. People fear cancer more than any other disease. This DVD shows you how to cure just about any disease through diet. I love that they show quotes from Nobel prize winners on the reality of the cancer industry. I've been trying to convince people for years about chemo. Most people just believe the medical establishment. You have to open your eyes to the reality.
SKU: 094922882523

Healthy Beginnings: The Revolutionary CHIP Prescription for Taking Charge of Your Health

After watching these fast-moving, motivational and entertaining videos, you won't be the same. Tens of thousands have been helped by putting into practice Dr. Hans Diehl's revolutionary life-style guidelines.

Heart Health

Unlocking the power of plant-based nutrition

Every day, thousands of people have heart attacks. Those who survive often have another heart attack later on. But this need no happen. Heart disease can often be prevented and even reversed with simple dietary and lifestyle changes. This empowering program offers new hope and scientifically supported guidance to set you up for success in health. (58 minutes)

Interview with Sergi Boutenko

This movie was created spontaneously from scratch, without any scenarios, or rehearsals. Watch Sergei being funny, serous, goofy, smart, at play, at work, and, of course, preparing and enjoying delicious raw food. (45 minutes)

Introducing CHIP

An 11-minute introduction to the CHIP program (Coronary Health Improvement Project) with founder, Dr. Hans Diehl. Inspiring testimonies and vignettes of CHIP graduates and medical experts about a lifestyle program that is dramatically improving the lives of thousands around the world.

Is Raw Food For You?

A Sincere and heart-warming Lecture with Victoria Boutenko

In this lecture Victoria tells her remarkable raw food story and explains the 4 levels of addiction to cooked food: chemical, biological, emotional and spiritual. Victoria believes being aware of our multi-level attachment to cooked food can help us transition effectively onto a raw food diet and stay on it successfully for a lifetime. (60 minutes)

Is Water Just Water?

Nutrition, Hydration and Athletics with Shan Stratton, Nutritionist to the Pros

Living on Live Food

An up-close and personal session with Alissa Cohen! Watch and listen as Alissa prepares over 20 delicious, mouthwatering recipes. You will be sitting in on a 3 ½ hour food preparation class and in-depth discussion of the raw and living food diet along with two of Alissa's clients.

Living Matrix

In this full-length film, *The Living Matrix-The New Science of Healing*, you'll discover the intricate web of factors that determine our well-being. From the quantum physics of the human body-field to the heart coherence and informational healthcare, explore innovative ideas about health. Scientists, psychologists, bioenergetic researchers and holistic practitioners share their knowledge, experiences and insights. (83 minutes)

Making A Killing

A documentary on the untold Story of Psychotropic Drugging.

…A tale of deception… Psychotropic drugs. It's the story of big money- drugs that fuel a $330 billion psychiatric industry, without a single cure. The cost in human terms is even greater- these drugs now kill an estimated 42,000 people every year. And the death count keeps rising.

Containing more than 175 interviews with lawyers, mental health experts, the families of victims and the survivors themselves, this riveting documentary rips the mask off psychotropic drugging and exposes a brutal but well entrenched money making machine.

May I be Frank

(90 minutes)

Frank Ferrante is a 54 year old Sicilian from Brooklyn living in San Francisco. A lover of life, great food, beautiful women and a good laugh, Frank is also a drug addict, morbidly obese, pre-diabetic, and fighting Hepatitis C. He's estranged from his daughter, single, and struggling with depression. Frank knows that life can be better than this, and is looking for a way out. *May I Be Frank* documents the transformation of Frank Ferrante's life. He unknowingly stumbles into a local restaurant in San Francisco, Café Gratitude, a raw, organic and vegan café. As he becomes friends with the staff, his life changes forever.

The Meatrix

Expose the truth behind today's industrial meat and diary production while using animation, action and humor to educate audiences. Join our heroes Moopheus, Leo and Chickity as they confront industrial agriculture and save small family farms.

Nicotine Bees

(53 minutes)

Nicotine bees gets to the truth of why honeybees of the world are in big trouble and why our food supply is in trouble with them.

Nutrition Detectives

Nutrition Detectives was developed by David Katz, M.D., and his wife Catherine Katz, Ph.D., as a strategy to educate elementary-age school children about good nutrition. The focus of this program is to teach children how to read nutrition labels, what to look for, and how to select the most nutritious foods. It is a fun program for children, but it is also a chance to improve the nutrition and health of the entire family by providing a "nutrition detective" as an expert guide. This video is creative, engaging and efficient--imparting crucial information in minimal time.

Overcoming the Food Imprint: The Origin of Our Cravings with Valya Boutenko

In this intriguing documentary, Valya interviews health experts, authors, teachers, psychologists, children and people on the street. The second half of this film looks at the reasons why children, loved ones and friends often respond to diet-related advice with resistance and even defiance. This section is dedicated to working with the defensive reaction, and communicating in a kind, loving manner that supports positive growth and change. (50 minutes)

Processed People

Featuring Financial Disaster and Obesity Epidemic features in depth discussions with leading health experts detailing why so many of us are sick, and others offers solutions to our current devastating health crisis. Tragically, many Americans are victims of a "health care" system and way of life which is devastating to our overall well-being. To those running our system, the bottom line on the dollars we're able to spend is more important than machine, unable to escape.

It's nearly impossible to be liberated when there's so much confusing, conflicting information, and when the "authorities" giving you advice – be they the government or industry – controlled organizations like the American Dietetic Association don't necessarily have your best interests at heart.

Raw Food Formula for Health by Paul Nison

Speaking from first-hand experience, Paul Nison shares his personal journey to vibrant health and his passionate belief in the healing powers of the human body. Focusing on life-enhancing raw foods, Paul presents sensible information about nutrition's role in preventing disease along with how to determine the root causes of illness.

Raw for Life: The Ultimate Encyclopedia of The Raw Food Lifestyle

It is our heartfelt with that watching this two-disc set will transform your life. The intention of "Raw For Life" is to empower you with the tools to have the happiest, healthiest life possible. Imagine what a few simple changes can do for you and your family, if after just one month the six participants in our feature film experience profound psychological and emotional benefits from following a raw food program. The interviews with medical doctors and raw food experts will give you and your loved ones the confidence you need to succeed. We envision that by viewing this DVS set, people around the world will be able to make positive lifestyle changes for themselves, their community and the planet.

Raw Gourmet Dishes Simplified

Raw Food Preparation Class with Victoria Boutenko

Victoria Boutenko is the author of *Raw Family, 12 Steps to Raw Foods* and several raw recipe books. She teaches classes on Raw Food all over the world. As a result of her teachings, many raw food communities have formed in numerous countries. She continues traveling worldwide sharing her gourmet raw cuisine and her inspiring story of change, faith and determination. Victoria touches the hearts of her listeners, assuring us that we can choose to live raw, be healthy and live the life we imagine! (60 minutes)

Raw Spirit Fest

Sedona Arizona, October 2006 with Viktoras Kolvinkas

Recipes for Life

Insights and Guidelines for Living Harmoniously

An exciting and rare compilation of the speakers, filmmakers and other highlights of the 2008 Raw Lifestyle Film Festival (now the Green Lifestyle Film Festival.)

Reversing the Irreversible

37 Testimonials of People Who Improved Their Health Naturally

In this eye-opening documentary, people present their amazing transformations to health from conditions such as: acid reflux, allergies, diabetes, cancer, heart disease, weight loss and osteoporosis and many more. (90 minutes)

Spiritual Awakening with Raw Foods

Victoria shares her unique perspective on the connection between spirituality and diet. Victoria addresses issues such as spirituality, clarity, choices and life mission along with others in one of her most inspiring talks, illustrating it with anecdotes from her own life. (60 minutes)

Spiritual Nutrition for Yoga and Liberation

Hatha Yoga and a Raw-Live Vegan Diet are the only initial foundations toward the health and transformation of the Self and the Planet. Here Dr. Gabriel Cousens shows us the way to integrate the ancient wisdom of yogic-liberation and new scientific discoveries within the context of our modern lifestyle. (135 minutes)

Supercharge Me

Ever wonder what the opposite of the film "Super Size Me" would be like? With a tip of the headdress to Morgan Spurlock of "Super Size Me", Jenna Norwood takes us on her journey to see what happens when she enrolls in a raw food detox center and consumes only organic, raw, enzyme-rich foods for 30 days. It's all in an effort to fit into a Las Vegas showgirl costume for Halloween, but the experience has some surprising results. Meet experts (David Wolfe), celebrities (Ben Vereen and Kathy Sledge) and others seeking to resolve serious health issues on a raw food diet. (72 minutes)

Supplements, Brian Clements, Hippocrates Institute,

(140 minutes)

Thrive

(132 minutes)

Thrive is an unconventional documentary that lifts the veil on what's really going on in our world by following the money upstream-uncovering the global consolidation of power in nearly every aspect of our lives. Weaving together breakthroughs in science, consciousness, and activism, Thrive offers real solutions, empowering us with unprecedented and bold strategies for reclaiming our lives and our future.

Two Angry Moms

(62 minutes)

In the face of a national child health crisis. Two angry moms ask: "What are our children eating in school and how is it impacting their learning, behavior and Health?"

Uncooking with Jackie and Gideon: Country Barbecue

Dedicated to teaching and promoting the living foods lifestyle for mind, body and spiritual awareness.

Understanding Qigong

The Chinese word Qigong (Chee kung) means 'energy work'. Qigong is the ancient art of using the mind to naturally develop the body's Qi (energy) for improved health and longevity. Dr. Yang, Jwing-Ming, Ph.D. explains the concepts of Qigong and the human energetic circulatory system.

Weight Control

Unlocking the power of plant-based nutrition

Many people try to lose weight with a punishing, low-calorie diet. Others try fad diets, such as low-carbohydrate diets. However, these diets can be both dangerous and ineffective. Luckily a much better and easier weight loss method, the plant-based diet, offers many added health benefits. (55 minutes)

Why Is the Good Life Killing Us?

A 47-minute interview with Dr. Hans Diehl, founder of the ground-breaking CHIP health improvement program to prevent and reverse many Western killer diseases. Learn how the good life is in fact killing us. Dr, Diehl shows us how we can live longer and die "younger" without succumbing to the hazards of the good life.

Why Kangen Water? Change Your Water...Change Your Life

Let Dr. Dave Carpenter along with others, explain what is happening today with our health care system and how Kangen Water tm is benefiting those who are drinking it. Complete with facts and statistics, animations and testimonials. Sit back and watch our water demonstration from start to finish with and onscreen pH scale mirroring the action, with no cuts or breaks, and no questions of "how'd they do that?"

Yoga in the Garden of Serenity with Kathleen Anderson

Kathleen Anderson, MA has a Master's degree in Dance Movement Therapy as well as a B.A. in Dance from SUNY. She has been certified to teach by the Kripalu Ashram is Massachusetts since 1896. Kathleen uniquely blends her dance, yoga and Pilates backgrounds to offer an exciting new way of working out. The DVD will strengthen the abdominals and muscles of the lower back while promoting suppleness, strength, relaxation, and flexibility.

Recipes for Life: Insights and Guidelines for Living Harmoniously

An exciting and rare compilation of the speakers, filmmakers, and other highlights of the 2008 Raw Lifestyle Film Festival (now known as the Green Lifestyle Film Festival.)

Eating Right for Cancer Survival (2nd Edition)

Each year, more than 1.3 million people in the U.S. are diagnosed with cancer, with this DVD you can learn how the right food choices can help you survive. Researchers have been investigating how food choices can help prevent cancer, and when cancer has been diagnosed how they can improve survival. Dr. Neal Barnard has nine presentations on this lovely DVD.

12 Steps to Raw Foods: An inspiring an informative lecture with Victoria Boutenko

This DVD is saturated with ground breaking information, and presented in a clear and simple way. Victoria addresses the issues of food addiction. She demonstrates many techniques that help to cope with attachments to cooked food and aids with the transition to the raw food life style.

Latest in Clinical Nutrition Volume 1

Michael Greger, M.D., reviews the latest in cutting-edge research published in peer-reviewed scientific nutrition journals and offers practical advice on how best to feed ourselves and our families to prevent, treat, and even reverse chronic disease. Learn how a humane diet is also the healthiest!

Latest in Clinical Nutrition Volume 2

Michael Greger, M.D., reviews the latest in cutting-edge research published in peer-reviewed scientific nutrition journals and offers practical advice on how best to feed ourselves and our families to prevent, treat, and even reverse chronic disease. Learn how a humane diet is also the healthiest!

Keys to Longevity, a CD by Craigh Sommers N.D

2 CDs with 90 minutes of content that discuss ways how to prolong your life.

Recipe Books

Amsden, Matt – RAWvolution

Boutenko, Sergei & Valya- Eating without Heating

Boutenko, Sergei & Valya – Fresh

Clement, Anna Maria – Healthful Cuisine (Book1 & 2)

Cohen, Alyssa – Living on Live Food

Cornbleet, Jennifer – Raw Food Made Easy for 1 or 2 People

Davis, Brenda, RD and Vesanto Melina, MS, RD, with Rynn Berry – Becoming Raw

Elliott, Angela – Alive in 5 – Raw Gourmet Meals in Five Minutes

Engelhart, Terces – <u>I am Grateful</u>

Esselstyn, Rip – <u>The Engine 2 Diet</u>

Jansz, Meg - <u>Salads</u>

Jubb, Annie Padden & David – <u>Life Force Recipe Book</u>

Kane, Sharon – <u>Create Restorative Foods for Optimal Health</u>

Keller, Jennifer – <u>The Best in The World II</u>

Kohler, John – <u>Living& Best Recipes for Health</u>

Meyerowitz, Steve – <u>Power Juices Super Drinks</u>

Meyerowitz, Steve – <u>Kitchen Garden Cookbook</u>

Nungesser, Charles, Coralanne & George – <u>How we all went Raw</u>

Panayi Gina – <u>The Raw Greek</u>

Rose, Linda Joy – <u>Raw Fusion, Raw Fusion Recipes</u>

Sarno, Chad –<u>Vital Creations</u> (not for circulation)

Shannon, Nomi – <u>The Raw Gourmet</u>

Sommers, Craig B. – <u>Raw Foods Bible</u>

Underkoffler, Renee – <u>Living Cuisine</u>

Verkade, Whitney – <u>Preserve It Naturally – The Complete to Food Dehydration</u> (not for circulation)

Young, Shelly Redford and Young, Robert O–<u>Back to the House of Health</u> (Book 1 & 2)

Reference Books

- Altman, Nathaniel – <u>Oxygen Healing Therapies</u>

- Anderson, Richard N.D., N.M.D. – <u>Cleanse & Purify Thyself 1& 2</u>

- Angier, Bradford – <u>Feasting Free on Wild Edibles and Edible Plants</u>

- Balch, James F & Phyllis A. – <u>Prescription or Nutritional Healing</u>

- Barker, David MD, <u>Nutrition in the Womb</u>

- Barnard, Neal D., <u>Dr. Neal Barnard's Program for Reversing Diabetes</u>

- Barnard, Neal D (& 6 others) <u>Nutrition Guide for Clinicians</u>

- Barnard, Neal D. - <u>Breaking the Food Seduction – The Hidden Reasons Behind Food Cravings and 7 steps to End Them Naturally</u>

- Barnard, Neal D. <u>The Cancer Survivor's Guide</u>

- Barnett, Libby and Chambers, Maggie – <u>Reiki Energy Medicine</u>

- Baroody, Theodore A. – <u>Alkalize or Die</u>

- Batmanghelidj, F. - <u>ABC of Asthma Allergies & Lupus</u>
- Bazler, Thor – <u>Raw Power!</u>
- Berger, Stuart – <u>Immune Power Diet</u>
- Berry, Joel – <u>The School of Self-Applied Prevention</u>
- Bisci, Fred, PHD – <u>Your Healthy Journey</u>
- Bohager, Tom – <u>Everything You Need To Know about Enzymes</u>
- Boutenko, Victoria – <u>12 Steps to Raw</u>
- Boutenko, Victoria – <u>Green for Life</u>
- Boutenko, Victoria – <u>Raw Family</u>
- Brazier, Brendon –<u>The Thrive Diet</u>
- Bragg, Paul C. – <u>Apple Cider Vinegar</u>
- Breiner, Mark D.D. S – <u>Whole Body Dentistry</u>
- Burroughs, Stanley – <u>The Master Cleanser</u>
- Byers, Dwight C. – <u>Better Health with Foot Reflexology</u>
- Burroughs, Stanley – <u>The Master Cleanser</u>
- Carmos, David & Miller, Dr. Shawn – <u>You're Never Too Old to Become Young</u>
- Campbell, T. Colin – <u>The China Study</u>
- Castleman, Michael & Lanou, Amy Joy – <u>Building Bone Vitality</u>
- Cichoke, Anthony Dr. – <u>The Complete Book of Enzyme Therapy</u>
- Clement, Anna Maria – <u>Health and Healing</u>
- Clement, Brian – <u>Exercise – Creating Your Persona</u>
- Clement, Brian-<u>Hippocrates Health Program</u>
- Clement, Brian-Hippocrates   <u>Killer Clothes</u>
- Clement, Brian-<u>Hippocrates LifeForce -Superior Health & Longevity</u>
- Clement, Brian- <u>Living Foods for Optimum Health</u>
- Clement, Brian <u>– Longevity – Enjoying Long Life Without Limits</u>
- Clement, Brian – <u>Spirituality in Healing and Life</u>
- Clement, Brian – <u>Supplements Exposed</u>
- Cobb, Brenda – <u>The Living Foods Lifestyle</u>
- Cooper, Carleigh <u>– Cell Phones & The Dark Reception</u>
- Cohan, Phuli, MD – <u>The Natural Hormone Makeover</u>
- Comby, Bruno – <u>Maximize Immunity</u>

- Connone, Jesse – The 7-Day Back Pain Cure

- Cooper, Kenneth – Preventing Osteoporosis

- Cousens, Gabriel, MD, Spiritual Nutrition

- Davis, Brenda RD, and Vesanto, Melina MS, RD – Becoming Raw

- Diamond, John – Your Body Doesn't Lie

- Diehl, Hans & Ludington, Aileen MD – Health Power - Health by Choice Not Chance

- Dina, Rick and Karin MDs, - Foundations of Raw Food Nutrition

- Ehret. Arnold – Mucusless Diet healing System – Scientific Method of Eating Your Way to Health

- Ehret, Arnold – Physical Fitness through a Superior Diet Fasting & Dietetics also Physical, Spiritual and Mental Dietetics

- Elliott, Melinda – Cancer as a Sacred Journey – Healing Breast Cancer Through the Arts

- Engelhart, Matthew & Terces, Sacred Commerce

- Esselstyn, Rip – The Engine 2 Diet

- Essene Gospel of Peace- Book One

- Essene Gospel of Peace – Book Three

- Finkelstein, Eric & Zuckerman, Laurie – The Fattening of America – How the Economy Makes Us Fat, If It Matters and What to Do About IT

- Francis, Raymond – Never Be Sick Again

- Gaby, Alan – Preventing & Reversing Osteoporosis

- Gerson, Charlotte – Arthritis, Bone and Joint Diseases

- Green, Wayne – Secret Guide to Health

- Greiger, Michael – Carbophobia

- Hanna, Thomas – The Body of Life

- Hay, Louise L. – You Can Heal Your Life

- Heung Lee, Seung - Brain Respiration

- Heung Lee, Seung - Healing Society,

- Hiatt, Judith – Cabbage, Cures to Cuisine

- Howell, Dr. Edward – Enzyme Nutrition - The Food Enzyme Concept (1985)

- Howell, Dr. Edward – Food Enzymes for Health &Longevity(1994)

- Huddleston, Peggy – Prepare for Surgery, Heal Faster

- Ingham, Eunice D. – Stories the Feet Can Tell Thru Reflexology

- Jensen, Bernard – Tissue Cleansing Through Bowel Management

- Kimbrell, Andrew – Your Right to Know

- Kliment, Felicia Drury – The Acid Alkaline Balance Diet

- Knudson, Eva – The Top 10 Foods

- Kravitz, Judith – Breathe Deep – Laugh Loudly

- Kulvinskas, Viktoras – Survival in the 21st Century

- Lapchick, J. Michael – Food Additives

- Lewis, Dio – Talks About People's Stomachs

- Lopez, D. A., Williams, R.M.. , Miehlke, K.-Enzymes – The Fountain of Life

- Lucier, Joe – Tam Healing System

- Ludwig, David MD, PhD – Ending the Food Fight – Guide Your Child to a Healthy Weight in a Fast Food/Fake Food World

- May, Jeffrey – My House is Killing Me,Healthy Home Tips,Mold Survival Guide

- McCabe, Ed – Flood Your Body with Oxygen – Therapy for Our Polluted World

- Meyerowitz, Steve – The Complete Guide to Sprouting

- Meyerowitz, Steve – Food Combining and Digestion

- Meyerowitz, Steve – Water – The Ultimate Cure

- Meyerowitz, Steve – Wheatgrass

- Mielcarski, Samuel A. MD – Revolutionary Rehab Manual – A Common Sense Approach to Optimal Health and Healing

- Moritz, Andreas – The Amazing Liver and Gallbladder Flush

- Moritz, Andreas – Timeless Secrets of Health & Rejuvenation,

- Nelson, Miriam – Strong Women Stay Young

- Nick, Gina L. – Clinical Purification

- Nison, Paul – Health according to the Scriptures

- Nison, Paul – Healing Inflammatory Bowel Disease – the Cause and Cure of Crohn's Disease and Ulcerative Colities

- Nison, Paul – Raw Food – Formula for Health

- Nison, Paul – The Raw Life

- Nison, Paul – Raw Knowledge

- Nutrition in Clinical Care – Official Publication of Tufts University, Vol 2, No. 3, May/June 1999

- Oasis, Happy – Bliss Conscious Communication

- Peace Pilgrim

- Phillips, Bill Body for Life

- Polland, Michael – In Defense of Food

- Ranzi, Karen – Creating Healthy Children

- Ross, Herbert and Keri Brenner with Burton Goldberg-Sleep Disorders

- Santillo, Humbart – Natural Healing with Herbs

- Sarno, John - Healing Back Pain

- Sarno, John – Mind Over Back Pain

- Schenck, Susan – The Live Food Factor – The Comprehensive Guide to the Ultimate Diet for Body, Mind, Spirit & Planet

- Siegel, Bernie – Love, Medicine & Miracles

- Shinya, Hiromi – The Enzyme Factor-Diet for the Future that will prevent heart disease, cure cancer, stop type 2 diabetes

- Store, Diana, Editor – Raw Food Works – Leading Experts Explain Why

- Stoll, Andrew L. – The Omega – 3 Connection

- Summers, Craig – The Raw Foods Bible

- Tapp, Teresa – Fit and Fabulous in 15 Minutes

- Tel-Oren, Adiel – Digestive Systems

- Tilton, Buck – Medicine for the Back Country

- Truman, Karol – Looking Good, Feeling Great

- Whang, Sang – Reverse Aging

- Wigmore, Ann – Scientific Appraisal of Dr. Ann Wigmore's Living Foods Lifestyle

- Wigmore, Ann – Spiritual Diet

- Wigmore, Ann- Why Suffer?

- Wigmore, Ann – The Wheatgrass Book

- Williams, Ron – Faith & Fat Loss

- Wolfe, David - Superfoods

- Young, Robert O. – Sick and Tired?

- Young, Robert O. – The pH Miracle

- Young, Robert O. Inner Light

- Zavasta, Tonya – The Ulitmate Elixir of Youth

Appendix
DVD Questions and Answers

DVD – Principles of Health

1. Who was the Hippocrates Institute named after and why (what were his primary beliefs)?

A: Hippocrates (ca. 460 BC - ca. 370 BC) was an ancient Greek physician of the Age of Pericles, and was considered one of the most outstanding figures in the history of medicine. He is referred to as the "father of medicine" in recognition of his lasting contributions to the field as the founder of the Hippocratic school of medicine. This intellectual school revolutionized medicine in ancient Greece, establishing it as a discipline distinct from other fields with which it had traditionally been associated, thus making medicine a profession."Let medicine be thy food" and "Do no harm" – the Hippocratic oath.

2. Who was the founder of the Hippocrates Institute?
A: Ann Wigmore

    a) What was her country of origin?
      A:Lithuania

    b)How was she healed and from what?
      A:Her legs were mangled in a horse-and-carriage accident. She chewed up grass and put it on the wound and saved her legs from being removed. In her 50s, she healed herself from colon cancer..

    c)When and where did she found Hippocrates?
      A: In 1955 she founded Hippocrates in her Red School House in Stoughton, Massachusetts

    d)What great book inspired her?
      A: *The Essene Gospel of Peace,* translated by Dr. Edmond Bordeaux Szekely in 1928.

3. Who were the key people who helped the founder make the Hippocrates Institute what it is today and what were their roles?

    a)J. Dudley White learned about Ann from his patients, who shared how they had been healed by wheatgrass

    b)Dr. Margaret Drumheller was a blueblood who provided her home at 25 Exeter Street, Boston, for Ann and became Ann's business manager

    c)Dr.Viktoras Kulvinskas contributed how it worked and why it worked, and helped to develop the program and why the use of living foods is so important.

4. What are the three major food groups of the Living Foods Diet?

    a)Sprouts: The most nutritious of land-based foods, 30 times more nutritious than other vegetables.

    b)Sea vegetables: The most nutritious in the ocean, high in trace minerals

    c)Freshwater algaes: The most nutritious in fresh water

5.Why are wheatgrass and sunflower greens the number one food group at Hippocrates?
A: They have the most chlorophyll, because they capture energy from the sun through the photosynthesis process.

6. How much wheatgrass is the recommended amount to have per serving per day?
A: 2 oz twice a day

7. How many pounds of vegetables is 2 ounces of wheatgrass said to be equivalent to?
A: 3 pounds

8. Name the five of the second group of healing sprouts with half the amount of chlorophyll?
> a)Clover sprouts (best purifier of blood helps liver function)
> b)Radish sprouts
> c)Chia sprouts
> d)Broccoli sprouts
> e)Onion sprouts and garlic sprouts kill cancer because of sulfur compounds.

9. What is in the Hippocrates Green drink?
A: Celery, cucumber, greens and sprouts

10. What is the third group of Living Food?
A: Grains

11. What is the process of sprouting grain?
A: Soak for 6-8 hours, and then rinse to sprout 2-3 days, or plant. In 5 days becomes grass about 11 inches tall, or you can use an automatic sprouting unit.

12. How is the pulp from juicing wheatgrass used and why?
A: Poultice from pulp with juice gauze pan will heal wound.Heals 3 to 5 times faster and it's also a disinfectant

13. What are the 5 most highly recommended grains?
A: 1.) millet 2.) buckwheat 3.) amaranth 4.) quinoa 5.) teff
They have 25 percent protein building and are energy givers

14. How should beans be eaten and why?
A:Sprouted because they are more digestible and it eliminates gas and bloating. More energy complex carbohydrates, fatty acids

15.The two kinds of beans not be eaten are:
A: Soy and black beans, because they are hybrids, which changed their molecular structure, making them very dense and hard to digest.

16.The two unique beans from Asia are:
> a)Mung – used for premature grey or balding, and prostate and breast cancer.
> b)Adzuki – used for kidney and bladder disorders.

17. What sprout makes body odor disappear?
A:Fenugreek

18.When you sprout, do you sprout inside or outside?
A: Inside

19. Which sprouts create more alkalinity in the body?
A: All sprouts create more alkalinity in the body.

DVD - Eating

Introduction

1. True or False? Health conditions caused by eating kill 2 out of 3 Americans each year.
A: True

2. What condition was not even included in medical textbooks in the 1800s?
A: Heart disease

3. Name 3 foods that were a major part of the diet of the people in the 1800s.
A: Bread, potatoes, corn, oats, rye, barley meal, beans, vegetables, fruit, whole grains

4. What foods were uncommon on the plates of the working class in the 1800s?
A: Meat, dairy products, eggs, and fish.

> 4a. Why were they uncommon?
> A: Working-class people could not afford them.

5. What was the biggest dietary change in human history?
A: People started to eat more animal products.

> 5a. Why?
> A: Because animal products became more affordable.

Heart Disease

6. What has become our #1 killer?
A: Heart disease

7. An animal-based diet causes arteries to open/close, while a vegetable-based diet caused arteries to open/close.
A: Open, close

8. What percentage of the populations will get some form of cancer:

> a)80%
> b)20%
> c)40%
> d)50%

A: c. 40%

9. The one thing an animal-based diet does best is _____.
A: Kill people.

10. What happens when you deprive the heart of oxygen?
A: A heart attack.

11. What happens when you deprive the brain of oxygen?
A: A stroke.

12. What happens when you deprive your tissues and cells of oxygen?
A: You set up the underlying cause of all cancers.

13. The vast majority of diseases today are caused by _____.
A: Clogged arteries.

14. More people die of _____ than from all other causes of death combined.
A: Blood vessel diseases.

15. The primary cause of clogged blood vessels is _____.
A: Cholesterol.

16. What is the only dietary source of cholesterol?
A: Animal Foods

17. What is estimated to be more deadly than all the wars of the 20th century, all natural disasters and all automobile accidents combined?
A: Cholesterol

18. How many varieties of fruits and vegetables did ancient humans eat?
A: More than 800

19. What has been called "animals' revenge"?
A: Cholesterol

20. How much cholesterol is required in our diets?
A: Zero

21. The Atkins diet causes a _____ reaction.
A: Toxic

22. What is the only thing that can reverse heart disease?
A: A plant-based diet.

23. According to U.S. Health Standards, a cholesterol level of under 200 is safe. What is the only safe level?
A: Under 150

24. It is not the type of fat (good or bad) but the _____ in your body.
A: Total fat

Cancer

25. What are two hallmark diseases of an animal-based diet?
A: Heart disease and cancer

26. What strengthens our immune system?
A: Plant foods

27. An animal-based diet has caused abnormal _____ levels in men and increased risks for _____ _____.
A: Testosterone, prostate cancer

Food Myths

28. Is protein deficiency a problem in the United States?
A: No

29. True or False: Fruits and vegetables have protein.
A: True. In fact, many plant foods have a higher percentage of protein than beef.

30. Is calcium deficiency of dietary origin?
A: No

31. What is the primary cause of osteoporosis?
A: Sedentary work and lifestyle

32. How do you make your bones stronger?
A: Exercise

33. Three glasses of milk have the same amount of cholesterol as ___ pieces of bacon.

A: 21

Food Politics

34. In the United States, what percent of raw materials and fuels are used to raise animals?

_____ _____ __ _____.
A: 33 percent

35. What would be the cost of beef, per pound, without subsidies?
A: $90

36. What percent of food subsidies are given for fruits and vegetables?
A: None

37. Who said "Let food be thy medicine and medicine be thy food"?
A: Hippocrates

38. What does the acronym R.A.V.E. stand for?
R_____A_____V_____ ¬¬¬¬E_____
A: No Refined Foods, Animal Foods, Vegetable Oils, Exceptions, Exercise

39. Name three of the long-term changes caused by a plant food diet.
A: Clearing of blood vessels, more oxygen in the body, stronger immunity, less cancer, disease friendly, less toxins & hormones, lower blood pressure, stronger bones, longer life

40. Is a plant-based diet old or new?
A: Old

Beyond Health

41. What is the leading cause of kidney failure in the United States?
A: Animal feces

42. How many wild animals are slaughtered each year to protect cattle in United States?
A: 1.5 million

43. What is Mad Cow Disease often misdiagnosed as?
A: Alzheimer's disease

44. What is the cause of 75 percent of all new infectious diseases?
A: Animals

DVD – Food Combining

1. How did our early ancestors eat and why? A, b, c

A: a - Nomadic people follow the food chain, food comes out when sun was new, over a 12 month period, anthropological b - Ate only when hungry, berries, spinach c - Ate only one food at a time – high quality, nutritious

2. What is the worst combination of foods?

A: Protein and starchy carbs do not go together

3. When is the best time to eat protein?

A: In the middle of the day 11:30 – 1:30 more hydrochloric acid activity, At night takes longer to digest it

4. How many hours does it take to digest protein in a healthy person?

A: 4 hours to digest protein

5. How many hours does it take for starchy carbs to digest?

A: 2.5 hours

6. When is the best time to eat starchy carbs?

A: At night

7. How much fruit should you eat if you are sick and why?

A: None, because of the sugar content and acidity.

8. What are the 3 categories of fruit? Give 2 examples of each.

        a)Acid: citrus, strawberries, pineapple

        b)Sub-acid: berries, mangoes, cherries, peaches, apples, pears

        c)Sweet: dried fruit

9. What are two major rules in buying fruit and why?

        a)Buy ripe fruit, because unripened fruit is highly acidic & sucks out the minerals

        b)Buy organic only, because non-organic sprayed up to 17 times, increases as soil gets worse

10. What two rules in eating fruit?

        a)Eat only 15% of diet 5 or 6 fruits a week

        b)Eat one fruit at a time – digest at different rates

11. On rare special occasions for an extremely healthy person, which fruits can be combined?

A: Sub-acid with acid or sub-acid with sweet

12. What's the rule about fruits and vegetables and give 2 reasons why?

        a)Never combine, 1. Do not neutralize your digestive fluids

        b) Do not slow down food that digests quickly

13. What are exceptions to this rule about fruits and vegetables?

        a)Avocados digest at same speed as whatever attached to

        b)Onions

        c)Garlic – anti-fungal part of flower family

        d)Flowers

14. What are the rules and facts about melons?

        a)Eaten alone or left alone

        b)Melons can be mixed with other melons – 98% water

        c)Lots of sugar

        d)15-30 minutes to digest

        e)When mix, decompose

15. Where do tomatoes fit into the food chart?

A: A sub-acid fruit, good cleanser for the liver

16. When do beans become starchy carbs?

        a)Mung and adzuki take 5 days and are not starchy carbs

        b)All other beans and grains are starchy carbs

        c)If sprouted, not a starchy carb

17. How do you feel about powdered and capsulated garlic sold in health food stores?

        a)Sprouts best, 45 times better

        b)Are some substitutes, kyolic

18. What are complete proteins? Are eggs, dairy and meat included?

        a)Eggs are not consumable – more blocking of the arteries

        c)Dairy

        d)Meat – 60% of world do not eat meat; not a complete protein

        e)All foods started as blue green algae

        f)When land became populated, first plant was grass – all essential amino acids, phytonutrients

DVD - *Why Kangen Water?*
20 minutes

1. What are the five types of water produced by the LeveLuk and the LeveLuk SD 501?
   a)Kangen water (for healthful drinking and cooking)
   b)Acidic water (for beauty)
   c)Clean water (for drinking)
   d)Strong Kangen water (cleaning and food prep)
   e)Strong Acidic water (for disinfecting).

2. Is the LeveLuk SD 501 a water cleaner?
   A: It is not just a water cleaner. It is a Kangen water machine that produces five types of water, and additionally cleans water.

3. What type of water can I use to produce ionized water?
   A: Regular tap water is best. Distilled water or water filtered by reverse osmosis does not have any minerals, therefore it cannot be ionized.
   3A: What if I have well water?
   A: Water ionizers can also be used with most well water. The two most common problems found in well water are hydrogen sulfide (rotten egg, sulfur smell) and high iron content.

4. What is active hydrogen?
   A: Active hydrogen has the ability to immediately neutralize free radicals and render it non-poisonous. The power of oxygen to cause rust is called "oxidizing power."

5. Is the Kangen water made in Japan effective in the U.S?
   A: Yes, it is effective.

6. What is the problem with bottled water?
   A: One of the problems with bottled water is the impact of plastic bottles on the environment. As far as water quality is concerned, the water loses pH and ORP (the oxidization reduction potential is the electrical potential needed to reduce or slow down rusting and decay (oxidization.) as time goes by.

7. Is Kangen water OK for pets?
   A: Kangen water is great for your pet.

8. Is it ok for children to drink Kangen Water?
   A: Absolutely. Even nursing infants. And since children have usually not accumulated toxins in their bodies, they experience no detoxification symptoms. (a few adults might).

9. What advantages does Kangen Water have over reverse osmosis or distillation?
   A: Reverse Osmosis (RO) and distillation, are considered dead waters because everything has been removed from them, including important minerals like calcium, magnesium and potassium. Kangen water concentrates health-giving alkaline minerals like magnesium and calcium, after removing all harmful contaminants. Water from RO and distillation is very acid (pH 4.5-5.7) and so contributes to the over-acidity of our bodies. Alkaline water helps counteract acid / alkaline imbalance. Because RO and Distilled waters are mineral deficient and strongly acid, there are warnings from a number of physicians not to drink them on a sustained basis.While RO and distilled waters are strongly oxidizing, alkaline ionized Kangen Water is a proven powerful super antioxidant with a ORP of -400 or higher.

10. The LeveLuk seems extremely expensive. Is it different from other water cleaners?

    A: Yes. In terms of the hardware, other companies offer clean water that will make three kinds of water (alkali, clean-water and acidic), while the LeveLuk additionally makes strong Kangen and strong acidic waters. Kangen Water has the highest recorded anti-oxidant or ORP then any other liquid source. LeveLuk also offers a strong service department and the LeveLuk SD 501 offers a five-year guarantee.

11. Is the LeveLuk electrolyzing tank different from competing models?

    A: The LeveLuk uses five titanium-anodized electrodes. The surface area of the electrodes is the largest in the industry. The LeveLuk SD 501 offers seven titanium-anodized electrodes. The surface area of the electrodes is the largest in the industry.

12. How often should the cartridge be changed?

    A: The cartridge is good for 12,000 liters. Depending on the quality of the tap water that will last for six months to a year.

DVD - Sprouting Seeds and Growing Wheatgrass
By Michael Bergonzi
1 hour and 7 minute

1. What 3 things are sprouts good for?
A: Nutrition, enzymes, and proteins

2. What are seeds?
A: Dormant forms of life

3. How should hulled seeds be kept and for how long?
A: They should be kept in the refrigerator for 1 month and up to 3 months

4. How should unhulled seeds be kept and for how long?
A: They should be kept cool and dry, and they last forever

5. What are hulled seeds?
A: Seeds without a shell

6. What are unhulled seeds?
A: Seeds with a shell

7. What temperature should seeds be kept?
A: Lower than 85°F

8. What is soaking?
A: Completely submerged under water

9. What is sprouting?
A: Already soaked and starting to grow

10. Name 3 sources to learn about the nutrients of different sprouts.
A: 1) Ann Wigmore's book, Sprouting Seeds, 2. Steve Meyerowitz book, Sprouts: The Miracle of Food 3) Google

11. How do you get enough protein and high energy on the "Living Food" diet?
A: From sprouts

12. How do you keep your energy up when traveling?
A: Eat sprouts

13. How long do you soak the seeds in group A?
A: 12 to 24 hours

14. What is the best type of container for soaking seeds?
A: Glass or stainless steel because they clean thoroughly

15. What can be used for draining seeds?
A: Non-metal screening or a colander with tiny holes

16. What percent of the jar should be filled with seeds?
A: One third

17. What kind of water should be used?
A: Filtered

18. What do you do after you soak the seeds and how often each day?
A: Rinse and drain 3 times a day and be sure all the water is out

19. How long will it usually take for the seeds to sprout before you can eat them?
A: 2 to 3 days

20. How long will sprouts stay fresh in the refrigerator?
A: One week

21. Where should the seeds sit in relationship to sunlight?
A: No sunlight, dark dry place (under kitchen counter)

22. What sprouts fight cancer?
A: All

23. How long should you soak Group B seeds and why?
A: 8 hours, because they are smaller

24. How many days does it take to sprout?
A: Usually 3

25. How often to rinse?
A: 3 times a day for 3 days.

26. Explain what is meant by the greening stage?
A: Lay it out, keep watering, and put it in direct sunlight on the 4th day

27. How long will group B's sprouts last in the refrigerator?
A: 7 days.

28. Should they be rinsed off before you eat them?
A: Yes

29. What kind of bags should they be stored in and why?
A: Evert fresh, because if kept in plastic or paper bag, they will absorb moisture and rot

30. Give 10 benefits of wheatgrass (see handouts) complete food, detoxer, and chlorophyll
A: 1) One of the riches sources of vitamins A and C
B: Contains a full balanced spectrum of readily-assimilated B vitamins, including laetril
   1)Has been credited with selectively destroying cancer cells without affecting normal cells
   2) Contains high-quality organic calcium, phosphorous, magnesium, sodium, and potassium in a balanced ratio
   3) Provides organic iron to the blood to improve circulation
   4) Contains 92 of the 102 trace minerals recognized as available to plants from the soil
   5) Is the most effective form of chlorophyll-therapy
   6)Assists in reducing blood pressure
   7)Is very similar to the chemical molecular structure of your red blood cells, thereby enhancing the blood's capacity to carry oxygen to every cell of your body
   8) Assists in eliminating drug-deposits from the body
   9) Purifies the liver
   10) Helps wounds to heal faster
   11) Counteracts metabolic toxins in the body

12) Combats blood-sugar problems

13) Has been credited with combating both loss of hair and graying

14) Aids in relieving constipation

15) Increases resistance to radiation

16) Acts as a disinfectant by killing bacteria in the blood, lymph and various tissues.

17) Because it incorporates all of the necessary amino acids, it is considered a complete food by many authorities

31. What temperature should wheatgrass be grown?

A: Above 50 degrees at all times

32. How often should wheatgrass be watered?

A: Twice a day

33. What other 2 conditions are important besides watering and why?

A: Air circulation to prevent mold and indirect sunlight

34. What kind of soil to use?

A: 1 part peat moss to 3 parts organic potting soil

35. How many large and small trays of wheatgrass can you fill with a 30 dry quart bag (the average large size?

A: Between 30 and 50

36. What is the difference between hydroponics and soil grown sprouts?

A: The color of the sprouts

37: What kind of seeds is used to grow wheatgrass?

A: Hard winter wheat

38: How long does harvested grass stay fresh in the refrigerator?

A: One week

39. How many cups of dry seed per tray?

A: 1 to 1.5 cups

40. How long do you soak the seeds?

A: 8 to 12 hours

41. When will they be ready to plant?

A: Immediately

42. How much soil do you put in the tray?

A: Half way up or does not matter

43. What do you do with a second tray?

A: Tamp it with a second tray to make it firm

44. How much wheatgrass should you drink a day?

A: 2 oz. twice a day, more is not better

45. How much juice can one get from a large tray?

A: Michael says 18-20 oz. per large tray

46. How do you sow the seed?

A: On top of the soil, cover the soil completely thick and heavy

47. How should it be watered and how often?

A: Water heavily, but gently until the tray drips, and for 4 to 6 days

48. After the seed is sown, what is the next step and why?

A: Put a tray on top to keep it warm, moist and dark so it thinks it is in the earth

49. What do you do for the next 3 days?

A: Water heavily in the morning and at night mist it and recover

50. When is it ready to harvest?

A: When it has a second blade

51. How do you harvest/cut it?

A: With a knife or scissors

52. If it is moldy, why?

A: Not enough air circulation

53. If it is yellowish in the middle, why?

A: It was planted too thickly

54. What way do you get rid of bugs?

A: If it is winter, put it outside for 20 minutes since cold kills the bugs, or flypaper in the summer

55. What kind of sunflower seeds to use and why?

A: Use black oil sunflower seeds, because you get more per tray and the husks fall off

56. What are the differences between planting wheat grass and sunflower seeds, and why?

A: Sunflowers cover with weighted tray filled with soil so it will grow evenly for 4 days. Put empty tray upside down for 2 more days and put in indirect sunlight for 4 more days

57. When should sunflower seeds be harvested?

A: Before they sprout a second one – if there are 4 leaves, it is too old. You should only see 2 leaves

58. How does buckwheat differ from sunflower seeds?

A: It takes only 3 days compared to 1 week

DVD - Delicate Balance

By Aaron Scheibner

1 hour 24 minutes

This movie is produced by the Physician Committee for Responsible Medicine, a non-profit organization with strong ties to the organization People for the Ethical Treatment of Animals. Thus, this movie has a relative bias against eating animal products and skews some information about the health benefits of an all vegan diet. The film states studies prove certain medical facts without providing adequate evidence to support many of the assertions that the film makes. Take this into account when watching the movie and formulate your own opinions on it for class discussion.

1. What is an HCA?

A: An HCA is a Heteorcyclic Amine. It's a carcinogen that forms on meat when it's cooked

2. Describe the China Study and its findings?

A: The China Study examined the amount of meat in the diet of people from rural china and examined the rate of disease in those people. It shows that people who eat a diet of solely vegetables are healthier than those who eat meat.

3. For optimum health how much protein do women/men need to eat per day?

A: Women: 35g

Men: 47g

4. What is Osteoperosis and what causes it?

A: Osteoperosis is a disease which the body takes calcium from the bones making them brittle and weak. Eating animal protein increases the metabolic acid in the body and facilitates the loss of calcium in the body

5. List some problems with fish

A: Lots of fat, mercury poisoning, fish act as filters for the water and take in toxins from the water …

6. How much of the land area of the USA is used to produce food?

A: 50%

7. The human body was made to digest meat? True or False

A: F

8. Why is Casein Bad for you?

A: Casein is a protein that has been shown to stimulate the growth cancer cells

9. What percentage of protein in dairy is casein.

A: 87%

10. What is the best way to absorb calcium

A: Eating Kale, collards, or Bok Choy

DVD – Fasting on Liquid Nourishment

1. What are two similarities of water and juice fasting? What are the differences?
A: 1. Cleanse the body and 2. Rest: Green juice nourishes the body and provides it with oxygen, complete protein, enzymes

2. How often does Hippocrates recommend fasting and what is its significance?
A: Once every week on the same day every week. In seven years, you will have fasted for a year and it takes your body 7 years to renew itself; seventh day rest theologically

3. What are our bodies' 3 areas of energy and describe each? What percentage of ourselves should each be and what percentage are they usually?

>a)Physical (sexual and food and feelings)
>
>b)Emotional
>
>c)Mental and spiritual (understanding of the universe and your part in it) 91% physical sex, food & hatred; 1% spiritual

4. How do we change the imbalance in our lives in these areas?
A: Fast and pray will change the physical, emotional and psychological

5. What percent of the brain do most people use according to MRI's?
A: 3%

6. What are the key elements for strengthening the immune system?
A: Oxygen, water, food, rest, sunshine

7. What is Dr. Kenneth Cooper famous for?
A: Aerobics

8. Why is weight resistance training important?
A: weight resistance training is important so to strengthen body, osteoporosis, and arthritis

 9. What are the two major factors why people die?

A: people die from lack of sleep (sleep deprivation—-young need 8 hrs and dehydration; loss of sleep is cumulative so cut life short with 28 hours of sleep/ 4 hours of sleep a night mentally like a 75 year old

10. What hours of the day should one fast? When begin and when end?
A: Begin in evening until following day until noon
11. Why is it called liquid nourishment instead of fasting?

A: Fasting is without any nutrients or enzymes. Liquid nourishment is the juice of green leafy vegetables filled with powerful enzymes and nutrients

12. What are the 3 S's?
A: Social, Sensual and Sexual.

13. What are some of the effects of fasting?
A: Faster thought patterns – mental clarity; focus; can do more in life – more time

14. On a green juice fast, is an enema recommended and can you explain the mechanics?
A: Can throw out the electrolytes; one in morning and one at night followed up by implants – hold 4 oz for 15 minutes to stabilize electrolytes; the following day do an enema or colonic followed up by an implant

15. Does fasting reduce the toxic load on the body?
A: Extremely; it's a terrific way to detox

16. What are the results of liquid nourishment for people with dementia?
A: Diet contributes to a healthier brain function; need more than diet

17. Should you take drugs (medications) on fasting day?
A: For psych drugs, recommend mono diet

18. Should you exercise or rest on fasting day?
A: Rest at beginning and eventually exercise; Olympians fast before a meal

DVD – Internal Awareness

1 .Why is it important to clear the intestinal tract when you are changing your lifestyle?

A: It is important to clean the toxins in the intestinal track so as to be free of toxins and gas as well as any build up of acid. You need to remove toxins in the intestines as the undigested matter solidifies and congeals in the intestines so you need to loosen it up and remove it in order to start to rebuild and replenish the system. Once the toxic matter is removed you can start to fortify it with nourishment and great nutrients.

2. When is it important to do an enema and why?

A: Enemas are important to cleanse the intestinal tract. Once the toxic matter is removed you can start to nourish the intestines.

3. What is the difference between an enema and a colonic?

A: The difference between a colonic and an enema is that the following.

A colonic is 20-30 enemas done in a time frame of 40 minutes and remove a lot more toxic matter than an enema.

4. How and what does an enema do in respect to cleaning the intestines?

A: Enemas are important for the following reasons: An enema loosens the toxic matter that congeals in the intestines. It breaks it up and cleanses the matter with irrigating the intestines with distilled water. It is best to you 30 drops of vegetable grade hydrogen peroxide to cleanse the intestines with oxygen.

5. How much water should you take in and why?

A: You should take in half your weight in water in ounces to keep your blood vessels flexible and cleansed.

6. What is the importance of an implant and what is the procedure in respect to performing an implant?

A: The importance of an implant is to nourish the intestines with excellent nutritional matter and to bring properties to help rebuild the intestines.

In order to do an implant you use an enema bag with a little water and four ounces of wheat grass juice and implant it in the intestines as you would and enema.

Sometime the implant stays in the intestines other times you must discharge the matter.

7. Why is it important to rub the belly when you are performing an enema and what is the procedure of how you should rub the belly in the areas above the intestines?

A: It is important to rub the belly to help massage the intestines as you do the enemas to help as you do the enema to help discharge the matter.

8. What is the difference between a molecule of hemoglobin and a molecule of chlorophyll?

A: The difference between a molecule of hemoglobin and a molecule of chlorophyll

is the following: Hemoglobin of the blood carries iron while chlorophyll carries magnesium.

9. What is the soup like matter called that is created by the small intestines?

A: The soup like matter created by the small intestines is cheml.

10. What happens to the intestinal tract over the years to create a stoppage by not doing its job and what causes the inflammation?

A: The intestinal track becomes very sluggish and doesn't do the job it should because it contains acid forming materials like dairy products. Antidepressant medication cause chromes disease or cialitis. Medication is tough on the intestines

11. What is a Villi?

A: Villi are hair like structures that are like filters to process the food through your intestines.

12. What is a hippatic vein?

A: The Hippactic vein is connected to the liver that can cause irritation due to poor digestion.

13. If you don't have wheatgrass for implants what else can you use?

A: If you don't have wheatgrass on you when you do an implant you can use 4 ounces of kale, parsley, or watercress. If you don't have that you can take a tablespoon of algae or five capsules with 4 ounces of distilled water

DVD – Detox and Elimination

1. What is detox and what is the cycle?

A: Detox means cleaning the immune system. Emotional detox happens at the same time. At first you may experience heavy detox; it lessens each time and eventually plateaus as you become healthier. The cycle is usually 10 days of heavy detox followed by 10 days of feeling better.

2. What are the filtering organs?

A: Lymph, liver, lungs and kidneys.

3. Which is the largest?

A: Lymph.

4. What moves lymph?

A: Oxygen. The diaphragm acts like a pump.

5. What does it store?

A: White blood cells.

6. Where are white blood cells made?

A: Bone marrow.

7. What is a good total white blood cell count?

A: 4.5 - 7.5

8. What is the differential?

A: Lymphocytes: T-cells and B-cells. They should be 33% of the total white blood cell count.

9. What are T-cells?

A: T-cells are the brain of immune system; they store memory and antibodies of what have been fought before.

10. What are B-cells and how long do they make antibodies?

A: B-cells make antibodies within 2 days of an infection.

11. What are the other components of white blood cells and in what percents?

A: Leucocytes 60%.

12. What are the different kinds of leucocytes?

A: Neutrophils scavenge waste 60%
Monocytes clean up viruses, usually only 4% of white blood cells.
Eosinophils 3% clean up yeast and parasites
Basophils .2%

13. What happens to the percentages of leucocytes when eating a highly processed diet?

A: A processed diet will make a high level of neutrophils and less of others that fight disease because all oxygen and resources goes to the neutrophils.

14. Where are lymph nodes?

A: Neck, armpits, groin

15. What should you do when you are detoxing (have swollen lymph glands)?
A: Eat 100% raw, rest, receive body-work (acupuncture or massage), use a trampoline, skin brushing

16. What does the lymph do?
A: It's a filtering system.

17. What are the liver enzymes?
A: Alkaline phosphatase has to do with the bones, should be between 40 and100, and higher in children.

> Total bilirubin - food related, should be <1
> GGTP
> SGOT
> SGPT gallbladder related, should be 10-15
> LDH heart related, should be 100-200

18. How much bile does the liver make and where is it stored?
A: 1 gallon, in the gallbladder.

19. How and where is fat digested?
A: small intestine with bile from gall bladder.

20. Where are carbohydrates digested?
A: Liver

21. What carbohydrates digest easiest?
A: Those from greens. Green drinks can control sugar cravings.

22. What do the lungs expel and where does it come from?
A: Carbon dioxide from the metabolism of all cells.

23. The Living food diet is important for the lungs because it's high in what?
A: Oxygen.

24. What are cilia and what do they do?
A: Cilia are tiny hairs in the nose and lungs that help move out viruses, bacteria and allergens from the lungs.

25. What foods are destructive to cilia?
A: Dairy and flour.

26. What is asthma?
A: Allergen infection.

27. What can dissolve phlegm in the lungs?
A: Garlic.

28. What do the kidneys get rid of?
A: Uric acid.

29. What are good levels for uric acid?
A: 3.5 for women 5.5 for men. If less, drink more.

30. How much water should you drink?
A: Drink 1/2 oz fluid per pound of body weight.

31. What causes high uric acid?
A: High protein diet.

32. What are the kidney enzymes?
A: Creatinine and B rin.

33. What should the Ph of your blood be?
A: 7.365

34. What number should your Ph be when you test your saliva with a Ph strip?
A: neutral, around 7.0- To balance the alkalinity of the body. Urine should be lower, more acidic

35. What is cranberry juice used for?
A: It is highly acidic and can be used to help urinary infection and flush the kidneys. Use organic cranberry concentrate and dilute 6 times. Take 1 tbl of apple cider vinegar 3 times a day. Don't drink anything alkaline, no green drinks or lemon. Don't use if you have gout or arthritis.

36. How long is the intestinal tract?
A: 7 times our height. Small intestine 26 ft long and large intestine 5 ft long and has bacteria to ferment and soften stool.

37. How long is the intestinal tract of a carnivore?
A: 2 X their height.

38. How often should you fast and cleanse?
A: Once every seven days fast and enema with implant for the first 7 years.

39. What is the largest elimination organ in the body?
A: Skin.

40. How does the skin eliminate toxins?
A: Skin brushing, sweating.

41. How do you detox with ginger?
A: Add 1 cup of powdered ginger to a hot bath. Take a cold shower after and go to bed.

42. What clothing fibers allow your skin to breathe?
A: Natural fibers such as hemp, cotton, silk and wool.

43. What types of oils should you only be putting on your skin?
A: Only those you would eat, minerals and plant based.

44. What emotions are stored in the organs?
A: Liver - anger
Kidneys - fear and worries
Lungs and large intestines - sadness and grief
Small intestines and heart - love and joy

45. What harm can coffee cause?
A: Causes an acidic body with can lead to arteriosclerosis - calcification of arteries, raises blood pressure and cholesterol; harms the prostrate.

46. How does fruit affect alkalinity?

A: Ripe fruit off the tree is alkaline. But fruit is hybrid now. 15% of the diet can be fruit if you're healthy.

47. What does garlic do for blood pressure and cholesterol?

A: Garlic balances blood pressure and cholesterol, increases HDL.

HDL should be 1/3 of total cholesterol or more. Ideal cholesterol is between 70 and 150. LDL should be < 100. Triglycerides < 100.

DVD - Hippocrates Supplements

1. Who was Dr. Lee and why was he important?

A: Dr. Lee started making vitamins that were bio-active. (They were food in a pill.) Because of the Industrial Revolution the middle class was not eating as well as in the past.

2. What does Bio-Active mean?

A: Completely alive, with trace minerals and proteins, hormones, oxygen, phyto-chemical, enzyme.

3. What does "HOPE" stand for?

A: Hormones, Oxygen, Phytochemicals & Enzymes.

4. What brought about the birth of chemical supplements?

A: People started sending their kids to college to become chemists. These chemists were looking for a more economical way to make money.

5. What problems arose with the birth of chemical supplements?

A: The immune system does not accept isolated vitamins; they weaken the immune system. Chemical supplements are isolated vitamins, isolated minerals, mixed together and called multivitamins. They are not like natural bio-active, which strengthen the immune system.

6. What affect did bio-active supplements have in the Hippocrates study of an ill population?

A: 26% more recovery from use of bio-active supplements.

7. What are the 4 legs of the table of health?

A: Physical (exercise and nutrition), Mental, Emotional and Spiritual

8. Why take whole food supplements even if well?

A: Healthy people can still be under stress; at these times the immune system needs an extra input to keep mind and body well.

9. What was the result of the 2-year Hippocrates study on use of taking bio-active supplements with both the well and the ill population?

A: They both achieved the same very high level of immunity. 80% have a choice of whether to use supplements or not; the other 20 % their condition makes it imperative to take supplements. 72% of young people have taken antibiotics and need supplementation; 3% of the population has mechanical deficiencies/dysfunctional organs, which need long term use of supplements.

10. What supplement should everyone take? Name 2 kinds of this supplement.

A: Fresh water algae because it changes the DNA. As we age, our DNA is devolving. Blue green algae from Klamath Lake easy to digest, and has a high mineral content. It will keep you young, vital, and strong. Chlorella (green) is digestible, but Spirulina has a hard cell wall. To take both Blue-green algae and Chlorella is wise and prudent.

11. How does it protect our DNA?A: It speeds the process of healing by creating activity and development of stem cells, first, by its pigmentation that collects chlorophyll and secondly by their polysaccharides, a form of protein.

DVD - Practical Living

1. Where is the best source to get nutrition to keep a healthy lifestyle?
A: You get your nutrients from wheat grass Sprouts and vegetables.

2. What kind of green drink do you make with the best nutrients? List the percentages of each of the two items.
A: The best drink to help balance your metabolism and to make your body more alkaline is the green drink made with 50% sprouts and 50% vegetables such as celery cucumbers.

3. Where do you get your amino acids from for living a healthy lifestyle?
A: You get your amino acids from Sunflower sprouts.

4. What are the green drinks you should make to best nourish the body for a healthy lifefood lifestyle?
A: You should make your green drink from the following: Sprouts from sunflower & buckwheat, a few stalks of celery, Half an English cucumber, Parsley and spinach.

5. If you are very anemic what is the best thing you can do for your body to create the best results to normalize metabolism?
A: If you are anemic you the best thing you should do or your body is to take in dark green vegetables.

6. What is the best way to nourish the body and why?
A: The best way to get the nourishment you need for your body is by juicing. Juicing gets the nutrients, enzymes and natural vitamins directly through your bloodstream and to the organs to help revitalize your organs to the best benefit possible.

7. What is the best investment you can make for your life in respect to your body in living a healthy lifestyle?
A: The best investment you can do for yourself is to purchase a juicer that will be an investment for your health that will help you revitalize your health and body.

8. What is the best type of juicer to purchase to obtain the best results for juicing?
A: The best type of juicer you can obtain is the masticating juicer (auger or grinding type of juicer).

9. Why is it better to use a masticating (grinder or auger) style than a centrifugal juicer?
A: The masticating or grinding type is better than a centrifugal one because the centrifugal juicer oxygenates the juice, breaking down the nutrients because the machine has a higher speed as it turns faster and also gets hotter breaking down the nutrition of the juice.

10. What is the temperature that enzymes break down?
A: Enzymes essentially start to breakdown around 118 degrees Fahrenheit.

11. Why is it important to use a juicer that doesn't heat up?
A: It is important to buy a juicer that doesn't heat up because the heat breaks down the nutrients in the juice as it is making the juice.

12. What are two ways to grow sprouts?
A: You can grow sprouts by hyrdoponically and by using the other method with soil.

13. Why is it better to use organic produce and support organic farmers than non-organic?

A: It is better to purchase organically grown produce because the produce that they grow non-organically uses pesticides and fertilizer that are synthetic and dangerous and get into our ground water.

14. Why is it better to drink the juices right away instead of making a whole lot ahead of time and drinking them later?

A: It is better to drink the juice right away because the juice starts to begin to lose the nutrients and starts to break down in nutritional value.

15. What is the importance and value of drinking juices and what does it do to your organs and blood stream?

A: It is important to drink juice because it is easier to digest and to get the nutrients right away to the blood stream and to every organ in your body. It therefore, gets the best absorption and nutrients the quickest and for the best results.

16. What is the best breakfast drink to drink on an empty stomach in this raw foods lifestyle and why and what drink would you follow up right after?

A: The best drink for breakfast is two ounces of wheat grass followed up with a green drink of sprouts and vegetables.

17. What are the heaviest detoxing hours in your body?

A: The heaviest detoxing hours in your body are between 3a.m. till about noontime.

18. What is another drink or helping to cleanse after the green drink?

A: Another drink to cleanse after the green drink is one lemon and ½ a quart of distilled water or purified water and a little cayenne, stevia.

19. What does cayenne do for the body?

A: Cayenne pepper opens up the capillaries and gets circulation going. It also has vitamin C.

20. Why is it better to toast bread before you eat it?

A: It is better to toast bread as it breaks down the carbohydrates and makes it easier to digest.

21. What is the Hippocrates salad dressing?

A: Hippocrates salad dressing is the following: Two tablespoons of olive oil, Two tablespoons of water, Herbs of either oregano, rosemary or dill, lemon juice.

22. Why is it better to dehydrate food than to bake it?

A: Dehydrating is better than baking because you keeping the food almost live as you are removing the water not heating it over a certain temperature which breaks down the nutrients.

23. List the four grains that they recommend to use when dehydrating.

A: The four grains we recommend to use for dehydrating are the following: rye, oats, spelt and kamut

24. Why is it unhealthy to use whole wheat?

A: It is unhealthy to use wheat as it causes a lot of allergies

25. Describe a recipe for making veggieburgers in the dehydrator?

A: Veggie burgers Recipe: Use rye oats spelt or kamut and take the pulp of these sprouts make a little veggie burger with fennel or cumin Use Lima pinto or lentils Add either Mexican or Indian spices for the final seasoning and there you have the veggie burgers.

26. Describe a recipe for potato chips in the dehydrator.

A: To make good and healthy potatoes chips slice a sweet potatoes with either Italian or Mexican spices or lay of dehydrator sheet and set the temp and done in 48 hours.

27. List the five gluten free grains that are recommended to use in this video?

A: The five gluten free grains are the following: Millet, quinoa, amaranth, teff, buckwheat &kasha.

28. Why is it important to purchase a dehydrator that you can control the temperature and why?

A: It is better to purchase a dehydrator that you can control the temperature so you won't overcook the food and have a better control of them.

29. Describe what irradiated spices are and are they healthy to consume?

A: Irradiated foods are foods that have essentially been nuked and lose their nutritional value. They are dangerous and unhealthy to consume because their molecular structure has been altered

DVD - Bringing It All Home

1. How do you implement a raw food program in the "real world"?
A: Commitment to your own health & self- esteem

2. What is being committed in a "living food" lifestyle?
A: Being committed to doing 8 % per month that will achieve 100% commitment by the end of your first year

3. How do we convince ourselves to make this commitment to follow this lifestyle?
A: By creating realistic goals a little at a time that are reachable

4. Do your family and friends discourage you from following a "living food" lifestyle and if so, why?
A: Yes because they are comfortable and habituated to following the SAD diet.

5. How do you deal with family if they are uncomfortable with your "living food" lifestyle when you are creating it?
A: Don't fight or argue. Take one step at a time. Create your own lifestyle privately. As you change gradually, you can go with them to Joe's Steak House and be satisfied with a salad.

6. What is the name of the lifestyle you wish to achieve which is also the name of one of Ann Wigmore's books?
A: To Be Your Own Doctor

7. What are the three steps in reaching your goal in a "living food" lifestyle?
A: 1. Focus on what is most important to you and what you want. 2. Follow the commitment to that. 3. Follow that until you achieve it.

8. This is the first time you were told that gas is good for you. What do the initials G.A.S. mean?
A: G = Goal, A=Act on Goal, S=success

9. Explain the regeneration in your body.
A: Your body regenerates in 7 years. The human heart regenerates creates a whole new heart in 30 heart. The human lungs regenerate in70 days. The brain also regenerates.

10. What is the foremost major challenge you'll have in creating a "living food" lifestyle?
A: Dealing with the physical and what you are made of.

11. What are the two basic areas in creating this lifestyle?
A: What you eat and how you exercise.

12. What are the challenges you'll face between the 7th and 14th year of this new lifestyle?
A: Emotional who you are.

13. What are the challenges you'll face in dealing with the years between 14 and 21 years and what is the largest scope of understanding that is limiting our own lack of awareness?
A: Spiritual Cycle

14. What is the Hippocrates implementation through a "Living Foods" Lifestyle for achieving health and wellness? (The following is from my Hippocrates notes during the Health Education course.)

       a)Sun

       b)Oxygen

       c)Water ½ your weight

       d)Living Food Diet

       e)80 % 60% sprouts & green; 15% rainbow

       f)15% steamed

       g)5 % fruit max no more than15% - 1-2 a day

       h)2 two ounce glasses green juice a day

       i)Drink and implant wheatgrass

       j)Blue green and green algae

       k)Soaked and sprouted seeds, grains and legumes before eating – sometimes acceptable once a day

       l)Handful of nuts or seeds 2 to 3 times a week during a meal

       m)Raw garlic in salads and juices

       n)Water with cayenne sprinkled on it 30 minutes before meals

       o)Limit oils to cold pressed

       p)Eat only when calm and relaxed between sunrise and sunset

       q)Exercise

       r)Rest

       s)Positive environment and Positive Thinking

15. Compare the environmental factors involved in produced a vegan diet versus animal-based diet? (The following is not in the DVD)

A: According to the late R. Buckminister Fuller – the internationally respected engineer, scientist and architect – the resources of our planet are sufficient to feed every man, woman and child at American middle-class standards if we utilize our resources properly. Cattle-raising requires much more land than plant-raising. It takes 12-24 pounds o vegetable-protein to generate a single pound of meat protein. 70% of the grain that is harvested in the US is used to feed animals rather than people. There is only one acre of farmable land per person on earth; and the average American meat-eater requires 1.6 acres per year to feed him while a vegetarian needs less than one-half acre. Vegetable protein sources are cheaper than the least expensive meats, and sprouted grains and seeds provide an excellent source of protein at even greater savings.

16. What's the difference between consuming salmon for Omega 3's versus obtaining Omega 3's in Blue-Green algae?

A: Salmon could contain bacteria along with the Omega 3's whereas plant-based Omega oils are much healthier.

17. Explain the conclusions of T. Colin Campbell's The China Study.

A: Everyone should be on a vegan diet with no animal meat or fat which is dangerous.

18. What do you think about the product "laetril" concerning cancer treatment?

A: Laetril is a pharmaceutical to treat cancer which the immune the immune system can not tolerate and is injurious to intestines.

19. What is the second evolution of the healing cycle called?

A: Emotional.

20. What is the third evolution of the healing cycle called?

A: Spiritual.

21. What is similar to hemoglobin in the blood and chlorophyll?

A: Seawater.

22. What is the main component of killing microbes and mutigens?

A: Oxygen.

23. Why is wheatgrass chlorophyll important?

A: Vegetables and other raw plants contain chemical elements ie. Photo-nutrients to remove disease from your body. It nourishes and protects from disease.

24. What are Phytochemicals? (Not in the DVD)

A: Phytochemicals are non-nutritive plant-chemicals that contain protective, disease-preventing compounds. More than 900 phytochemicals might be in just one serving of vegetables! Although phytochemicals are not yet classified as nutrients –substances for sustaining life – they are known to embody properties that assist the prevention of illness and disease. Phytochemicals are associated with the prevention and/or treatment of at least four of the major causes of death in the United States-cancer, diabetes, cardiovascular disease, and hypertension. In the DVD, Brian, however, refers to phytochemicals as phytonutrients.

25. What happens to phyto-nutrients when heated over 115 degrees Fahrenheit?

A: All are neutered and destroyed.

26. Where are phytonutrients found?

A: Plant life.

27. What are the 3 types of sprouts that are anti-microbial, anti-carcinogenic and anti-cardiovascular?

A: Broccoli onion and garlic.

28. What is the chemical "MTBE" and where is it used? And why is it dangerous to your health?

A: Chemical compound used in gasoline that if spilled enters our water supply and causes cancer.

29. What are the two forms of filtration to create the best water and explain each type?

A: Distillation and wellness filtration. Distillation is a process of distilling water (heating water to eliminate all the toxins and everything else) Wellness filtrations a Japanese method of organizing molecular structure of water and uses a super mass filtration system that charges the water.

30. Does anything happen to vegetables if you freeze them and defrost them for consumption?
A: If flash frozen, it contains some life in it. After 10 days the life force is dissipated totally. If you deep-freeze vegetables, 24 to 48 hours, all the nutrients are destroyed.

31. Describe a recipe with the gluten free grains they recommend?
A: The recipe they recommend is the following: Take 2 ½ quarts of water, heat to boiling and cool to 115 degrees and put a half a cup of anyone of the gluten then add vegetables on top for a nice dish with grains and vegetables.

32. Describe the difference between white potatoes and sweet potatoes?
A: The difference between white potatoes and sweet potatoes is the fact that those white potatoes are very starchy and acidic, while sweet potatoes are much easier to digest and full of more nutrients.

33. Describe the noodles that are recommended in this video as well as why tomatoes are not a good sauce to use on pasta?
A: Soba noodles and Quinoa noodles are good for digestion, not wheat noodles. It is not healthy to use tomatoes sauce on pasta as once they are cooked they are too acidic.

34. What is an excellent spaghetti sauce to use on pasta?
A: A good pasta sauce using fresh red peppers basil, oregano and garlic is an excellent raw sauce to use.

Made in the USA
Charleston, SC
04 June 2013